Learn the truth &,

diet failure...

the Naked Truth

THE BRAIN CHEMISTRY KEY TO LOSING WEIGHT—AND KEEPING IT OFF!

Discover Why 98% of All Diets Inevitably Fail.
Learn What Causes Cravings and Food Addictions—Moreover,
How to Control Them.
Learn to Live Longer, Look Younger, and Be Healthy for Life!

The Crucial Serotonin-Insulin Connection Exposed!

Phoenix Gilman

G&G PUBLISHING

This book is dedicated to
my father, mother, and grandmother,
and to my ever-loyal and loving friends,
Peggy, Billy, Janene,
Scotty, Eric, Karen, and Loretto.

— Phoenix Gilman

Acknowledgements

Long ago, I discovered the indescribable bond that is shared with a true friend. For me, it is those special few who come into your life and completely accept you for who you are, without ever feeling the need to change you, judge you, or treat you less than. They don't pretend to have your back—only to find out that they are the ones you need protection from. Instead, they support you. Believe in you. Respect you. They love you unconditionally. And all without ever betraying that sacred bond of friendship. This, however, is sadly very rare. I, therefore, feel extraordinarily blessed to have such wonderful friends throughout my life. To those who have shared their lives with me so selflessly, I am eternally grateful. And, to those who have helped and encouraged me along this venture, thank you.

To my father, Frank Gilman, thank you for your many sacrifices so that your children could have a better life. Though you gave to us above and beyond, I've come to appreciate most, all those not-so-little things we often take for granted, i.e., clean clothes, a warm bed, never knowing hunger, regular medical/dental checkups, access to unlimited athletic opportunities, and a good education. And while I believe our character evolves as we grow, you gave me a strong foundation in which to grow from. Through the many years since then, thank you for being there for me, loving me, and most of all, for finally coming to understand that all I really want from you is to be heard. And, though, you most certainly don't always understand or agree, thank you for respecting my free-spirit and desperate need to live a life that is true. I love you.

My mother, Barbara Holcombe-Gilman, though you were, regrettably, taken from me at such a young age, I am so thankful that I'm now able to spend time with you and get to know you, not only as my biological mother, but also as a friend—and as a loving, compassionate human being. You are an amazingly kind, caring, funny, and sensitive soul. Your love, your sense of pride in me, is truly overwhelming! I love you.

Peggy Collins, who has since passed on, there is not a single day that goes by that I don't miss you. Since the day I first met you at merely 18, and you, stunning at 64, you showed me nothing but respect, kindness, and a love I had never before known. You were far more than my best friend, you were the mother I never had. You loved me completely. Without conditions. You guided me. Cared for me. Nurtured me. You took such pride in who I was as a person, as a young lady. *I love and miss you forever!*

To my grandmother, Harriet Vander Molen-Gilman, who has also passed on, you were an incredible woman, a woman so far ahead of your time. Thank you for showing me what living a healthy lifestyle is all about. Thank you for showing me that life is meant to be lived to the absolute fullest, regardless of age. I love and miss you.

Billy Ciampo, we're far more than best of friends, *we are family!* You love me like I'm your own. You care for me. You respect my spirited nature. You watch out for me, as I do likewise for you. You're one of my greatest blessings! Thank you, as well, for giving *soooo* much of your personal time and artistic talents to help me bring to life my endless creative visions over the years, particularly this book. (I know it wasn't easy, but thank you for letting go and allowing me to create.) I love you and I am *forever* grateful for our friendship!

Janene Bogardus, my wonderfully loyal, ever-so-protective friend of over 25 years, I cherish you! Our friendship, our love for one another, is one of the purest bonds of all. No matter my joy, no matter my sorrow, you have always been there for me. And all without judgment, only loving and accepting me for all that I am, and all that I am not. I love you!

Eric Hewko, thank you for always gently consoling and guiding me. Besides being a truly incredible, compassionate friend for over 16 years, you've shown me nothing but the utmost respect. I hope you know just how much I admire all that you are: from friend, lawyer, to a loving, devoted husband and father, and as a man with such profound faith. How often I've wished there were more men with your strength of character.

Scotty Christensen, your unadulterated interest in my work—and unrelenting faith in who I am as a person—is exceedingly touching. Your forever-encouraging friendship and shoulder to cry on when I'm feeling overwhelmed has equally meant so much to me. And, how can I *ever* possibly thank you for donating such extraordinary funds to this venture! You're an amazing man with so much heart. I am extremely grateful! I love you! *("Stage right!")*

Karen Lukeman, my oldest, most beloved, and loyal friend since 6th grade. What wonderful memories we share! In a time that was often terribly painful for us, we gave each other hope and comfort. We're connected far beyond the physical form. I love and adore you!

Loretto Kraft, you have been one of my dearest friends and biggest supporters for over 20 years! Oh, how I miss our days at the pool! I love you! Dream big—and never give up!

Vicki Gesmundo-Marcinek, I forever cherish our friendship of those years long ago.

Robert Grimes, my high school creative writing teacher and confidant, I have never forgotten all that you did for me. You were a man who, though twice my age, always respected me, believed in me, and gave me tremendous emotional strength through the toughest years of my young life. I am infinitely grateful.

Christine Salvo, thank you for your friendship and loving support. I love you.

To Billy, Janene, Scotty, Christine, Karen, Sam, Roberto, Mary, Jolie, Keven, Tony, Raven, Layla, Dr. Johnson, Damion, and my many other loyal clients, thank you for making the commitment to living a healthier lifestyle! Thank you for allowing me to help you.

Copy editor, Martha Sigwart, thank you for all your hard work. Though I wrote for another 6 months after you edited, your expertise added a much-needed touch to my manuscript.

Jerry Davidson, my photographer, and his assistant, Young Cho, thank you for allowing me to create my cover photo *exactly* the way I envisioned it. Your dramatic lighting, professional excellence—and patience in making sure I got the image I so badly needed—were crucial to the success of this photo shoot.

Kevin Kotowski, Chief Creative Officer of Olson/Kotowski, thank you so much for lending your copy expertise to my cover. Your advice was greatly appreciated!

Michael Murray, ND, celebrated naturopathic doctor, speaker, and best-selling author, thank you for taking the time to read my manuscript—and being willing to offer such a generous quote. Your genuine, encouraging support is appreciated more than I can say.

Stephen Scheinberg, PhD, MD, one of my most loyal, successful clients, I'm so proud of all the changes you've made. I'm equally grateful for your endless support and willingness to endorse my work. Thank you, Stephen.

Chuck Yesson, thank you for your friendship and powerful, thought-provoking quote.

Dr. Glass, a man with such impressive medical credentials, I'm humbled by your review.

Rex Licklider, I'm honored by your belief in my work—and who I am as a person.

Diana Schwarzbein, MD, leading endocrinologist, speaker, and best-selling author, thank you for taking the time to meet with me in 2001. Thank you for sharing my passion and encouraging my efforts. Your support was enormously flattering.

G & G Publishing, how very grateful I am.

Norm Morales, President/CEO of Vineyard Bank, thank you for affirming my vision.

Orange County Printing, your sincere intentions to deliver only the most exceptional quality of work is unsurpassed. Thank you for making sure my book does not fall short.

Web designer, LewRay Rosado, clean, simple, yet classy; you delivered all that I envisioned—and more. Exceptional talent! Thank you for your efforts and patience.

Jay Haldeman and Mr. C, two perfect strangers, who believed enough in my work to make donations—I'm appreciative. J.J. and B.D., thank you for your compassionate support.

My chemist, Philip Bromley, thank you for allowing me to expect nothing but perfection.

Special thanks to PETA, Vegan Outreach, and Viva USA! for their support and for allowing me to use their photographs for chapter 23.

Higher Power, Infinite Intelligence that has blessed, inspired, and guided me throughout my life—and particularly this journey—I'm eternally grateful for your quiet, yet constant presence in my life. I'm only sorry that I haven't always paid close enough attention.

Kashif, Greta, and Gunther, my beautiful Rottweilers and loyal companions who have all sadly passed on, I miss your sweet, loving, and ever-protective souls! There is no greater, no purer love than that which I shared with each of you. Your selfless, oh, so innocent souls reminded me each and every day to live in the moment; moreover, that nothing else really matters except to give love—and be loved—by man or animal. I love and miss you!

CONTENTS

Acknowledgments vii

Disclaimer xv

Introduction: *Managing Expectations*. xvii

Attention, Reader! xxi

PART I

diet failure...
the Naked Truth
The Crucial Serotonin-Insulin Connection Exposed!

1   Why 98% of All Diets Fail 7
    The missing link needed to overcome obesity

2   An Extraordinary Brain Chemical 11
    A carb addict you are not!

3   Oh, the Many Diets We've Tried! 21

4   This Is NOT a Diet! 29

5   Conditions Associated with Low Serotonin. .33

6   How to Naturally Boost Your Serotonin. 35

7   Health Benefits of Serotonin-Enhancing Supplements 39

8   Unheard of, but Why?. 45

9   Storing Fat, One of Insulin's Many Roles. 51

10 Type 2 Diabetes Running Rampant 55

11 Sugar & Its Sweet, Addictive Nature 59

12 The Many Faces of Sugar 63

13 WARNING: High-Fructose Corn Syrup 65

14 Aspartame—A DEADLY TOXIN!. 69
Making us fat, depressed, & deathly ill!

15 Obesity, an Alarming Epidemic 75

16 Fat Cells Gettin' Fatter! 79

17 Stimulants Not Needed. 83
But freedom of choice is a MUST!

18 Direct Link: Depression & Our Diet. 87
Sugar, high GI carbs, caffeine, nicotine, etc.

19 Insulin & How It Affects Cholesterol. 105
The key to helping cure heart disease

20 Insulin & How It Affects Blood Pressure 111

21 Eating Healthy Without Ever Feeling Deprived. 115

22 Marketing Scams That Are Making Us Fatter Than Ever! 121
Not to mention sick as hell!

23 From Petting Zoo to Dinner Table 129
When did it go so terribly wrong?

24 Exercise & Its Many Glorious Benefits .137

25 Genes. 151
Use 'em or abuse 'em!

26 Expect More from Yourself. 157

27 Pharmaceutical Drugs & Their Side Effects 169
Weight gain, depression, liver & heart failure, new disease, even death!

PART II

Carbohydrates & the Glycemic Index

28 What Is a Carb?. 187

29 Good Carb? Bad Carb?. 189
Which is it?

30 Glycogen's Role 195

31 Crucial Carbohydrate Facts 199

32 Excellent Low GI Carbs 203

33 Suggested Foods. 205
    My personal choices

34 How to Read a Nutritional Panel. 209
    Don't be fooled! Know what you're eating!

35 Summary of Health Tips 217

PART III

300+ Personal Health Tips

36 Physical Health Tips. 223

37 Mental, Emotional & Spiritual Health Tips. 243

PART IV

In Closing

In Appreciation/Order. 254

Research/References/Recommendations. 255

Company Profile/Consultations/Webinars
Wellness & Anti-Aging Center/Wellness Retreat. 259

Author 261
Journey of Discovery

In Loving Memory 267

"As a consumer, this book is, at minimum, enlightening, but more so alarming. As a businessman, I discovered a whole world of underexposed, unethical possibilities. As a human being, Phoenix created new hope for a better life. More than a case study of the diet question, this book is an extensive discovery of everything that is good for you. Well worth reading. Well worth memorizing."
—C.J. Yesson, Retired Life Insurance CEO, Investment Banker

DISCLAIMER

No particular product is being promoted, sold, or endorsed in this book.
It is, instead, about certain individual ingredients. Any references made
by the author, including, but not limited to R&D, products, supplements, trial testing,
clients, client's results, etc., were done entirely for the purpose of conveying a point
of expertise. Any principles and/or health benefits discussed can be easily achieved
with similar products. This book's sole purpose is to educate the consumer
as to the research within. And, to reiterate, this book is not intended to diagnose, treat,
cure, or prevent any illness. This book is the sole opinion of me, the author. It was written
merely to inform the reader. It is not intended as medical advice. It should not be used to
replace any medical care or any therapeutic program recommended by a medical doctor.
The author (and publisher) disclaim any and all liability arising directly or indirectly from the
use of the information contained within this book.

IN ADDITION...

This is not a diet.
It is, though, a lifelong solution to help you achieve your long-term weight loss
goals and excellent overall health—physically, mentally, and emotionally.
Discover why this book offers you the safest, most effective solution to reach all
your health and fitness goals. Plus, learn hundreds of fascinating health tips, alarming
facts, and warnings that the FDA, AMA, FTC, pharmaceutical companies, and
food manufacturers don't ever want you to know about!
If you want to lose weight, alleviate depression, anxiety, insomnia, ADD, PMS,
reduce your risk for type 2 diabetes, high blood pressure, even cancer and heart disease,
so as to live a long, happy, and healthy life, this book is an absolute
MUST-READ!

"Phoenix explains, in explicit yet simple detail, the underlying cause of cravings, carb addictions, even ADD, depression, and heart disease. Serotonin is truly the crucial link to overcome obesity—and numerous other health issues. As a physician, scientist, and formerly overweight person, I recommend everyone read this book, especially parents. It will change, if not save, your life and the lives of your children."
—Stephen Scheinberg, PhD, MD

INTRODUCTION:
Managing Expectations

I've written this book with the sincerest desire to help others finally understand why 98% of all diets fail—and equally why depression, ADD, type 2 diabetes, high blood pressure, even heart disease—are so disturbingly prevalent. This breakthrough information is based on clinical research, not diet or marketing hype. To help insure you get the very most from the information presented, I respectfully ask that you first carefully read the following:

1) This is NOT a diet or a quick fix. I am not promising, "Lose 30 pounds in 30 days!" My suggested lifestyle program is, though, about how to live a much *healthier lifestyle*. So please, don't stress over losing the excess weight. It will come. I promise you. Focus instead on healing your body and mind. Just remember, it took a lifetime to damage your body, it will equally take time to reverse the damage. It will also require effort and consistency to achieve your various goals. You must be willing to do what it takes.

2) I wrote my book in a Q&A format, as it best reflected the actual dialogue exchanged between me and my clients, and even total strangers simply seeking advice on any given day. It was also crucial that I represent the average consumer, that I directly voice *their* viewpoints, concerns, and countless frustrations. Some questions may seem trivial to one, but extremely helpful to another. In addition, I needed to challenge my own viewpoints, play the devil's advocate, so to speak.

3) Based on the far too confusing information provided by the AMA, FDA, and our very own doctors, I felt it was absolutely necessary to address all such issues in an easy-to-comprehend and personal tone, *minus* the usual over-the-top medical jargon that tends to confuse people even more.

4) I was intentionally a bit repetitive, because, just as in real life, it often requires saying something repeatedly, and in various ways, before someone truly begins to grasp the information in its entirety.

5) To further assist you in reaching your health/fitness goals, read each chapter twice before going on to the next. Also, as you read, stop and ask yourself how the information relates to you and yours. Underscore those points of interest. It's essential that you then apply the knowledge in your daily life. Review this book often. Once you get it, your life will *forever* be changed! Then, help me, help others, by sharing this book with others!

6) Set realistic weight loss goals. Don't set yourself up for failure.

7) You will lose inches long before you actually lose pounds—particularly if you begin weight training, as muscle weighs more than fat. Hence, please do not judge your weight loss by the scale, as it's not an accurate way to measure your success.

8) Throughout the book, I use both the terms "weight loss" and "fat loss." My focus, though, is always about losing excess body fat. Another good reason to avoid the scale, as it's not so much about a number, as it is about losing excess body fat, while gaining lean muscle tissue. And, unlike what most weight loss programs claim, it is genetically impossible, not to mention unhealthy, to lose more than 1 to 2 pounds of fat per week.

9) This book is giving you the solution, as to why diets most often fail. It is, on the other hand, up to you what you will do with this information. *Will you take advantage of it? Are you ready to make the commitment?* I sincerely hope so.

10) With respect to designing my book, <u>everything</u> I did (along with Billy's graphic touch), was for a very precise reason, from selection of colors, font size, format, title, to interior photos, cover image, etc. I chose *diet failure...the Naked Truth*, as I needed a name that would best convey this extraordinary research. It needed to be raw. Direct. To the point. It was imperative that I let the reader know the truth, the NAKED TRUTH behind their many failed diets. I equally needed to create a cover that would capture the consumer's attention, to make them curious enough to reach out and review the book more closely, and, moreover, make them want to read it! I also knew it had to somehow stand out from the other thousands of diet/health/fitness books. So I asked myself: What are we attracted to, especially those individuals who are seeking to improve their health, their bodies, their minds? We're attracted to other beautiful bodies, bodies that inspire us to push ourselves harder, bodies that make us expect more from ourselves—strong, lean, attractive physiques that let us know that *all things are possible* when it comes to our fitness goals, no matter our age. With those marketing strategies in mind, it was important to play off the name, to make it eye-catching, inspiring, thought-provoking, and, yes, sensuous, yet not offensive. To increase the impact, *to hopefully inspire others*, the couple featured on the cover, and throughout the book, are simply two ordinary, middle-aged people. The man posing is one of my long-time clients and dearest friends, Billy Ciampo. He looks incredible for any age, even more so, because he's 53! And, being a very proud woman, a woman who feels I absolutely <u>must</u> reflect that which I kindly expect from others, I am the woman featured. I'm 46. Now, if you'd like to find out how we're able to look like this at our age—and WITHOUT dieting, ever feeling deprived or hungry, or having to live in the gym—all you have to do is <u>read</u> <u>this</u> <u>book</u>. I promise you, it will change your life forever!

11) To those who have asked, "Who are you? Are you a doctor? What is your degree?" I modestly reply: I'm a woman who seeks the truth. Always have. Always will. I'm a woman who wants to make a difference. I want to teach others how to help *save their own lives* by living a healthy lifestyle. I'm a woman who, after 20 plus years of being involved in various degrees in Health & Wellness, was fed up with the misinformation, deceit, and marketing scams running rampant within the diet, food, and pharmaceutical industries—deceit that borders on the criminal, and, at bare minimum, makes Americans fat, depressed, and sicker than ever! I freely admit I'm not a doctor; nor do I need to be. This also means I'm not driven by greed or profit margins. I don't have a college degree; nor is it necessary.

Equally, my professed expertise does not come simply from reading medical journals or passing some exam. I am, however, proud to say that my expertise comes instead from an insatiable desire to educate myself; spending nearly 6 years diligently researching this precise subject. But that wasn't enough for me. I needed to actually test the many remarkable claims. So, I also developed dietary supplements based on the research. What I witnessed firsthand throughout the trial stages of my company's various products is what prompted me to write this book. I knew, *without a doubt,* that all the clinical studies that I had read, all the amazing research that I had studied for years was, in fact, true.

12) I humbly exposed myself throughout the book, as it was important that the reader know I'm not just a researcher, but have actually experienced most of what I speak of— both good and bad. And, as such, the book will be at one moment serious and scientific, the next provocative, challenging, and in your face, to then playful and sexually frank. The very next second it may make you cry, get angry, or dare you to rethink your life. All such honest emotions expressed will hopefully help keep the reader's attention from cover to cover. My motive? I want to force you, the reader, to think, to feel, to reach outside yourself—and to live a healthier, more compassionate life. And, to those who may be offended by my candor, please don't be. There are plenty of serious health books, but the story I needed to tell goes *far beyond* science.

Furthermore, I'm hoping that by sharing so much of my very private world, it will give you a better idea of who I am as a human being, as a female with that certain edge, more so as a passionate, sensitive, strong-willed individual—so that, hopefully, in some small way, it will *encourage* you to live a happier, fuller, more determined life. One that is true to you, and those you care for. To help you find the emotional, mental, and physical strength when you feel less than. And, to hopefully inspire you to discover your own unique passion and go after it. Because you see, throughout my life I have endured many struggles and heartaches. But I am also a survivor. I believe in myself. I've never allowed others to drag me down or abuse me—be it verbally, mentally or physically. And I never give up. Ever. All things are possible if you believe in yourself and persevere!

And, finally, my intentions with this book are pure and simple: To educate. To inspire. To empower. (Especially women.) To give hope. To make a difference. I sincerely hope it helps you live a much longer, happier, and healthier life!

Wishing you the greatest of success in health—in love—in life.

Phoenix Gilman, CPT, CSN
Nutritional/Medical Researcher, Motivational Speaker, Consumer Activist, Author

xix

ATTENTION, READER!

Before you begin this journey,
and to help insure you get the most from this book,
you must first, please, read and understand the following:

Those of us in the alternative healthcare industry are severely restricted by the FDA, pharmaceutical companies, and the FTC as to what we can say about any and all illness and/or disease. We are not allowed in any way, to attempt to diagnose, suggest treatment and/or cures, or make any medical claims. Though I would love to believe this is out of genuine concern for the welfare of the public, it is not. Instead, it's unfortunately due to the fact that our all-natural, alternative remedies—remedies that are highly effective, affordable, and come with little, if any, side effects—are a serious threat to the actual survival of the drug companies and the medical industry as we know them today. Without disease, without a need for the drug companies' millions of senseless, cost-prohibitive, and often deadly pharmaceutical drugs, they would be out of business—a business that was founded, and is solely dependent on our getting and remaining sick.

Worse yet, even as these drugs are <u>killing</u> well over 100,000 innocent people every year, the FDA turns a blind eye, due to their far too close (if not illegal) tie to the drug companies—drug companies that they are supposed to be protecting the Americans from. They also sit back quietly while the drug companies bombard the media with false and unethically inaccurate reports regarding the safety of dietary supplements, hoping to frighten the consumer away—and back to their DEADLY DRUGS!

My goal here is simply to educate the consumer as to the many extraordinary health benefits that come from a very precise brain chemical, and beyond that, but with no intentions whatsoever to diagnose, cure, or above all, cause harm to another. But I must walk an extremely fine line. Whether it pertains to the causes and/or treatment of obesity, depression, insomnia, ADD, heart disease, etc., or explains how dietary supplements may help alleviate, treat, and/or cure such illnesses, I am harshly restrained in what I can say.

My sincere desire is to help others, but, at the same time, avoid fines and retaliation by these frighteningly monopolized, yet equally powerful, government agencies. Hence, it will require that you, the consumer, read my book with your eyes and mind wide open. You will need to read, analyze, and research further on your own. You will then be much better prepared to make your own decisions. Do not allow me, the FDA, AMA, FTC, drug companies, or your personal physician to tell you what is best for you or your loved ones. That is your right. That is your choice. Please use it wisely.

Enjoy the journey...

PART I

diet failure...
the Naked Truth

The Crucial Serotonin-Insulin Connection Exposed!

The time has come.
Time for change.
Starting with this book.

So,
are you tired of being overweight?
Are you fed up with failing at every diet you've tried?
Are you sick of being called fat, lazy, & weak-willed?
Are you done crying yourself to sleep at night?
Are you through being ashamed to go out in public?

Wouldn't you like to know why food controls you?
Wouldn't you like to know why certain foods give you such emotional comfort?
Wouldn't you like to know why your willpower is never enough?
Wouldn't you like to know why, no matter how hard you work out,
you still don't have the body that you desire?

Wouldn't you also like to know why you are so often
depressed, unable to sleep, or suffering with
ADD, high blood pressure or heart disease?

Are you ready, though, to make a change,
to put forth the required effort?
Are you ready to make the commitment?
I sincerely hope so, as this is the answer you've been waiting for.

Be prepared.
Your life is about to be forever changed.

1

WHY 98% OF ALL DIETS FAIL
The missing link needed to overcome obesity

You have certainly caught my attention, but let's get right to the point, shall we? What is this "Naked Truth" you speak of?
It is a fact, and an alarming reality, that 98% of all attempts to lose weight be it—low-cal, low-fat, or low-carb diets, even stomach stapling—inevitably fail. The Naked Truth that I speak of, however, is that these diet failures are not due to lack of willpower, food addiction, or emotional attachment. The Naked Truth is that diet failure is not your fault. That's right. It's not your fault. Do you really think anyone chooses to be overweight? Fat? Obese? Do you really think anyone would intentionally keep failing at every single diet? Of course not. Diet failure, in most cases, is not your fault.

Yeah, right! It's not my fault? Please! Are you kidding or what?
First of all, please understand that the mere word "diet" implies someone is, in fact, at least trying. And no, I'm not kidding. I'm very serious. To be able to tell someone that diet failure is not their fault is so empowering. Whereas everyone else would love for you to believe it's about willpower/mind control, determination, starvation, deprivation, or food addictions, I'm going to tell you something that will change your life forever—and free you from the tortured guilt of having failed at so many diets in the past.

Haven't you ever wondered *why* it's so hard to stick to a healthy way of eating? Haven't you ever wondered *why,* no matter how many times, in how many ways, health experts tell you what to eat to lose the weight, you simply cannot stick to their diets? Haven't you ever wondered *why* cravings are always your downfall? Haven't you ever wondered *why* all your diets have failed?

Of course you have. We all have. Time after time, you start a diet with all the passion, conviction, and promises that you'll succeed. You vow to do *whatever* it takes, and as *long* as it takes, to lose the weight! Considering you're far from being a quitter, you begin each new diet with this same intensity. You're off to a great start. Eating low-calorie, then low-fat, now it's low-carb. You're not really sure what to eat anymore, but you are committed like never before!

Sadly, only weeks, maybe months into it, you find yourself sabotaging this diet as well. Chip by chip. Cookie by cookie. You find it *impossible* to resist the foods that have always given you such comfort. With each loss of control, the pounds start to creep back on.

Whatever weight you lost, you've gained back—and more! *But why?* Why is it so hard? It's not like you're incompetent. After all, you're successful in your career. You have a happy and fulfilling marriage with three beautiful children, so *why* is it that you can't succeed at losing some lousy weight—and keeping it off?

Wouldn't you like to know why all your best intentions have *never* been enough? Wouldn't you like to know why food has *always* controlled you? Wouldn't you like to know why, no matter how hard you train, you still *don't* have the body that you really desire? Aren't you tired of people assuming you're overweight because you're weak-willed, lazy, or unwilling? *Don't you want to know why all your diets have failed?*

Yes! Of course I do!
First of all, diets fail for two simple, yet crucial, reasons: cravings and appetite. Most of us hopefully realize by now that our shocking rate of obesity is not due to eating healthy fats, but due instead to eating the wrong type of and/or simply far too many carbohydrates. And though we can be told all day long what NOT to eat to stay lean and healthy, it is entirely another matter to *control* the insatiable carbohydrate/sugar cravings and overall appetite. Hence, the astounding 98% rate of diet failure.

You're exactly right. I have no willpower! I feel like I'm addicted to certain foods! But *why* can't I control my cravings?
Unlike what so many others have told you through the years, it's not your fault that you can't stick to those diets. In most cases, it's not your fault that you're overweight. While you'll most certainly have to at least make an effort to eat healthy, successful dieting has absolutely nothing to do with a lack of willpower, nor is it about food intolerances, having to starve yourself, or using stimulants. And it is most assuredly <u>not</u> about being addicted to certain foods.

Can't I just not worry about my lack of willpower and get my stomach stapled like so many others are doing?
I suppose you can do anything you want. But unless your weight has gotten to the point where it means life or death, I would seriously recommend you reconsider. Gastric bypass surgery is an extremely risky procedure and should be considered only if you need to lose 100 pounds or more. And while its goal is to severely reduce the amount of food the patient can take in, you need to realize that it is only a *temporary* fix. It is only masking the underlying problem. (I discuss this in greater detail in chapter 3.)

So, what is your solution? What is the missing link? *Please tell me!*
Are you sure you want to know? Are you really ready to take this information and utilize it? With all due respect, even though I've shared this research with hundreds of people, there is a certain percentage of those who sadly choose to totally disregard it, who are basically unwilling to make the necessary changes in lifestyle, and who, instead, keep silently praying for that ever-elusive magic diet pill. I'm sorry, but if you don't know it already, that

magic pill does <u>not</u> exist! Therefore, your success will require effort. So, again I ask: Are you ready to take this information and utilize it?

Yes, I'm very serious. I'm ready! Please, I want to know!
The Naked Truth is that successful, i.e., *long-term* weight loss is, in fact, based on "BRAIN CHEMISTRY." The answer, the solution, the missing (and crucial) link that most experts have missed, is that 98% of all diets fail due to the depletion of a very precise brain chemical.

Excuse me? *A brain chemical?*
Yes, a brain chemical. That extraordinary, extremely powerful major neurotransmitter is called *serotonin*. Stronger than any street drug, it is the most important neurotransmitter, the master communicator among the many other brain chemicals. For your mind, and therefore, your body, to work at its very best, *to function as effectively as possible*, serotonin levels <u>must</u> be maintained. Serotonin, though, is also the brain chemical that has clinically proven to control the two major reasons why diets inevitably fail. To finally understand that successful weight loss is based on brain chemistry, NOT willpower or addiction, is <u>the most empowering</u> information that I can share with my clients. Without a doubt, it's the research everyone needs to learn about. It will empower people as never before! It will free them of the endless and senseless shame over all their failed diets!

***Are you serious?* Are you saying my inability to stick with a diet is not about being weak-willed?**
This is exactly what I'm saying. Successful weight loss is based on maintaining healthy levels of serotonin. And healthy levels of serotonin will subsequently lead to controlling insulin levels. This **"Serotonin-Insulin Connection"** is the crucial link for achieving successful weight loss. (I explain this in much greater detail in the following chapters.)

All this time, I've felt like such a loser! A fat one, at that! I'm so ashamed at how many diets I've tried and failed at. I'm sure everyone who has ever failed at a diet feels like I do. But why isn't anyone else talking about this?
I have no idea. Most people only know of serotonin and its relation to depression. They have no clue as to its amazing abilities to control carbohydrate cravings and overall appetite. Nor do I hear anyone in the media discussing the direct correlation to low serotonin and insomnia, ADD, PMS, migraines, etc. All these reasons, and many more, are why it's so important for me to get this information to the masses. It gives people the answer, the *solution* they've been searching for. It explains in precise, yet simple, detail exactly *why* all their past diets have failed. It also explains why they may be so moody, anxious, unable to concentrate, sleep, and so forth. And while the information I am about to share with you is based on sound clinical science, it's extremely easy to comprehend. When I share this research with my clients, the light suddenly goes on. *They finally get it!*

2

AN EXTRAORDINARY BRAIN CHEMICAL
A carb addict you are not!

Can you please tell me again what serotonin is?

Serotonin is the most important neurotransmitter (a brain communicator) that regulates food cravings, satiety (appetite), mood, sleep, pain, aggression, anxiety, and much more.

What causes cravings?

Cravings are due to low serotonin levels. When this brain chemical gets depleted, we *subconsciously* crave the types of foods that break down quickly into blood sugar, i.e., high glycemic index (GI) carbohydrates. These particular carbs range from bagels, white bread, pasta, (yes, pasta) pastries, chips, crackers, candy, cereal, sodas, fruit juices, etc. These foods spike insulin levels. Insulin, in around about way, allows tryptophan to enter the brain. Tryptophan transforms into serotonin. And serotonin, *makes us feel good!* These foods have subsequently become known as "comfort foods." This is why people tend to eat out of emotion. This chemical shift in the brain, though subtle, makes us feel good! Simply put, people eat these particular foods to feel better. They are, in fact, self-medicating. So you see, there is indeed an emotional attachment and reward to this eating pattern. Unfortunately, this is exactly why our obesity rate is as high as it is.

That's ironic. Isn't this how low-fat foods make you feel?

Yes. While fat-free/low-fat foods may be low in fat, they are, instead, loaded with sugar, causing the same response. Furthermore, though foods like bagels, bread, cereal, and pasta are usually fat-free/low-fat—and generally considered complex carbs—they're highly refined so as to give them that oooh, so delicious taste; especially bagels to make them *ever so moist!* It's this process that makes them high GI carbs. *Why?* Because refined/processed foods need relatively no digestion time. Therefore, the minute you eat them, they immediately break down into blood sugar. This causes your insulin levels to rise rapidly. You're actually better off eating foods that still have healthy fat in them. Also, these fat-free/high-carb foods contain little, if any nutrition, no fiber, and minimal protein.

Once again, when serotonin is depleted, cravings sneak in. Eating these high GI and/or excessive carbohydrates causes a rapid release of insulin. While one of insulin's roles is to carefully regulate the amount of blood sugar going to the brain, the increased levels of insulin will also boost serotonin levels. And it's serotonin that makes us feel so damn good. But, this feeling of comfort we get from these foods is merely temporary, lasting an hour or so. To get that feeling again, our brain forces us, on a subconscious level, to eat more of these foods. Once again, insulin spiking leads to the production of serotonin. This cycle is repeated over and over. Day after day. Month after month. While the effects of serotonin are short-lived, the excess calories consumed are not. The result: a nation that is 65% overweight—and depressed. FACT: 98% of all diets will inevitably fail, unless you're able to maintain healthy levels of serotonin.

I swear I'm addicted to bread! And I sure do love my chips!

Unfortunately, there are far too many people who believe it's about being addicted to these foods. This is not true. It is instead about this vital brain chemical being depleted. The only addiction is wanting to self-medicate by eating foods that trigger the increase of serotonin. All of which is done on a subconscious level.

With all due respect, and with no desire to ever speak out of turn, I can't begin to tell you how many times I've heard Oprah speak of her carbohydrate addiction. She once admitted that she was "no different than any other type of addict." She went on to say that this was simply who she was and she'd have to accept it. When I heard this, I wanted to cry in frustration. *Why?* Because, as you now know, her addiction to carbs is due to her serotonin being depleted. I was desperate to share my knowledge with her, to help her understand why she craves certain carbs and how to control her carb addiction, once and for all.

There are millions who feel like Oprah! Most of us, though, have pathetically given up! We're fatter than ever! We've come to believe it's something we must live with.
You're exactly right. But after you read this book, you will most definitely realize it is NOT something you have to live with. I would also ask that you use Oprah as an example of all that is possible if you put your mind to it—and I mean really put your mind to it! Truth be told, and if I may be so bold, far too many people bitch and moan endlessly about being overweight, but they aren't *willing* to "make the commitment" that is required to achieve the leaner, sexier, healthier body that they dream of. Oprah, on the other hand, has finally figured it out—and she is committed. She, with the guidance of her trainer Bob Greene, knows what it takes to get the body she desires.

Oprah is an inspiration in so many ways, to so many people, but when it comes to what she has done with her body, she is, without a doubt, a phenomenal example of what someone can achieve by eating a healthy diet—at the very least, that which is void of refined/high GI carbs—along with a consistent and intense workout routine combining both weight training and cardio. And while I have never seen anyone make such a total and glorious transformation as she has, I'd like to think her weight loss journey might have been slightly easier had she been aware of this information. Maybe one day I will be fortunate enough to share my expertise with her. I think she would be absolutely astounded to realize just how easily her "carb addiction" would disappear, and to learn that her past failed diets were most often not her fault.

Oprah is definitely an inspiration for what can be achieved if someone really gets serious. I'm ready to make the commitment, but I just need help getting over the cravings that have always kept me overweight.

After you read this book, you will be armed with the knowledge required to live a much healthier lifestyle. At the very least, you'll learn how to maintain your serotonin levels, thereby controlling those ever-powerful carbohydrate cravings.

What else does serotonin control?

Serotonin is a major neurotransmitter that not only controls carbohydrate cravings, but also naturally reduces appetite, as it's the satiety control mechanism for the body.

Really? Serotonin controls my appetite, as well as my cravings?

Yes. It's one thing to control cravings, but your total caloric intake also plays an essential role in long-term weight loss. The most basic concept of weight loss is: *Eating more food than your body requires will be stored as fat.* This is predominantly true with an excess of carbohydrates, because carbs cannot be used for anything except to fuel the body and mind. Thus, if they're not used, they will be promoted to fat storage. Whereas with protein and fats, the body can utilize these foods for rebuilding the body's cells, hormones, enzymes, muscles, neurotransmitters, etc. Once again, serotonin naturally controls the two key reasons why diets fail: Carbohydrate cravings and appetite.

Does serotonin control anything else?

Healthy levels of serotonin are also crucial to alleviating depression, anxiety, stress, migraines, pain, PMS, ADD, OCD, etc. Once you're able to achieve and maintain healthy serotonin levels, you will not only start to lose the excess weight, but your mood will also be fantastic. You'll feel less stressed. Sleep patterns will improve greatly. You'll be slower to anger, calmer, and more focused. Body aches and pain will be reduced. You'll have far more energy, without having to use harmful stimulants. Your entire life will be more focused and energized.

Cravings are merely a side effect of low serotonin.

Serotonin controls all these things?

Yes, and believe it or not, serotonin controls many other amazing functions within the body. I insist, though, that my clients do not take my word for it, but, instead, research it on their own. Then, they will truly understand serotonin's extensive health benefits.

How does serotonin become depleted?

Basically everything in life seems to deplete serotonin, ranging from stress, lack of deep restorative (quality) sleep, poor nutrition, sedentary lifestyle, low-fat dieting and dieting in general, high GI and excessive carbohydrate consumption, processed/refined foods, sugar, and artificial sweeteners. Caffeine, nicotine, ephedra, chocolate, alcohol, over-the-counter meds, and prescription and nonprescription drugs all deplete serotonin, as well.

Oh, my! All of those things deplete serotonin?

Yes, and it's a vicious cycle. *Why?* Because who doesn't have stress in their life? How often do you eat balanced, nutritious meals? When's the last time you had a quality night's sleep? And who doesn't drink coffee or alcohol? All these things, plus numerous others, deplete serotonin. We then become depressed. Irritable. Anxious. Stressed. Quick to anger. Tired. We look for emotional relief. Anything to make us feel better! Our minds then *subconsciously* force us toward the types of foods or substances that it knows will stimulate the production of serotonin, thereby making us feel good. Most of us don't even know why we crave chocolate cake, mac' and cheese, potato chips, bagels, or even caffeine and alcohol. We just assume we're weak, addicted, or without willpower. Not true! Cravings are a side of effect of low serotonin. Critical fact: Elevating serotonin in this manner, requires a spike in insulin. And insulin is the hormone that causes the body to store fat.

Is this why I find myself craving carbs after a long, stressful day?

This is exactly why. In addition to the high stress level, you've probably also consumed many of the other things that equally deplete serotonin. By day's end, your serotonin has plummeted. Your brain then begins to create noise, i.e., cravings. And it will continually force you to seek the foods that it knows will once again trigger the production of this ever-comforting brain chemical. For all those who have ever had a craving, including myself, you know only too well just how powerful they can be. They are <u>not</u> to be ignored. To reiterate, brain chemicals are stronger than any street drug, and when the brain thinks it's starving, it will do anything and everything to save itself. Hence, it forces you to consume the foods and/or beverages that break down <u>quickest</u> into blood sugar. Its other critical goal is to boost serotonin, no matter how brief, so as to help the body/mind function properly.

Lack of sleep and the cravings that will surely follow.

Another example is when you don't get enough sleep. (Insomnia is another side effect of low serotonin.) Haven't you ever noticed when you're tired, maybe after a night out or merely a restless night's sleep, and the only foods you seem to be hungry for are carbs? No matter how hard you try to avoid them, *nothing* satisfies your appetite. That is, not until you finally take a bite of your favorite carb. Maybe it's pizza. Cereal. Sweet potato pie. Toasted bagel. Pretzels. French fries. (And, my dear Sam, you know just how good those fries can taste!) Or maybe you lean more toward ice cream. Dried fruit. Yogurt. Raisins. Oreo cookies. Chocolate bar. Nonetheless, whatever your carb selection, once consumed, *once you've spiked your insulin*, the increase in serotonin is soon to follow. Ooooh, that feeling of comfort is only moments away! Like magic, the cravings suddenly stop. Your hunger ceases. You sit back, take a deep breath, you feel soooo good! Well, at least for an hour or so. But there they are. Once again. The cravings come gently knocking. Then pounding! Until you give in. The cycle repeats. Over and over.

This is so true! I can't believe it! This is exactly what happens to me when I don't get enough sleep. It's only after I eat one of my favorite carbs that I feel content.

The comfort you derive from eating high GI carbs is definitely short-lived. And once your serotonin drops again, which it will within about an hour, your brain will start the craving cycle all over again. Don't forget, each time that you give in to these cravings, you are causing your body to store *more* fat.

Where does serotonin come from?

Neurotransmitters, i.e., serotonin, are derived from dietary proteins. Tryptophan is an amino acid naturally found in dietary protein—and tryptophan is essential for the production of serotonin. When you eat a fat-free/low-fat diet, the often feared, but so-called fatty foods such as red meat, eggs, nuts, avocados, poultry, butter, and cheese (which are healthy sources of protein) are often eliminated from your diet. By doing this, you have robbed your body of the raw materials needed to produce adequate amounts of tryptophan. Without enough tryptophan, your body can't *naturally* produce enough serotonin.

What are the side effects of serotonin deficiency?

There are numerous side effects when serotonin is deficient. However, the side effects that contribute to diet failure are, of course, cravings and binge eating, particularly for the kind of carbs that break down quickly into blood sugar. And as you've just learned, those carbs are known as simple or high GI carbs. Depression is also an extremely common side effect when serotonin is low.

Depression, as well? Any other side effects?

Depression, no matter the underlying cause, is due to serotonin being depleted, especially when it's low on a constant basis. As for other side effects, most people I share this information with are shocked to realize just how many health conditions are directly related to low serotonin. (Or as the FDA and drug companies would like to call them: *diseases*.) Nevertheless, people need to understand that serotonin is a "MAJOR NEUROTRANSMITTER" and as such, when it's out of balance—your entire body and mind will suffer in various ways. So, yes, in addition to carb/sugar cravings, binge eating, insomnia, and depression, other side effects would include obesity, rage, sudden outbursts, mood swings, ADD, ADHD, extreme agitation, anxiety, panic attacks, PMS, alcoholism, headaches, migraines, repetitive behavior, chronic body pain, low energy, lack of creative focus, decreased sex drive (yes, *decreased* sex drive!), irritable bowel syndrome, memory loss, schizophrenia, and suicidal behavior.

I would never have believed that serotonin could control so many things! I guess it makes perfect sense, considering it is, after all, a major brain chemical.

Yes, serotonin undeniably controls all these things—and many more. Therefore, when this brain chemical is depleted, countless health conditions will arise. Side effects will vary from person to person. They also vary in degree depending upon whether or not serotonin levels are fluctuated quickly versus if they're constantly low. Either way, be sure to read chapter 5 for a more detailed list of the health conditions caused by low serotonin.

The next important question has to be—how do I achieve and maintain healthy levels of serotonin naturally?
For starters, you need to provide your body with balanced nutrition, regular exercise, and quality sleep. These things will help provide healthy serotonin levels. A diet that contains plenty of foods rich in tryptophan, i.e., fresh fish, meat, milk, eggs, cottage cheese, turkey, wheat germ, and nuts, may also be helpful in boosting serotonin. Unfortunately, it would be extremely difficult to eat enough of these foods to supply the needed tryptophan. In addition, you must also eliminate all stress, stimulants, recreational drugs, high GI and excessive carbohydrate consumption, sugar, artificial sweeteners, prescription and non-prescription drugs, nicotine, caffeine, alcohol, and any other insulin-releasing factors. Add to that the fact that most people live sedentary lives, and it's easy to understand why it's nearly impossible to maintain healthy serotonin levels on our own. Based on the lifestyle of most Americans, we are a nation that is, without a doubt, suffering from what is now being recognized as "Serotonin Deficiency Syndrome."

What are the benefits of healthy serotonin levels?
The health benefits are truly endless. To begin with, when the brain has healthy levels of serotonin, it will stop demanding outside substances, i.e., high GI carbohydrates, sugar, caffeine, nicotine, alcohol, etc., that stimulate a quick release of serotonin.

It seems low serotonin levels are displayed in different ways?
This is precisely what happens. Through the years, our brains have become conditioned to know exactly what will elevate our serotonin. Some people will crave corn bread, chips, biscuits, or cereal. Others may crave chocolate, juice, or sodas. Some will crave alcohol or caffeine. Still others may crave cigarettes. Each person exhibits low serotonin levels in their own unique way. To reiterate, we each have *unknowingly* conditioned our brain's through our lifetime of eating habits. To crave anything is a sign of low serotonin. It's also a sign of being unhealthy. And to those who say they "don't have cravings," it doesn't necessarily have to be an overwhelming urge. It's simply the types of foods you are *drawn* to—and they'll most often be high GI carbs, i.e., foods that trigger insulin.

What are some other health benefits?
Properly balanced serotonin levels will also provide a tremendous sense of well-being, contentment, and happiness. It will energize your life, promote deep restorative sleep, diminish anxiety and stress, alleviate pain, ADD/ADHD, PMS, as well as enhance your sense of focus, mental clarity, creativity, productivity, and sexual behavior. As you can see, serotonin is absolutely crucial to your mental and physical health.

Is this why I feel so depressed when I diet?
Most often, yes. Fat-free or low-fat dieting is the biggest contributor to this, as it eliminates the precise foods the body needs to make adequate amounts of serotonin.

How will low-carb dieting affect my mood?

People will unquestionably feel their moods spiral downward, as they will no longer be consuming the high GI carbs that so easily triggered the production of serotonin. They'll also feel more stressed, anxious, unable to concentrate, etc. And this is when the cravings kick in. Because the brain is perfectly conditioned to know what it needs, it will literally force you toward the foods and/or beverages that it knows will elevate this powerful brain chemical. Your brain will create this noise until you give in. It will force you to eat the types of carbs, i.e., bread, chips, candy, sodas, fast food, etc., that will once again elevate serotonin. The result: you'll feel great! Unfortunately, it will also make you FAT! Now, more than ever, people need to realize that unless they're able to maintain adequate serotonin levels, all attempts at dieting will fail, *especially low-carb dieting!*

Is this why so many diets fail?

This is *exactly* why most diets fail. It's one thing to tell people what not to eat; it's another matter entirely for them to adhere to that diet regimen if their serotonin is low. This is particularly important when it concerns controlling cravings and/or desires for high GI carbs, because it's these precise carbs that cause the body to store fat.

My eating habits are fine in the morning. In fact, I rarely eat breakfast.

Your first mistake is skipping breakfast. Most people, especially women, feel that the less they eat, the thinner they will be. Not true. This is a far too common misconception. This is a classic example of low-calorie dieting—and low-calorie dieting will only set you up for more weight gain. (I discuss this further in the following chapter.) Then, there are others who complain that by eating breakfast, they're much hungrier throughout the day so they, too, skip breakfast, eat a late lunch on the run, and then, come dinner time, when they're basically starving, they inhale whatever is put before them.

More often than not, either scenario will lead to people consuming far too many calories for that late hour. Regardless, that one large meal at the end of the day is not generally enough to make people fat. Those who attempt to lose weight this way must wonder *why* they're gaining weight. After all, they only ate one meal, and even though the meal was late in the day, it was far from an "excess" of calories. So, why can't they lose weight? Moreover, why are they gaining weight so fast? Allow me to explain:

1) When you don't properly fuel your body throughout the day, your serotonin will plummet. Low serotonin will cause cravings for high GI carbs and binge eating. Hence, your only desire at the end of your long stressed out day will be to eat processed/refined carbs and lots of them. *Why?* Because the body is desperate to raise this crucial brain chemical—and the quickest way to achieve this is by eating high GI carbs. Unfortunately, these particular carbs will spike insulin, forcing them directly into fat storage. And even if you were to work out with hopes to burn off the excessive sugar caused by these high GI carbs, it's never healthy to spike your insulin.

2) In addition to eating the <u>wrong</u> types of foods at that late hour, *even if you were to eat healthy,* this food will also be encouraged to be stored as fat. *Why?* Because by not having properly fueled your body on a regular and consistent basis, your body has long been in the starvation mode. By the time you finally get around to eating, your body will be ravenous and fearing when the next meal might come. It will, therefore, instinctively hoard whatever food it gets and store it as fat instead of using it as fuel. Hey, the body's goal is simple: Stay alive! So, what's the moral of the story? It's a *good* thing to be hungry. Your body is telling you that you need to fuel it—and on a regular basis. So, please, stop depriving your body the nutrition it needs to sustain you.

Chocolate is *your* drug of choice!

No wonder I can't lose weight! I'll definitely start eating breakfast. But I'm still confused. Why do my cravings for chocolate only come late in the day?
Depending on your quality of sleep, your cravings generally should be nonexistent upon rising. This is because your body is able to replenish some of your serotonin as you sleep. As a result, when you get up, you should feel rested, ready to go, minus any cravings. As the day goes on, though, you will endure endless degrees of stress. While stress alone can play complete havoc on serotonin, you'll be exposed to many other contributing factors. They can range from cereal, skim milk, fruit juice, donuts, bagels, mocha frappuccino, latte drizzled with a sugary syrup, toast, sodas, chips, pizza, fries, a midday candy bar with a cigarette, and another latte. All in the same day, you find out your teenager has been skipping school, your boss is on a rampage, your car needs work, and your husband is going out of town—again. As you prepare to tackle the long commute home, you drink some orange juice, taking three extra strength Excedrin with the hope that they will help alleviate your throbbing headache! *Ahhh, another day!*

Whew! That sounds just like my life!
I know. Unfortunately, this is a very common description of how most Americans get through their day. It is also a mere example of some of the many things that we ingest, and endure, from day to day. Nonetheless, each and every one of those things depletes serotonin. This is why, by day's end, your serotonin is bottomed out. It's amazing chocolate is all you reach for.

And I go for sweets because?
You go for sweets because your brain is long conditioned to know that chocolate is *your* drug of choice, so to speak. Your brain knows that chocolate is what will boost your serotonin. I'm sure you started this behavior many years ago, probably as a young girl. Consequently, your brain starts to create this craving, and it will *continually* force you toward chocolate, because it knows, from years of experience, that this is what elevates your serotonin. Your comfort food just happens to be chocolate.

You're right, chocolate has always been my comfort food. Now I finally know *why* **I can't live without it. I guess serotonin really is the key to successful fat loss!**
Without a doubt, you need to maintain healthy levels of all your brain chemicals for optimum health, but serotonin, the master communicator of all brain chemicals, is the crucial link to successful weight loss, as it controls the cravings for the types of foods that cause the body to store fat, while at the same time controlling overall appetite.

This is all so fascinating, but I really love my chocolate! What if I'm not ready to give it up?
Ah, L-O-V-E! Or so you think. This is an excellent comment, as I have counseled many a client who has said the exact same thing. And while you may think you "love and need" your chocolate, what you're actually so in love with is the feeling of *comfort* you get after eating it. It is the emotional relief that always follows after you eat chocolate that has you so attached to this sweet, creamy delight. It is this act of self-medicating that gets you into this addictive behavior pattern. It is the elevation in the wonderful, mood-altering brain chemical serotonin that makes you hesitant, if not fearful, to give it up. You need to understand, though, there is a huge difference between simply wanting something versus *having* to have it at all cost. Those costs are your health and well-being. I'm not saying you can never eat chocolate again. I'm trying to make you understand "why" you feel so attached to it. It's the same for someone who is attached to pasta, pastries, chips, dumplings, soda, alcohol, caffeine, and nicotine.

How will I know the difference?
Easy. One of the most rewarding aspects of maintaining healthy levels of serotonin is that you will no longer be controlled by these cravings. You will be able to get through the day and night <u>without</u> needing (*or even thinking about!*) these insulin-producing foods. Your once insatiable desire or "love" for chocolate will simply vanish. You'll be amazed at how easily this happens. I guarantee you.

Are you sure I won't miss my chocolate? With all the diets I've tried, I've never been able to give it up.
The only reason your mind continuously tempts you with chocolate is because your serotonin is unquestionably, deficient. But once you maintain healthy levels of serotonin, your craving for this comfort food will disappear. *Why?* Because your brain will become satiated. Hence, the noise, i.e., craving, will stop. Your brain will no longer need to force you toward this high GI carb that has faithfully boosted your serotonin for years. And unlike every other diet you've ever tried before, your cravings and appetite will be controlled *without* any sense of frustration, deprivation, or starvation. You will be in complete control. Without effort. Without the usual emotional drama and struggle. You will come to fully understand that this desperate, so-called love affair with chocolate is NOT about love, after all. It is, instead, merely a "side effect" of low serotonin. It is at this time that you will finally be free of this food addiction. It is, once again, the **"Serotonin-Insulin Connection"** that is absolutely vital to achieving and maintaining your weight loss goals.

3

OH, THE MANY DIETS WE'VE TRIED!

All this time I thought eating low-calorie or low-fat were the answer.
Didn't we all. Contrary to these theories that the AMA (American Medical Association) and FDA (Food and Drug Administration) preached to us for nearly 30 years, they just did not work. In fact, as a nation, we got fatter than ever before. This diet regime has caused an epidemic of alarming obesity-related health conditions, i.e., type 2 diabetes, cancer, heart disease, stroke, etc.

And why don't these diets work?
<u>Low-calorie dieting:</u>
As I just mentioned, your body interprets a low-calorie diet as starvation. This includes skipping meals and eating bare minimum. BTW: Meal replacement bars/drinks fall under the bare minimum category and they are perfect examples of severe caloric restriction. You'll lose weight at first, as your glycogen stores are depleted, but your weight loss will plateau. And then the real damage begins. Your body instinctively reacts with a survival mechanism that is intended to prevent loss of lean muscle and bone mass. Instead of burning fat, your body will actually start to *hoard* fat. The less you eat, the slower your metabolism, the slower your bodily functions become. Your body will eventually start consuming its own tissue in order to get the nutrients that it needs to sustain the most vital body part: *your brain*. This type of dieting actually changes the overall composition of your body. With each diet, you'll <u>lose</u> more lean muscle and bone mass, while at the same time *increasing* fat storage. The less lean muscle tissue, the less efficient your body is at burning fat. Thus, the all too common diet scenario: "Lose 10/gain back 20!"

So skipping meals is obviously not good?
Skipping meals is definitely not good. When you don't properly fuel your brain, *which will do whatever it takes to stay alive*, it basically says, "Look, I have no idea when you're going to feed me again, therefore, I'd better hold on to whatever food you do give me. I will store it in the form of fat to be used later." So, you see, skipping meals and eating bare minimum is not healthy for a variety of reasons.

<u>Fat-free/low-fat dieting:</u>
There was not one, long-term study that verified the efficacy of such a diet. First of all, eating healthy fat does NOT cause the body to store fat. Plus, if you're eating a low-fat diet, you're definitely eating too many carbs/sugar. It's by eating high GI carbs (and processed/refined foods), and an excess of carbs, that is the underlying cause of obesity.

21

You're saying eating butter and cheese won't make me fat? This is exactly the opposite of what we've been told for so many years!
Precisely, which is why people are so confused as to what to eat. Once again, eating good healthy fat does not make you fat, because it does not trigger the release of insulin, the fat-storing hormone.

FAT FACTS: You must eat good dietary fats to maintain optimum health. Your body needs fat to burn fat. Fat is a fantastic fuel source. Fat provides more energy than sugar. Fat slows down the transient time of food, hence lowering the GI. Fat-free/low-fat dieting accelerates the metabolic aging process, slows down your metabolism, can cause insulin resistance, which can lead to type 2 diabetes and other diseases. Fat-free/low-fat dieting actually *makes* you fat. Eating good fats is, unequivocally, vital for good health!

Eating healthy fat does NOT make you fat!

What is considered a good dietary fat?
Good dietary fats are found in nature, i.e., plant and animal sources. They include lean meat, real butter, cream, eggs, olives, tofu, poultry, fish, nuts, seeds, and avocados. You should try to eat a good dietary fat with every meal. Extra virgin olive oil and flaxseed oil are also recommended. Good fats are known as the essential fatty acids (EFAs), which include omega-3s, omega-6s, and omega-9s. Each of these is crucial to maintaining good health. Mackerel, tuna, sardines, salmon, flaxseed and walnut oils are all wonderful examples of omega-3s. Eggs, sunflower, safflower and canola oils, turkey, and chicken are all excellent sources of omega-6s. Omega-9s include oleic acid, which can come from olive and avocado oils. Fats to avoid: man-made fats such as hydrogenated/trans fats and oils which are found in foods such a fries, chips, cookies, pastries, certain meats, margarine products—and even some so-called health products.

I hear all this talk about avoiding "trans fats," but I'm not sure what they are?
Trans fats are basically fats that are "transformed" from their natural state. They are unsaturated fatty acids formed when vegetable oils are processed and made more solid. This processing is called hydrogenation. Avoid trans fats!

WARNING: Fat-Free/Low-Fat Food Alert: Fat-free/low-fat foods are loaded with sugar! When you take the fat out of food, you take out the flavor. To enhance the flavor, food companies add sugar. They add a lot, and they add the worst kind: high-fructose corn syrup. (They also add chemicals and salt. Salt causes water retention, which equals more weight gain.) High-fructose corn syrup is more harmful than table sugar. It accelerates the metabolic aging process more than any form of sugar. It depletes serotonin. Encourages the body to store fat. Perpetuates carbohydrate cravings. It's addictive. A vicious and unhealthy cycle of cravings, excessive fat gain, and low serotonin levels is perpetuated by fat-free/low-fat diets.

What about foods like fat-free yogurt? Aren't they okay?
Not exactly. All you have to do is read the nutritional panel to see just how much sugar is in one of those tiny containers. Dannon, for example: A 6 oz. container has 33g of carbs. As if 33g of carbs aren't bad enough, a staggering 30g of those carbs are SUGAR! And because most yogurts are "fat-free," they will affect your blood sugar response that much quicker. Without any fat and all that fruit sugar, it's going to spike your insulin, putting your body into a fat-storing mode.

What about the new drinkable yogurts?
Drinkable yogurts are even worse, due to the mere fact they're a *liquid* carb. Liquid carbs affect your blood sugar levels much faster than solid carbs. They also have just as many carbs/sugars, if not more, than the original yogurts. Example: Dannon's Fruision, 10 oz., has 52g of carbs; 49g of those carbs are sugar. Yoplait Nouriche, another liquid yogurt, at 11 ounces, has an astounding 60g of carbs; 46g of those carbs are sugar! It also contains high-fructose corn syrup! This product is one of the worst. And with absolutely zero fat, it's nothing more than liquid sugar. Yoplait's marketing campaign would like us to believe that this is the perfect healthy breakfast food for those on the run. Wrong. This is not a healthy choice for a meal, let alone the first thing you put into your body.

That being said, women need the health benefits that come with an occasional yogurt. But it must be plain and with live/active cultures to get the health benefits. (Read the labels to insure it contains live cultures.) Better yet, buy live, organic soy yogurt, those lowest in carbs/sugars, highest in protein, with some fat, and then don't eat them alone. Instead combine them with a quality protein and healthy fat to help lower the blood sugar response. I like to mix a little yogurt in with my cottage cheese or serve it over sliced tomatoes. It can also make a nice dessert.

Fruit contains fructose, i.e., FRUIT SUGAR!

And smoothies, aren't they a healthy choice?
Be careful of smoothies and any other fruit drinks. Smoothies should be limited, because they're generally nothing more than a ton of fruit blended, creating a delicious, but nonetheless, purely liquid candy beverage. Drinking a smoothie or a glass of fruit juice along with a healthy, balanced meal, i.e., healthy fat, lean protein, and low GI carb, will help lower the blood sugar response. It is generally, though, way too much sugar going into the blood stream. This surge of sugar will spike insulin levels, putting the body into a fat-storing mode. It will also deplete serotonin levels, cause mood swings, affect the body's energy levels, etc. (Adding a scoop of protein powder or organic peanut butter to these drinks will slightly help lower the blood sugar response.)

But isn't fruit healthy?
Yes, fruit is indeed healthy. But fruit contains fructose, fruit sugar, just as milk contains lactose, milk sugar. And when you blend fruit, you break down the fiber, turning it into

pure sugar water. As a liquid carb, it affects blood sugars levels even more dramatically than solid carbs, due to the fact the body doesn't have to break it down. Liquid carbs are basically sugar, as they go directly into the blood stream, quickly spiking insulin levels. Therefore, the best way to eat fruit is in its natural state. (An apple versus apple juice.) Don't blend it or break it down, and don't eat it first or alone. And whether it's a smoothie, fruit juice, pre-bottled, or you get one from Jamba Juice, they should all come with nutritional information. Read it. You'll see they are extremely high in sugar. Remember, the best way to eat fruit is in its natural state, which keeps the fiber intact, hence lowering the GI. Also, when trying to shed excess body fat, eat only one serving of a low GI fruit per day.

Okay, so avoid low-cal and low-fat. How do you feel about low-carb dieting?

What most people don't understand about low-carb dieting is that it is about being "carb conscious." It's about eating the *right* carbs versus not eating, or eating too few carbs. Remember, our brain needs sugar to survive. And the brain can only get this blood sugar from carbohydrates. Carbs are also the best fuel source for our bodies. This is why it's essential to eat a continuous and healthy source of carbs throughout the day. The key is to eat enough, based on your individual needs. Eating too many, or eating too many of the *wrong types of carbs*, is the leading cause of our obesity rate. It is precisely the cravings for these carbs that trigger insulin—and cause the body to store fat. It is, therefore, these cravings that must be controlled.

And serotonin is the crucial link to controlling those cravings?

Exactly! I don't want you not to eat carbs, I want you to eat the *right* carbs. This research is about helping people understand why 98% of all diets fail. This research is about helping people understand that their inability to adhere to any such diet is NOT their fault, but instead due to *cravings* caused by the depletion of a brain chemical. And these particular cravings are for the precise carbs that spike insulin levels, causing the body to store fat. By boosting and maintaining your serotonin—the brain chemical that governs carbohydrate cravings and overall appetite—you will finally be able to control the cravings for those insulin-producing carbs. No longer will you be controlled by the foods that have always kept you overweight. To sum it up: If you want to reach optimum health, it's not about dieting. It's not about eating low-cal, low-fat, or low-carb. It's about fueling your body and mind with the best *real* foods possible, by eating five to six meals a day, and never skipping meals. It's also about living a healthy lifestyle.

It makes sense, but I'm still confused. What do you eat?

My day religiously starts with a dose of product that will elevate, moreover, *maintain* my serotonin. Followed shortly thereafter with a protein drink made with filtered water and either a vanilla or banana whey protein powder. (I avoid using chocolate-flavored powder, as it contains cocoa, which is a stimulant.) I then take my few select supplements at this time. Next, I'll have two eggs with a handful of spinach, sprinkled with feta cheese. Or maybe I'll have a turkey patty with sprouts, cottage cheese, and avocado. From there, I like to graze, basically eating 5 (more often 6) smaller meals throughout the day. It is about keeping my body fueled, yet never overeating. I also have much more constant energy if I eat often—and light. With my serotonin balanced, it's effortless.

I just have to ask—did you ever have cravings?
Sure I did. My craving was for sourdough toast. Not just the bread—it had to be toasted with butter and/or cheese. And, as I would stand in my kitchen, taking that first ever-so-delicious bite, I asked myself a dozen times: *"What is in this toast that makes me feel soooo damn good?"* Seriously, I was truly amazed at how quickly my mood lifted, as I ate this treat. I could literally feel my body and mind relax, almost like a drug. I felt so calm. I swear I could have lived on sourdough toast, along with, of course, a few protein drinks.

Did you gain weight from this habit?
I definitely felt my pants get a bit tighter based on how many pieces I ate. But, if and when this happened, I simply worked out harder, and got back to eating healthier. Ironically, this is exactly *why* I came to believe I wasn't meant to eat. After all, other than a few lousy pieces of toast, I wasn't eating that much, and yet I felt bloated and fat! (I now realize my mind forced me toward this carb due to low serotonin—and, thus, perpetuated my cravings, spiked my insulin, caused water retention—and all by eating this particular carb.)

And the butter?
Truth of the matter is, the butter, real butter, and cheese, not fat-free cheese, were actually a good thing, as they're both healthy fats. As such, they lowered the blood sugar response caused by the bread. (Sourdough is a low GI carb, but with 20g of carbs per slice.)

What do your groceries look like now?
As I write this, I'm having a wonderful salad with mixed herb greens, topped with succulent fresh crab, pearl tomatoes, shaved cucumber, cilantro, drizzled with extra virgin olive oil, and fresh lime. Delicious—and so easy to prepare. And no, I do not live on salads. Nor will you have to. (Please read chapter 33, Suggested Foods.)

Unfortunately, my kids love junk food. As a parent, what am I supposed to do?
Don't buy it. Don't have it in your house. Why tempt you or your kids with food that you know is unhealthy? Far too many parents use their children as an excuse for why they can't stick to a healthy way of eating. I can't tell you how many times I've heard: "Oh well, you can stay thin, because *you* don't have kids! *I have children!* And they love Happy Meals, hotdogs, Doritos, fries, and ice cream! They <u>want</u> this kind of food! I can't deny them their favorite foods!" Sorry, yes you can. With all due respect, this is merely an excuse.

First of all, why would you want your kids to eat this junk food to begin with? It's only a matter of time before they, too, end up with weight issues. You'll also be wondering why they're so moody, depressed, suffering from ADD, etc. You need to start them on a healthy diet from day one. If not, then please start today! I don't care what they think they want. As their parent, it's your role to try and make sure they eat healthy. As their loving and devoted parent, your responsibility is to avoid buying the foods that you know are unhealthy. Don't forget, supplements that boost serotonin can easily help you and your children control the cravings for these fat-promoting carbs.

Your thoughts on gastric bypass surgery are what again?
Gastric bypass surgery is unfortunately, nothing more than a band-aid, a poor one at that, as it only masks the underlying problem. From what I've seen, there are far too many doctors performing this procedure who don't even begin to properly educate their patients on how to avoid putting the weight back on once they leave the operating table. For those who have had this surgery, many continue to eat the same junk food that put the weight on to begin with. I know a woman who had it done, and, yes, she lost a lot of weight, but her eating habits have not changed in the least bit. She basically lives off a few sips of soda with a handful of chips. You see, her cravings have not gone away, nor does she know *why* she craves this junk food to begin with. So she continues on the same destructive path that got her fat in the first place. With each passing day, she is able to eat just a little bit more. A few more chips. A little more soda. And an extra bite of her oh-so-favorite chocolate cake that faithfully comes calling by day's end. Now does this sound healthy? Of course not. Not only is this woman eating far too little to sustain her bodily functions, but the food she is taking in has absolutely no nutritional value. Furthermore, she may be thinner, but what has she learned to keep it off? Nothing! Unless these patients learn "how and why" their mind keeps forcing them to eat these particular foods, unless they're able to control their cravings and appetite, this radical attempt to lose weight will inevitably fail. Guaranteed!

Based on the obvious misinformation being provided to many of these patients, and realizing my expertise could help this unique area of weight loss, I looked into bariatric surgery centers, those who specialize in gastric bypass and the lap-band system. Although I already knew that there were doctors and/or aftercare providers who were not properly educating their patients, I was shocked to see just how overweight some of the surgeons and nutrition counselors were. Several needed to lose at least 50 pounds themselves! And yet these are the so-called *experts* in charge of helping others lose and maintain long-term weight loss? I'm sorry, but if they can't even do it for themselves, how can they possibly ever help others?

Furthermore, it was what they were actually recommending with regard to nutrition that concerned me the most. On one particular Web site, under FAQs, the patient's question was, "How soon can I drink sodas?" Now, instead of responding with, "Sodas are to be avoided, as they are not part of a healthy diet—or sodas are nothing but toxic sugar water and harmful to your health—or sodas will perpetuate your carbohydrate cravings and spike your insulin, both leading to more fat gain—and sodas will cause mood swings, water retention, etc." But instead of any of one of these excellent health/nutrition tips, their answer was: "Patients should not drink carbonated beverages until at least 3 months post operatively, as the carbonated beverages may cause excessive amounts of gas and balloon the pouch." That's it? That's all these "experts" could offer? Shameful. Absolutely shameful! Even more alarming is that they approved using aspartame, Sweet & Low, and Splenda! All artificial and all terribly unhealthy—aspartame in particular!

I must say I find it disturbing—and highly unethical, that the AMA allows this procedure to be done with so little consideration for the long-term care of these desperate, yet trusting, patients. Gastric bypass surgery or otherwise, these insulin-producing carbs will continue to control them. Not only is this an unhealthy, if not dangerous, way to live, but it will only be a matter of time before their newly designed stomach is stretched out, as before. Not forgetting they will be risking their very life with this surgery. Nevertheless, if you're still serious about having this procedure done, please read this book thoroughly, so you will at least be better prepared to keep the weight off long after your surgery.

How do you feel about the various weight loss organizations?
Never wanting to speak ill of another, I am, however, here to hopefully educate you so that you can make better choices. That being said, I first and foremost respectfully applaud anyone who at least takes the initiative to try to lose the excess weight. My biggest concern is that after reading the nutritional panels on most of these companies pre-packaged foods is that they contain some of the worst ingredients, including aspartame, high-fructose corn syrup, corn syrup, and saccharin! These ingredients will deplete serotonin, thus perpetuating cravings, weight gain, bloating, and depression. But due to their many harmful side effects, weight gain is the very least of your concerns!

My next concern is that one particular diet program has you eating based on points, each food being worth a certain amount of points. Their commercials show their clients blissfully eating such foods as pizza, bagels, desserts, pasta, cereal, etc. This clever marketing strategy is to appeal to those who don't want to live without their comfort foods, but they're not healthy choices, nor are they teaching them "why" they crave these foods to begin with. (I just met a woman on this plan. Her pre-packaged meal was mashed potatoes, mystery meat, and an approved diet soda! I wouldn't have fed that food to my dog!) By encouraging their clients to eat these processed/refined foods, they will encourage insulin levels to spike, followed by serotonin levels rising, then falling. At the very least, this program will perpetuate the craving cycle, further fat gain, water retention, and mood swings. This diet plan rarely works long-term. If someone is able to lose weight, their first 10 pounds lost will be from water weight. After that, their weight loss will start to plateau. This is because these plans are so often based on low-calorie dieting. The bigger problem is that once these people go off the carefully designed, pre-paid eating programs and back to their normal eating habits, they most often will gain all the weight back and more. *Why?* Because once again, the consumer has not learned *why* they have these cravings to begin with, or how they can control them. Without knowing *why* their brain keeps forcing them to consume those insulin-producing carbs, without knowing *why* they are so emotionally attached to these foods, diet failure is sadly inevitable. And another failed diet will sadly lead to a greater sense of failure, which will lead to a deeper state of depression, more weight gain, and with all of this combined, it will surely keep them coming back to these weight loss centers for years to come. Great for their business. Bad for their clients.

4

THIS IS <u>NOT</u> A DIET!

Isn't this just another diet?

No, absolutely not. This is not a diet. Diets don't work. What I'm sharing with you through-out this book is about a "healthy lifestyle." But that lifestyle is completely dependent upon whether or not you can maintain healthy levels of serotonin.

Diets, as we all know only too well, are associated with starvation, deprivation, and frus-tration. Eventually you'll end up with your head in the bag of whatever it is you crave. Cravings will always lead to diet failure! On the other hand, taking a dietary supplement that helps safely boost serotonin, can so easily control your cravings. When you control the cravings, you simply won't have the desire to eat as much—specifically high GI carbo-hydrates, which spike insulin levels and encourage your body to store fat. You'll no longer eat from emotion. Your professed carb addiction will be gone. You'll eat healthier. You'll eat less. (No more binging!) And all of this will be possible *without* ever feeling cheated, deprived, or stressed. It will be effortless. I promise you.

Equally as astonishing is that once you maintain healthy serotonin levels, you'll start stabi-lizing your insulin levels as well. Your body will then begin to utilize, to burn its fat stores, instead of storing new fat. Once you truly understand this critical serotonin-insulin con-nection, the so-called secret to fat loss is yours. Never will you have to diet again. You will now know exactly what to do to maintain your ideal body weight.

One of the most powerful aspects of achieving healthy levels of serotonin is that your mind will become quiet—the cravings will stop. Amazingly, you will then be able to have the foods you once craved, *foods you thought you couldn't live without,* you will be able to have them right in front of you, but you will no longer have the desire for them. Those comfort foods will no longer have control over you. You will finally be free of the cravings that have always controlled your life and kept you overweight. And that is exceptionally powerful—and empowering!

But how does this happen?

To reiterate, once the brain is able to maintain healthy levels of serotonin, it will stop forc-ing you toward the foods and/or substances that it used to depend on for this comforting elevation in brain chemistry. Where my clients once thought they couldn't live without their chocolate, sodas, donuts, caffeine, cereal, etc., they now find they simply no longer have the desire for them. This shift in eating habits is unbelievably subtle. And because of how subtle the changes are, you will need to reflect on just how much your eating habits have changed over time. In addition, there is never any sense of feeling deprived, hungry, or stressed. It is, then, only a matter of time before you lose the excess weight. Adding some sort of exercise program will help you reach your weight loss goals even faster. Exercise is a vital piece to a healthy lifestyle.

Never forget that all of this is a process. It takes time. It requires effort. No matter the product, there is no magic pill. (And Propolene is most assuredly NOT the answer! How that company gets away with that over-the-top diet BS ad is beyond me!) Nor will it work overnight, or work effectively if you don't make a conscious effort to eat healthier. With your cravings controlled, it's now up to you to break the old, unhealthy habits. Again, add-ing a regular exercise program will double your efforts. Sadly, there are many who expect to take a product and wake up with a perfect body. They keep eating the processed junk food that put the fat on in the first place. They continue to drink their daily caffeine, sodas, fruit juice, cocktails, etc., and yet wonder *why* they aren't losing the weight. All these things negate what any such product is trying to help them overcome. Once again, you must be *willing* to make the effort.

But aren't most people looking for that magic pill?
Yes, this is exactly what most people would love to find. Even though there is no such thing, unfortunately this truth doesn't deter the production of far too many fat loss products (and weight loss programs) that claim a lean, healthy body can be achieved in "only 48 hours," or by "eating anything and everything you want," or by merely taking a pill at night to wake up thinner. PLEASE! While it is alarming that companies market such useless and often harmful products, it shocks me even more to realize that the consumer actually still believes these products will work.

First of all, the *only* thing you'll lose in 48 hours is water weight. Secondly, you can never "eat anything and everything" you want and expect to achieve good health. Stop lying to yourself! It is possible, though, by reading this book, to learn how to eat delicious foods such as real butter, cheese, nuts, eggs, etc., and not gain body fat. It is also possible to lose excess body fat and yet NEVER feel hungry or stressed! All of this—and you will finally understand how to achieve and *maintain* long-term fat loss.

Amazing information! It's all finally starting to make sense. Is this similar to how Fen-Phen worked?
Fen-Phen was an extremely successful pharmaceutical drug treatment for obesity and binge eating disorders. Two drugs, fenfluramine (fen) and phentermine (phen) were taken together, in order to work in what was hoped to be a balanced fashion on two of the body's neurotransmitters: serotonin and dopamine. Phentermine blocked the absorption of dopamine, while fenfluramine worked on blocking the reuptake of serotonin. Fen-Phen made people lose the desire to eat, particularly carbohydrates. It gave people hope. They

lost weight like never before! Fen-Phen was *the most successful pharmaceutical diet drug in history!* In its prime, drug companies were selling 20 million prescriptions every month. That's about $500,000,000 a month, or $6 billion a year! However, as with all pharmaceutical drugs, it eventually proved to come with life-threatening side effects such as primary pulmonary hypertension and irreversible damage to brain neurons. To reiterate, and I can't possibly say this enough: All pharmaceutical drugs come with harmful side effects, as they alter the "natural" course of the body and mind.

Nonetheless, the medical industry is forever trying to duplicate Fen-Phen's success, minus the horrific side effects. Unethically, doctors were even prescribing the various SSRI (Selective Serotonin Reuptake Inhibitor) antidepressants as not only a way to treat their patients' depression, but also help them lose weight. The FDA finally put a stop to this profitable, highly unethical, if not illegal, practice.

In May 2004, yet another pharmaceutical drug was introduced to help fight the war on obesity. It's based on elevating the "feel-good" brain chemical, serotonin. *Really?* They're claiming their new diet drug is a "dual-action" product, able to control both carb and nicotine cravings. And, of course, this is true based on the fact serotonin controls both of these cravings. But beware! This is a DRUG! All drugs come with serious health risks. On the other hand, products that are derived from all-natural ingredients (such as those I'm speaking about) can give you the same control <u>minus</u> the above-stated health risks. So I must ask: *Why would anyone choose to take a DRUG that comes with so many serious side effects when you have a variety of dietary supplements that offer a safe, far more effective, and affordable alternative?*

What should I look for when buying a dietary supplement?
Read the supplement panel carefully; review all the claims the product is making; look for precise extracts used, doses of each per serving, quality of the ingredients, amount of product required to be effective, delivery system used to actually get the ingredients into the body, i.e., pills, tablets, capsules, or liquid time-release; look for the quality rating of the finished formula, purchase price, and number of servings per bottle. These are all things you need to consider before purchasing. Furthermore, if the type on the packaging is too small to read, don't buy it. I find it insulting that so many manufacturers use type that is so darn small you can't even read it. How am I, as the consumer, able to educate myself about their product if I can't read the ingredients or directions, and more importantly—the WARNINGS?

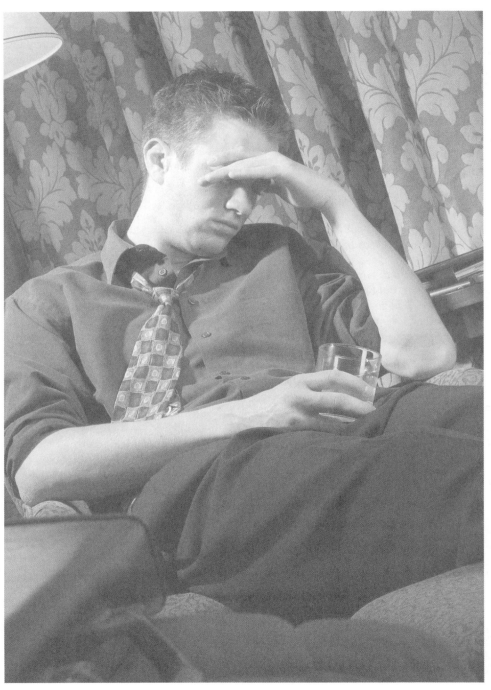

5

CONDITIONS ASSOCIATED
WITH
LOW SEROTONIN

What are the known health conditions related to low levels of serotonin?
As numerous medical studies reveal, when serotonin levels are low, the following health conditions can arise. As you can see, as a major neurotransmitter, serotonin regulates so many things within the human mind and subsequently the body. All the more reason to make sure you do whatever it takes to maintain properly balanced serotonin levels for yourself, your spouse, and your children.

- Aggression (quicker to anger, sudden outbursts, temper tantrums)
- Alcoholism (a disease, physical dependence on alcohol, insatiable alcohol cravings)
- Anxiety (feeling of apprehension, fear, or worry that interferes with life functions)
- Attention Deficit Disorders (severe difficulty in focusing and maintaining attention)
- Bulimia (binge eating followed by fasting, self-induced vomiting)
- Cravings (overwhelming desires for certain foods, primarily high GI carbs)
- Chronic Pain Disorders (complex chronic pain of joints, muscles, etc.)
- Depression (constant feelings of doom, gloom, inadequacy)
- Epilepsy (brain disorder involving recurrent seizures)
- Headaches (ranging from tension, chronic to migraines)
- Hyperactivity (excessively active)
- Insomnia (the inability to sleep for a duration of time and/or fall asleep)
- Lack of libido (decreased sexual behavior, ability, desire)
- Mood Swings (extreme changes in mood)
- Myoclonus (brief, involuntary, random muscular contractions)
- Obesity (excess of body fat that is 20% or more over ideal weight)
- Obsessive-Compulsive Disorder (persistent thoughts, ideas, repetitive behavior)
- Panic Attacks (unpredictable attacks of intense fear, discomfort, shortness of breath)
- Premenstrual Syndrome (symptoms prior to menstruation)
- Schizophrenia (mental illness; mood changes, withdrawn, regressive, bizarre behavior)
- Seasonal Affective Disorder (form of depression/mood disorder with seasonal pattern)
- Suicidal Behavior (actions/thoughts by those contemplating taking their own life)

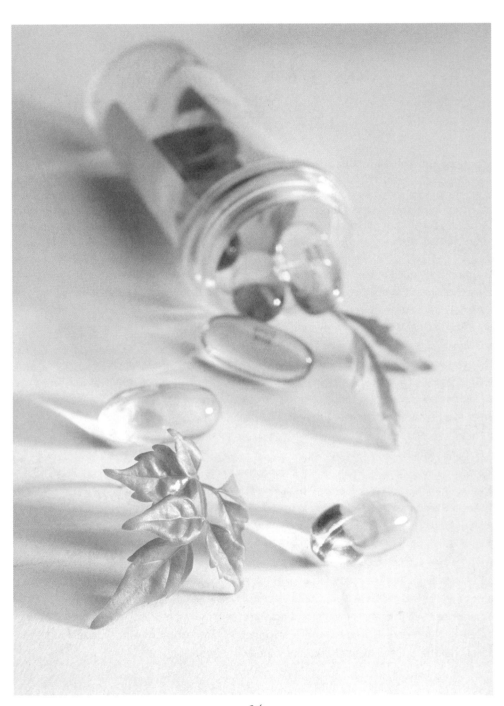

6

HOW TO NATURALLY
BOOST SEROTONIN LEVELS

All this talk of serotonin and its many amazing health benefits, but what dietary supplements do you recommend to boost my serotonin?
After several years of researching various extracts, and the subsequent results from having tested those extracts, I suggest the following:

My personal favorite, by far, is the *Griffonia* seed extract which is rich in 5-hydroxytryptophan, otherwise known as 5-HTP. I highly recommend 5-HTP, a natural amino acid, because it's a clinically proven serotonin precursor. This means it easily crosses the blood-brain barrier (the curtain that separates and protects the brain from the bloodstream) and effectively increases central nervous system synthesis of serotonin. 5-HTP transforms into serotonin once in the body. (Vitamin B6, also called pyridoxine, is often suggested to help further facilitate the proper conversion of 5-HTP into serotonin.)

To reiterate, clinical studies have shown that serotonin, the major neurotransmitter that is crucial for both the brain and body to function at their best, also controls cravings, primarily for carbohydrates, and satiety, the body's appetite-control mechanism. Serotonin also promotes mental and emotional well-being, encourages deep restorative sleep, and reduces stress. And 5-HTP has clinically proven to be exceptionally effective in treating the dozens of conditions associated with low serotonin. Based on all my studies, 5-HTP, is by far, the safest, most effective ingredient to boost serotonin.

Where can I find 5-HTP?
Thankfully, it's inexpensive and available at most drug and health food stores. You can purchase 5-HTP as is, or some companies like to develop more of a blend, a more effective, multi-action formula combining 5-HTP with several other extracts. Make sure you read the supplement panel carefully for doses required per day for maximum benefits. Furthermore, if you buy a blend, do NOT get one that has any stimulants in it. *Why?* Because stimulants deplete serotonin. They will negate what the product is trying to do, i.e., elevate and maintain healthy levels of serotonin.

Furthermore, 5-HTP is known worldwide as "Nature's Prozac." Unlike antidepressant drugs that come with so many harmful, potentially life-threatening side effects—ranging from nausea, dry mouth, diarrhea, headaches, loss of sex drive, insomnia, to seizures, liver damage and/or failure, severe withdrawal, suicidal thoughts and actual suicide—5-HTP can actually help *enhance* mood, sleep, and libido, while helping to relieve stress, anxiety,

35

and pain. In addition to those many extraordinary health benefits, research from the NCRR (National Center for Radiation Research) found that 5-HTP may also be a powerful antioxidant. The studies suggest that 5-HTP may protect our bodies from free radical formation and oxidative damage, thus slowing the aging process. Wow! *What more can you ask for?* I'll tell you this: If I were for some reason, restricted to taking only one supplement, my choice, *without a doubt*, would be 5-HTP. That is how much value I put on it.

What is the best, most effective way to take 5-HTP?
Great question, because, unlike so many other supplements, anything that is designed to boost (and maintain) brain chemicals must be taken on a regular and consistent basis throughout the day. With regard to 5-HTP, the typical dosage is anywhere from 50mg to 300mg, 2 to 3 times a day. For maximum effectiveness, it needs to be taken on an empty stomach. Therefore, you'll need to take it either 30 minutes before—or an hour after—eating. I suggest you also find a delivery system, i.e., pills, capsules, tablets, or the latest polylymphatic time-release liquid, that best suits your individual needs. Personally, if I can't get what I need by taking a supplement once in the morning, I don't want to bother with it. I have no desire to be one of those people carrying around a bag of pills that I have to take every few hours.

I hate taking pills, so the less, the better. But whether I take pills or a liquid, my cravings seem to be worse between 4pm and 10pm. Will they be controlled if I take something so early in the day?
Yes, due to the unlimited factors like stress, caffeine, sugar, processed foods, etc., that you'll encounter on any given day, depleting this crucial brain chemical, cravings will generally come calling late afternoon through the evening hours. If you take 5-HTP in the form of pills or capsules, you'll definitely need to make sure you take them 3 times a day, and, again, on an empty stomach. It's not always convenient or the most effective way to achieve the full benefits, but that being said, taking them *whenever* you can is far better than not taking them at all.

I suggest you start with the smallest dose of 50mg/3 times a day. (In case you're not aware, less is *more* when it comes to herbs.) Take your first dose as soon as you get up. Shower, then eat breakfast. Take your second dose at midday, followed by another around 5 or 6pm. Again, just make sure you take it on a regular and consistent basis. If, after a week, you find your cravings aren't controlled, I want you to first take a closer look at what you're consuming. Remember, if you aren't at least willing to make better choices, including avoiding caffeine, sodas, candy, bagels, fast food, and so forth, you'll negate what the product is trying to do for you. But if you have, in fact, been dedicated to eating healthier and your cravings have yet to subside, increase your dose to 100mg/3 times a day. Stay at that dose for two weeks. The maximum dose you should take is 300mg/3 times a day. That being said, 300mg is far more than I have ever needed to control my clients' cravings or my own.

What is the polylymphatic delivery you mentioned?

The polylymphatic technology is a cutting-edge process that insures the extracts are delivered in a *sustained* release directly into the bloodstream over 12 hours via the lymphatic system. (The only thing that is more direct is an injection.) Just one of the many extraordinary benefits is that you'll only have to take it once a day. Better yet, it has shown to increase bioavailability by over 50%, i.e., the extent to which the ingredients are absorbed—and become available to the body. Nevertheless, you still need to be consistent to help insure you maintain healthy serotonin levels. This will lead to helping control your cravings, as well as enhancing your mood, sleep, etc., 24/7. Although this technology is a far more advanced, convenient, and effective manner in which to deliver ingredients into the body, it's also more expensive. The choice is up to you.

Any other suggested extracts to boost serotonin?

Vinpocetine is a periwinkle plant extract (Vinca major) that has also been shown to improve brain function. It's been used successfully in Europe since 1983. Studies show vinpocetine increases the brain's turnover of serotonin and norepinephrine. It's also a powerful memory enhancer, commonly used in stroke patients. It's shown to increase cerebral blood flow and enhance the glycolytic and oxidative glucose break down in central nervous stimulation. It facilitates cerebral metabolism by improving cerebral micro circulation, stepping up brain cell ATP production (ATP is the cellular energy molecule) and increasing utilization of glucose and oxygen. Vinpocetine is also able to cross the blood-brain barrier. A series of studies conducted by researcher Gedeon Richter, involved 882 patients with neurological disorders ranging from stroke to cerebral insufficiency. Significant improvements were found in 62% of the patients. Richter also claims that vinpocetine selectively increases blood flow to the brain, improving blood flow to the impaired area without lowering blood flow to other parts of the body.

Another, but more expensive option to safely boost serotonin is SAMe (S-Adenosyl Methionine). It's an amino acid that naturally occurs in the cells of our body. It's known to be essential to at least 35 biochemical processes in the body, including maintaining the structure of cell membranes and balancing serotonin and dopamine. Studies have shown SAMe to be effective in alleviating nearly every type of depression.

And finally, noni, a tropical fruit, used successfully for thousands of years by the island people. It's the highest serotonin-binding plant of the Rubiaceae family. Hence, it produces nearly the same health benefits as 5-HTP. Regrettably, it's very limited in clinical studies to support its various claims. It is, nevertheless, another option to help elevate serotonin. That being said, my problem with most noni products is that they're loaded with fruit juice, which equals lots of sugar. Plus, I have no idea how much active ingredient I'm really getting. In addition to the sugar, this, too, is a concern for me.

To conclude this chapter, no matter how phenomenal an extract proves to be, it will only be as effective as the effort you devote to making healthier choices.

7

HEALTH BENEFITS
OF
SEROTONIN-ENHANCING SUPPLEMENTS

How long before I start to feel the benefits from boosting my serotonin?
Whether you take SAMe, 5-HTP solo, or a more advanced blend with 5-HTP, vinpocetine, etc., in it, the many amazing health benefits will vary in how quickly you actually begin to feel them. The control of your cravings can come as quickly as in one dose, or it may take several days. Once again, the various health benefits do not come all at once. It is a process. It takes time. You must be willing to take any such product on a regular and consistent basis for at least 30 days before making a judgment. (I actually prefer you stay on it for 90 days before drawing any conclusions.) Please keep in mind that the way in which this type of product works, i.e., affecting brain chemistry and without stimulants, is very subtle. But please know this: The longer you stay on any SES (Serotonin-Enhancing Supplement), the *greater* the benefits.

Furthermore, results will vary tremendously depending on "your" state of health and life-style habits. As I stated earlier, if you continue to consume processed foods, sugar, caffeine, alcohol, etc., you'll negate what any SES is trying to do for you. Though I consult my clients with regard to what they should eat and drink, it's ultimately up to them. If they choose to ignore me, they must realize each of these factors will greatly affect their progress. While SESs are formulated precisely to control cravings, you must still put forth an effort. You must be willing to break the old, unhealthy habits. If you keep eating sugar and high GI carbs, even though the cravings are gone, no product will work. This is *why* I say "effort" is required. You must also realize that if you want a lean, healthy, and sexy body—a body that looks terrific in and out of clothes—you must exercise. Training with weights is the most effective way to achieve such a body. The reality is, the key to achieving successful weight loss and overall good health is based on a "lifestyle."

Once you realize that this is not a quick fix, but rather a solution, it's up to you what you want to achieve. Is it a sleeker, stronger, sexier body? Would you like to alleviate cravings? Control appetite? Enhance mood? Be happier? Feel less anxious? Reduce body aches and pains? Improve concentration and ability to focus? Maybe you have issues with sleep or need more energy? Or maybe you'd like to enhance your libido or slow the aging process? Boosting your serotonin can help you with each of these concerns. But because serotonin is depleted by basically everything in life, the key to alleviating these numerous health problems is to *maintain* this brain chemical.

Are there any side effects from taking 5-HTP?
No, but I suppose there could always be potential side effects if someone were to misuse a product, ignore the warnings, dosage, or directions. Therefore, carefully read all the information found on the product label for full details. That being said, some claim they've felt a bit nauseous when first taking 5-HTP. Though it's extremely rare (less than 1%), it's nothing to be alarmed about. This is primarily from the 5-HTP getting into their system. It will subside after a few moments. It should also not be an issue after a couple of doses. Regardless, to help ease the nausea, I suggest taking your dose with a protein drink. If that doesn't work, eat something healthy within 20 to 30 minutes.

Is it safe for children? Both my teenagers could benefit from taking an SES.
Based on the clinical studies; my six years in R&D; plus my personal experience and that of my clients—I would say absolutely. However, the FDA requires supplements to contain a standard warning. Part of that warning states: "Keep away from children." Nonetheless, as their parent, this is your decision. I will say this: If I had a child, I would, <u>without</u> hesitation, have them take an SES daily.

How much weight can I expect to lose?
This research, along with a quality SES, is giving you the solution for long-term weight loss. Thus, there is no limit. But, once again, it does not happen overnight. It's not a quick fix or a magic pill. This is a process. It will take time, effort, and commitment on your part. And while no such product will ever work overnight, I guarantee you there is no safer, more effective way to achieve your lifelong health and fitness goals of both body and mind than by properly maintaining your serotonin.

How will I know it's working?
You will first feel a huge improvement in your mood and sleep patterns. And then, because the primary actions of an SES is remarkably subtle, you will slowly, and only in deliberate reflection, look back and suddenly realize how much your eating habits have changed. You will realize how you no longer need that caffeine or soda to get you going. You will no longer miss that chocolate bar that once consumed your every waking thought. No longer will you crave those scrumptious, extra large oatmeal cookies at midday. (I'm so proud of you, Scotty!) You will no longer find yourself reaching for the basket of bread or bag of potato chips. No longer will you need that bowl of cereal after dinner to finally feel satisfied. When you drink a soda (diet or otherwise) out of mere habit, it will taste awful and way too sweet. You will be able to go into a restaurant and not want to order everything on the menu. You will effortlessly lose the cravings for those high GI, insulin-producing carbs. You will find yourself wanting to eat healthier foods, while also being content with eating less. And *never* will you feel deprived.

While cravings and appetite are starting to be controlled, many also feel a huge relief in anxiety, feeling less overall stress. They're much slower to anger. They feel more relaxed, more energized, and a whole lot happier. At the same time, they find their sleep patterns are also greatly improving. All of these things add up to a much healthier body and mind. Moreover, you will, in all your glory, feel as if you have FINALLY—after all these years of struggling with diets—figured out how to harness and <u>control</u> your addiction, emotional eating, binging, or otherwise. This is because SESs are designed specifically to affect brain chemistry. With your serotonin levels now much healthier, your brain will stop forcing you toward those terribly unhealthy foods. It's perfectly natural that you will feel like "you" have finally been able to conquer, to overcome those cravings with pure and simple WILLPOWER! This is why an SES makes it all seem so wonderfully effortless, because it comes from *within* you! There is absolutely no effort to live a heathier lifestyle, once you are able to achieve and maintain adequate serotonin levels. Again, all of this takes time. It also requires effort to break the old, unhealthy habits. But it will happen, I promise you. Just remember how long it took to get your body (and mind) out of shape. You need to be patient in reaching your goals. And remember, you will lose inches long before you actually lose pounds, so please stay off the scale.

Why don't you want me to weigh myself?
Feel free to weigh yourself when first starting. Use that number as a marker. But then <u>forget</u> about the scale, as it is NOT an accurate way to analyze your overall body composition. Furthermore, measuring only your body weight will most often discourage you. Personally, I rarely ever weigh myself. I don't even own a scale. I've learned to not only listen to my body, but also to know exactly where I am, within a few pounds, simply based on how I feel and how my clothes fit. In time, you'll be able to do this, as well. To measure your success, take your various measurements, record them along with your body weight, more importantly, your percentage of body fat, then use these measurements as a guide.

How do I measure my body fat?
Rather than judging your potential heath risks based on the once highly acclaimed BMI (Body Mass Index), a method that does not take into consideration those who weight train and who will consequently have more muscle mass, I use a specific machine that will test my clients overall body composition. However, using a measuring tape to track your waistline is one of the most effective ways in which to measure your body fat. Remember, your "waistline" is your insulin gauge. It's a direct and immediate reflection of how well your diet is working, or not. Whatever the method, don't stress about it. Record the initial measurements and then let it go. Put your full attention on getting healthier.

What is the danger zone for my waistline?
Anything greater than 40" in men and 35" in women is considered the danger zone. The following chart, though bare minimum, as a healthy level of body fat changes with age, will at least give you an idea of where your body fat should be. Though I'd rather you hire a qualified personal trainer to perform this test, in the meantime, there are numerous Web sites that offer various methods in which to measure your body fat, BMR, EER, etc. (Go to csgnetwork.com/bodyfatcalc.html to get a quick assessment of your body fat.) Just remember, not only are their dozens of ways to test all such data, but the subsequent

results and the preferred "healthy numbers" will also vary greatly from person to person depending upon their age, height, weight, body composition, level of activity, etc.

Body Fat Chart		
Fat Level	**Men**	**Women**
Very Low	7-10%	14-17%
Low	10-13%	17-20%
Average	13-17%	20-27%
High	17-25%	27-31%
Very High	25%+	31%+

What does BMR and EER stand for?
Both numbers are extremely important and here's why: BMR (Basal Metabolic Rate) represents the actual number of calories your body needs to sustain your bodily functions without exercise. It accounts for about 75% of total daily energy expenditure. And the more LBM (Lean Body Mass), the *higher* your BMR. The higher your BMR, the higher the rate your body will burn calories/fat at rest. This is precisely why I keep saying you need to lift weights to build LBM, while also eating properly. LBM will help you not only lose body fat, but also keep it off! EER (Extra Energy Requirements) refers to the *extra energy* needed for a person to perform various physical activities. Although I don't want you counting calories to lose weight, you'll need a base number to work from. Once you determine your BMR and EER, you'll then be able to reduce your caloric intake (*based on science*) to force your body to burn stored fat. (And because BMR needs to be based on "LBM" versus overall body weight, the most accurate way to determine these numbers is by getting a Body Composition Analysis done.)

Fascinating! I've never heard of this, but it makes perfect sense. Eat too little, my body goes into starvation mode. Eat too much, it stores the excess as fat.
Very good! While an SES will control your cravings and appetite, the other crucial key is finding out precisely the amount of fuel your body requires so as to control your weight.

I can't wait to get started! Should I stop taking the product once I lose the weight?
While this is of course up to you, I would say no—merely because the health benefits of maintaining serotonin goes far beyond just losing excess body fat. An SES will, yes, help support healthy levels of serotonin, which will thereby help control cravings, stabilize insulin, and help reduce appetite. But this is only the beginning! Based on the many extraordinary health benefits that come with boosting serotonin levels, *benefits that are truly life-changing,* I suggest you use an SES as long as it serves you well. As for me, I take mine eagerly every day and will continue to do so for the rest of my life.

What happens if I go off the SES? Will my old habits come back?
Please allow me to answer that by sharing the following quick story: Because this type of supplement affects brain chemistry, and in such a gentle, subtle manner, it's only natural that my clients suddenly felt as if their newfound willpower was based on them alone. In

fact, as we were going through the trial stages, several clients were reluctant to give the product any credit at all. They truly believed that they alone were finally able to conquer their cravings. While I'm thrilled that no matter what they believed was the catalyst in the dramatic change in their eating habits, it was only when they ran out of product that their viewpoint changed. They were fine for the first few days. But once they were off it for about a week, to their dismay, their old and unhealthy eating habits came creeping back in. Their cravings for cookies, rice, sodas, caffeine, chocolate, corn bread, even cocktails, were suddenly back in full force. Their sleeping patterns suffered greatly. Their moods shifted downward. They were once again quick to anger, highly irritable, stressed, and, worst of all, they were back to eating the foods that had always given them such emotional comfort. Those foods were unfortunately, the same ones that got them fat and miserable in the first place. They knew it wasn't good, but no matter how hard they tried to control the cravings, they were once again helpless. Their newfound willpower was suddenly gone. My phone began to ring off the hook. My clients were in a panic. They were upset with what was happening to them. They were desperate for more product. I hated to see them suffer, but as a product developer—this was all-telling for me. This unequivocally confirmed the impressive clinical evidence supporting 5-HTP, as well as vinpocetine.

But this experience wasn't limited to my clients. You see, throughout R&D, there are untold changes involved in the formulation process. It was inevitable that I'd be without product at times, as I was forever making advances in the formula. (I expected nothing short of perfection, due to the diet industry being saturated with so many ineffective, over-hyped products.) So, to insure accurate testing, I had to periodically go off any and all ingredients that stimulated the production of serotonin. I, too, was fine for a few days, maybe even a week without cravings, anxiety, or mood swings. But then—*there it was!* While my so-called weakness was never for sweets, my craving for a piece of sourdough toast suddenly came knocking. Like clockwork, my mind started to force me to consume the carb it knew would elevate this vital brain chemical. I didn't panic, as I knew exactly <u>why</u> I was suddenly back to craving this particular carb, and why I was also feeling anxious and unable to be as creatively focused. I, therefore, reflected on my life to see why my serotonin would be low. I can easily answer this: My life is pretty stressed, and stress, as you recall, is one of the primary reasons why serotonin becomes depleted.

I *finally* understand why my mood and weight has never been stable. I can't wait to put to use the many things you've taught me! All I need now is your product.
Nothing gives me more personal satisfaction than knowing I've inspired someone to live a healthier life. As for my product, sorry, but it's only available to my private clients. *Why?* Because whether you take my product, 5-HTP solo, or another SES—no product will work, especially long-term—if you don't truly understand *why* you crave these insulin-producing carbs, or why you're depressed, anxious, always needing meds, etc. Therefore, it was imperative that I first educate others as to this incredible research. Remember, knowledge is power. So please, keep reading. *Empower yourself!*

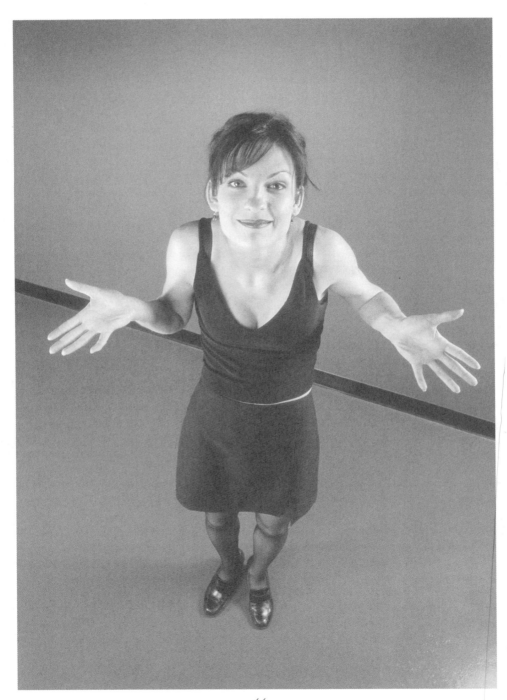

8

UNHEARD OF, BUT WHY?

If what you say is true about serotonin, this information could, in theory, change millions of lives. So why, then, isn't anyone else talking about it?
First of all, it's true and based on sound clinical research, not diet hype. Secondly, if this information was exposed as effectively and with the same intensity as any given blockbuster movie—better yet, as the drug companies promote their drugs—it would indeed change millions of lives. Furthermore, there are scientists and a few select health experts talking about it, with excellent books written about it, and most importantly, with impressive clinical studies to support it. Ironically, other than the authors/doctors listed below, I haven't met anyone, be it a doctor, psychiatrist, celebrity trainer, or layman, who was aware of this research. *Why?* Well, for one, less than 2% of all doctors are educated in nutrition. Even the many RDs (Registered Dietitians) and CNs (Clinical Nutritionists) that I've either spoken to, or heard being interviewed, are completely unaware of serotonin.

Speaking of RDs and CNs, I want to share my concerns: I have over two decades in the fitness industry, specifically the last six years devoted to nutritional/medical research alone, but it was while writing this book that I decided to further my education by earning my Sports Nutritionist certification. (I'll actually be taking an additional SN course to give me an even broader scope.) The rather unsettling aspect for me, however, with regard to the course that is so highly rated by the industry, is that what I'm forced to study and agree with is terribly far from what I know to be true. Their teachings with regard to diet are very old school. And I quote: "There is no good evidence that high insulin levels make people fat." (Liebman, 1996) If that statement isn't alarming enough, most of their research is from the same time period, *nearly a decade old*, which clearly explains why they still fear dietary fat. And, as such, they recommend <u>only</u> fat-free foods (which = too many carbs!), avoiding cholesterol, i.e., eggs, cheese, butter, etc., while fruit juice, skim milk, nonfat yogurt, cereal, bread, rolls, English muffins, pasta, pretzels, bananas, and potatoes are their preferred foods—and primary *protein* sources. Worst of all, they classify Coke and diet soft drinks as "sports drinks," and recommend eating margarine! *They can't possibly be serious?!*

I certainly grasp the concept of carb-loading (and needing to quickly fuel an athlete's body), but all that sugar is a false and unhealthy way to get energy. Their suggested meals consist mostly of simple and complex carbs, but those complex carbs are *refined* carbs. And without any dietary fat and very little protein to help lower the GI, let alone balance the food groups, those so-called complex carbs will affect blood sugar levels dramatically—and deplete serotonin. For those who work out, those carbs may supply fuel, but if they're not used, they'll be stored as fat. While some may be able to burn off the sugar, the more serious concern is the damage that will be done due to the overload of insulin required to control the sugar. High insulin levels are never good, burned off or otherwise. Even if one still believes in carb-loading, why not <u>low</u> GI carbs? They're far healthier, a more efficient fuel source, i.e., slower burning/longer lasting, and with no insulin spiking. And what about dietary fat? Where's the olive and flaxseed oils or avocado? Our bodies need fat to burn fat. It's also a far more efficient fuel than sugar. Moreover, why not eggs, fish, or tofu as a protein versus "cereal" or "two slices of bread?"

But hey, who the hell am I to doubt their expertise? I mean, after all, they have a "college degree" and I'm merely self-taught. Well, let me just say this: If this 30-year approach to nutrition was correct, if the nutritional advice that the colleges and various nutritional organizations are passing on to their students is accurate/nutritionally sound (which they then pass on to their clientele), *why* is our obesity rate at 65% and ever-growing? Why are those who are under the care of a RD and a personal trainer still struggling with their weight? And why are the majority of those individuals in the nutritional/educational/medical positions overweight themselves? It concerns me because these educators will continue to spread this information—and with no end in sight. All the while, what they're teaching with regard to diet is going to make the average person gain body fat, <u>not</u> lose it. And, just as I assumed, no mention whatsoever of serotonin.

Now, as for why most consumers are not aware of serotonin, how could they be? After all, if those in charge of educating others are completely unaware of it, how would the typical consumer ever be expected to? This is precisely why I spent the last year and a half of my life writing this book, with a passionate—and somewhat desperate desire to bring it to the forefront of society's consciousness. I won't be content until every man, woman, and child is aware of this information! You can help me by giving a book to your family and friends!

What prompted you into this area of research?
Through the many years of training and nutritionally consulting clients, I watched them frantically try to lose weight with whatever the latest diet craze was. And yet, no matter how good those diets sounded, no matter how many so-called impressive studies or raving testimonials they produced, many of my clients were simply unable to control their cravings so as to achieve long-term weight loss. Temporary weight loss was easy. Keeping it off was another matter. All because they couldn't resist certain sinful high GI carbs. My own sporadic craving for toast also astounded me. I knew without a doubt, cravings were something *far beyond* willpower or emotional attachment. Nevertheless, it wasn't until years later when I was a partner in a failed infomercial project that I shifted my focus from the gym and went extensively into R&D. And the more I learned, the more disgusted I was by the blatant and endless deceit within the diet, food, and pharmaceutical industries.

Where did you actually learn about serotonin?
I've read literally dozens of clinical abstracts, various medical studies, and health journals, but by far the best books I've read on this subject are the following:

5-HTP, The Natural Way to Overcome Depression, Obesity, and Insomnia by Michael Murray, ND, a highly respected naturopathic doctor, best-selling author, and speaker. This book is very detailed and exact, complete with clinical studies to support all such claims, yet it's equally reader friendly. It will reconfirm all that I say about serotonin and 5-HTP, plus much more. I recommend everyone read this book. For the record, there is no one in the alternative healthcare industry that I respect as much as this man.

The Schwarzbein Principle by Diana Schwarzbein, MD (and Nancy Deville), has over 14 years of extensive medical training in endocrinology, biochemistry, and physiology. More importantly, her work is supported by impressive clinical studies. She is an exceptional doctor, as well as respected speaker, radio host, and best-selling author. This celebrated book discusses, among many things, serotonin and its fundamental role in good health. And for those who will most assuredly question my opinions regarding low-fat diets, eating cholesterol, etc., I insist you read this book. While the results from her numerous controlled studies are truly impressive, I've also lived by her exact principles for years—and long before I ever read her work. I'm living proof, that at the very least, eating fat does not make us fat. We need to eat good dietary fat for our minds and bodies to function at their best. And as gifted and cutting-edge as Dr. Schwarzbein is as a physician, her compassion exceeds that exponentially. I was fortunate enough to have met with her back in 2001 to discuss my research and initial product. I was exceedingly humbled that she was impressed enough with both that she considered conducting a private study with some of her patients, while also wanting to private-label my formula. Due to her hectic schedule, this never came to fruition. Nonetheless, I'm still one of her biggest fans.

The perspectives set forth by the above two doctors with respect to what it takes to achieve overall excellent lifelong health are, undeniably, some of the most accurate of all the experts I've come to know. But, considering I'm a woman who questions everything, clinically proven or otherwise, no amount of clinical studies or books was enough for me. The last thing I would ever want to be part of was another weight loss marketing illusion. Based on the all-encompassing time I dedicated to R&D, the subsequent trial tests with approximately 50 clients, along with, of course, my own personal experience, I am confident, *without any hesitation,* in sharing this extraordinary information with you.

All the more reason why I'm shocked to see that not one of the major companies has focused their attention on this remarkable research, subsequently developing products that would address this essential link. Instead the diet industry's only focus is forever on using stimulants for weight loss. Considering our obesity rate, that approach is quite obviously not effective. And even though ephedra was pulled from the market, consumers beware: product developers are simply using every other type of stimulant, hoping to promote weight loss. That weight loss, if any, will be temporary and terribly unhealthy.

My sense of urgency to bring this information to the mainstream also comes from the fact that nearly every day I hear yet another health expert blaming the public for being "fat because they choose to be, they're too lazy, addicted, lack willpower, no control over their emotions, or they use food to comfort themselves." But to make matters even worse, when you berate someone, when you so cruelly judge them, it only fuels their sense of failure and hopelessness, and deepens their sense of worthlessness. Of course I realize there are always going to be those individuals who are simply unwilling or interested in losing weight. Too lazy? Maybe. Confused? More like it. But no one chooses to be fat! No one chooses to fail at every diet they try! No one chooses to comfort themselves every night with a bag of cookies and a liter of soda! No one chooses to be weak-willed! No one chooses to be addicted to anything that would bring them such emotional pain! No one intentionally chooses the many health risks that come with being obese, let alone the unfair public scrutiny!

The fact of the matter is, there are thousands of health experts, telling people a thousand different ways to lose weight (me included). But it's up to you to educate yourself about the various options and determine which ones are based on science, not diet hype. Nonetheless, it's entirely another matter when people, especially people with platforms that reach millions, share their opinions in a hurtful and demeaning manner. It worries me, because with this tremendous power, they can affect millions based on their commentary. I hate to think about just how many people will come to believe they're fat because they're too lazy, without willpower, or they merely—on a subconscious level—*choose to be.* Although I believe these particular people are sincere in wanting to help others, their comments are often brutal and unjustified. No disrespect intended, but I would only hope that those individuals who step into the weight loss arena have the required expertise. And, at bare minimum, they should equally reflect their expertise via their own physical body. No matter the profession, we should each be able to proudly represent what we expect from others.

I will, though, most certainly agree that people frequently use food to comfort themselves and, likewise, they often seem to lack willpower. No argument there. But it's "why" they eat this comfort food, moreover, "why" they can't *stop* using it as a crutch, that most health experts are unaware of. If they were aware of serotonin, the major neurotransmitter that governs cravings, appetite, depression, etc., I'm quite sure they would never make such insensitive comments.

You're right. I've heard quite a few people claim that diet failure is due to being lazy, weak-willed, and so forth. I struggled with this, because I was successful in every other part of my life, but failed miserably when it came to sticking to a diet. You and a million others. Bottom line, no matter how many times or in how many ways anyone—be it Dr. Sears (the Zone), Dr. Agatston (South Beach Diet), Dr. Atkins, or even Dr. Phil—tells you to stop eating processed/junk food or other high GI carbs, it is entirely another matter to actually *adhere* to that diet regime. Statistics don't lie: 98% of all diets fail. They fail because of cravings. *The crucial link to long-term weight loss is being able to achieve and maintain healthy levels of serotonin.*

I read Dr. Atkins' latest book, and he never mentioned serotonin. I often heard him say cravings were about people being addicted to certain foods.
You're exactly right. As I read Atkins' 2002 revised book, I was amazed to discover that he, too, was unacquainted with serotonin and its role in successful weight loss. Based on his books and numerous interviews, his expert opinion was that cravings were directly related to "individual food intolerances/allergies or a drop in blood sugar." He also claimed cravings were caused by being "addicted to certain foods/beverages." Due to his own admission that he couldn't control his patients' cravings, I knew he was unaware of the serotonin-insulin research. It was in January 2003 that I decided to write him a letter. Within weeks, ANI's (Atkins Nutritionals, Inc.) VP of Business Development called. They were eager to talk to me. Regardless, and to quickly summarize: After the pain-staking process of insuring their non-disclosure/non-compete documents were going to protect me, I signed. I then promptly offered to fly to New York. I knew it was necessary that I speak directly to Dr. Atkins. But I was told he was "not involved in the day-to-day business of ANI." Ah, the corporate veil. The first red flag. My only option was to disclose to an ANI senior VP. Only after I reconfirmed with her that Atkins/ANI was indeed unaware of this research did I agree to move ahead. This hour-long disclosure went so well, in fact, that she expressed interest in ANI private-labeling my formula. But first, she requested I send a copy of my clinical studies and my formula ASAP. I agreed to a partial submission of the clinicals only.

You must have been thrilled to see where this opportunity would take you!
Yes, absolutely. But, to my dismay, only days after the Atkins group received my research, my phone calls and emails were no longer returned. The VP I had dealt with was suddenly nowhere to be found. I'm far from a pessimist, but I knew these signs only too well. When I was finally able to reach her, she apologized for not getting back to me sooner and then claimed, "I'm sorry, but there has been a *slight* mistake. Dr. Atkins has long been aware of this research. He simply chose not to 'publish' it at this time. We are, nonetheless, still interested in possibly private-labeling your formula."

Without wanting to air any more dirty laundry, let's just say I felt it was in my best interest and that of my company to severe any and all negotiations. My lawyer was informed, as was ANI's in-house legal counsel. I was further guaranteed ANI would respect the terms of our NDA. My documents were returned, and I quickly moved on.

Please understand, however, that the only reason I share this story is that it reconfirms just how extraordinarily unique this research truly is. Furthermore, above any and all professed legally binding contracts, *listen to your inner voice.* That soft, yet not so subtle little voice, is there to protect you, to guide you. Please, learn to listen to it. This was a perfect example of me—ignoring mine.

9

STORING FAT
One of insulin's many roles

You've mentioned insulin numerous times, but what is its role?
Insulin is an extremely important hormone, secreted from the pancreas, that lowers blood sugar levels and builds and stores fat. Insulin tightly regulates the amount of sugar going to the brain. It is responsible for putting nutrients (fat, sugar, protein) into cells. Insulin regulates how much blood sugar (glucose, which is energy for the cells) will be allowed to enter the cells. Without insulin, blood sugar rises to harmful levels.

What happens when insulin is released quickly?
Among many things, the rapid release of insulin stimulates the production of serotonin, which makes us feel good, temporarily. This change in mood is so subtle that we are not *consciously* aware of it. The subconscious desire to feel good causes people to eat more carbohydrates. That same desire causes people to eat more food than necessary, which leads to weight gain. It's very simple: Calories in excess of our energy needs will be stored as fat, especially carbs, as carbs need to be used immediately as energy, or they will convert into fat.

Where does all this sugar come from?
For the last several decades, the American diet has been far too high in carbohydrates, primarily processed and refined carbohydrates, which means *too much sugar*. In addition, numerous types of sugar are hidden in thousands of foods. And, as we age, the body's metabolic system naturally slows down. The energy that carbohydrates provide are consequently diminished, yet our eating habits do not reflect this change.

What role does insulin play with regard to fat storage?
Insulin is the fat-building/fat-storing hormone. Fat cannot be stored without the presence of insulin. Let me repeat this, as it's extremely important: Fat, i.e., HEALTHY DIETARY FAT, CANNOT BE STORED WITHOUT THE PRESENCE OF INSULIN. Insulin is the trigger that opens fat cells. Once fat cells are opened, they're like hungry little Pacmen, ready to feed, to gorge, to fill up! Furthermore, once insulin is spiked, it will put the body into a fat-storing mode for several hours. Not only is the body now *storing* new fat, it will <u>not</u> allow stored fat to be burned as fuel. Once insulin is spiked, by caffeine, stress, high GI carbs, sugar, alcohol, etc., it encourages the storage of body fat from *whatever* nutrient group you eat. Controlling insulin levels is, therefore, vital to achieving successful long-term fat loss.

51

Are you saying that once I trigger insulin, no matter how healthy I'm eating, those foods will be encouraged to be stored as fat?

Exactly. This is why you have to be very aware of what you're eating and drinking. Example: Having a cup of coffee with your breakfast will trigger your insulin. *Why?* Caffeine is a stimulant. And all stimulants spike insulin levels. Stimulants can also cause insulin resistance. (Let's not forget, that most people rarely drink their coffee black; they add either sugar, nonfat milk, flavored creamer, or artificial sweeteners, all of which spike insulin.) Or maybe you have a chicken breast with white bread, or a side of white rice, with an iced tea. The white bread and rice are both high GI carbs, and both are recognized as sugar by the body. Plus, the iced tea with caffeine. Either scenario has the same result: If you spike your insulin, there is a much greater chance that this food will be stored as fat. Your body will also stay in this fat-storing mode for about two hours.

What else causes insulin to rise?

In addition to the many items listed above, excessive carbohydrate consumption, high-fructose corn syrup, dieting, fat-free/low-fat diets, stress, prescription and nonprescription drugs, processed and refined foods, nicotine, steroids, alcohol, candy, sodas, fruit juices, flavored drinks, iced tea, and lack of exercise will all cause insulin levels to rise.

Wow! Sounds like basically everything can spike it. But don't we need insulin?

Sure we do. Insulin makes sure our cells receive blood sugar (glucose) necessary to sustain life. It also increases glycogen storage which provides fuel for our muscles. Nevertheless, high levels of insulin also cause the body to use carbs for fuel instead of utilizing the body's stored fat. Once again, the key to long-term fat loss, *and numerous other health issues*, is to stabilize insulin levels.

Can increased levels of insulin be harmful?

High levels of insulin over a long period of time are extremely detrimental to your health. Increased insulin can cause fat gain by encouraging the storage of fat, and further weight gain due to salt and water retention. Continuous high levels of insulin cause abnormal and harmful cholesterol production, which leads to plaqueing of the arteries. Plaqueing of the arteries is the cause of heart disease, heart attacks, and stroke. The over-production of insulin causes insulin resistance, which can lead to type 2 diabetes. It also causes high blood pressure, and cancer—even death.

What is insulin resistance?

Years of excessive consumption of sugar start to take their toll on our cells. As cells become filled with sugar, they're unable to let any more in. To protect against any additional sugar overload, cells reduce the actual number of insulin receptor doors. Insulin is no longer able to unload as much sugar into the cells. Hence, *insulin resistance*.

WARNING: The fat we carry around our midsection is a pretty good indicator of insulin resistance. This type of stored body fat is considered the most harmful to our health.

Why is belly fat more harmful?

First of all, belly fat is closest to your vital organs. Researchers believe the culprit is visceral fat, and excess inches around the waist often suggest the presence of visceral fat. This fat contains more metabolically active fat cells. This is in contrast to subcutaneous fat, which is directly under the skin. Studies show that visceral fat is more active, releasing toxins into the body. In addition, its secretions go straight to the liver and may interfere with its functions, which include helping to regulate blood glucose and cholesterol. Anyone with a belly has visceral fat. And the more you have, the worse off you are.

A recent study published in the *New England Journal of Medicine* gave further support to the notion that visceral fat is more of a threat than fat found just under the skin. Doctors found that liposuction, which removes only subcutaneous fat, amazingly had no affect whatsoever on health, even when surgeons sucked out 20 pounds of subcutaneous abdominal fat. But a person who loses that much weight through dieting and exercise sees significant changes in blood pressure, cholesterol, and insulin resistance.

Liposuction may fail to improve health for another reason. While liposuction removes billions of fat cells, it does not shrink the billions more left behind. Obese people have huge fat cells, with 50 to 75% more mass than fat cells in lean people. Large fat cells are not a good thing to have, because researchers have found that they are more active metabolically than small ones, and more likely to produce harmful substances.

What do you suggest?

The best way to get rid of excess body fat, visceral or otherwise, and shrink fat cells is through proper eating habits and regular exercise. To reiterate, there is no magic pill or cosmetic procedure that will deliver long-term results when it comes to getting the lean, healthy, and attractive body that you desire. You have to be willing to make the effort through a healthy lifestyle. You can reach all your goals if you simply come to understand it is about the choices you make, and about being able to control your cravings and appetite. Nonetheless, if one year of being truly committed to a healthy lifestyle has yet to give you the results you want, then, and only then, consider a minor touch-up with liposuction or any other type of cosmetic procedure.

On a personal note: I waited until I was 43 before I had my breasts augmented. Not only am I a woman who has no desire to follow the crowd, but I also never had a problem with my small breasts. But, after 40, and with so little body fat, my size B cup was suddenly less than a hopeful A. My chest looked like that of a 12-year-old boy. Once I decided, though, to finally do something, I took that decision very seriously, consulting with about six different surgeons over a period of three years. But I'll tell you this, had I been able to sculpt my breasts through weight training, as I do with the rest of my body, I would <u>never</u> have gone under the knife. All I ask, lipo, breast implants, or otherwise, is that you do it for yourself, choose your doctor with the greatest of care—and please do not use these surgical options as a quick fix or an alternative to a healthy lifestyle.

10

TYPE 2 DIABETES RUNNING RAMPANT

What is type 2 diabetes?
In trying to overcome the cell resistance to excess sugar, the pancreas secretes even *more* insulin. This causes too much insulin in the bloodstream. The cells react by shutting even more receptor doors. At this point, any sugar in the bloodstream is directed into fat storage. When the fat cells become impacted, the sugar is no longer allowed to enter the cells. It remains in the bloodstream. Hence, *type 2 diabetes*.

What is adult-onset diabetes?
Adult-onset diabetes, or AOD, is just another name for type 2 diabetes. But because there are now so many cases of type 2 diabetes in young children, they actually stopped referring to it as adult-onset. It is once again known as type 2 diabetes.

What factors lead to diabetes?
The overwhelming number of those being diagnosed with diabetes is fueled by various factors, primarily being overweight. Poor diet, lack of exercise, smoking, and alcohol also contribute to this disease. To lower your risks, a significant change in lifestyle must be made. Instead of the AMA or FDA looking to reduce and even eliminate the *underlying causes* of diabetes, the actual treatment of diabetes has become a billion-dollar industry! But please understand, treating diabetes does NOT cure diabetes. Most treatments may extend life and possibly postpone many of the health issues associated with the disease, but diabetes itself will ultimately take its toll.

Why are so many people becoming diabetic?
I strongly believe this recent surge in diabetes is due to poor diet and lack of exercise. Some interesting facts to consider: A poor diet is due to the inability to adhere to a healthy diet. The inability to adhere to a healthy diet is due to insatiable cravings. Insatiable cravings are due to low serotonin. Lack of exercise is due to simply being too tired, unwilling, or too overweight, which are all due, once again, to poor diet. All of these elements play off of one another.

When serotonin levels are depleted, no amount of willpower or motivation in the world will overcome carbohydrate cravings. For most, the only relief is to consume the foods or beverages that trigger the quick release of this brain chemical. Unfortunately, the same foods (and beverages) that increase the production of serotonin equally trigger insulin. And insulin is the hormone that causes your body to store fat. Don't forget, this is all occurring on a *subconscious* level.

You see, most people really have no idea why they find themselves grabbing a bag of Cape Cod potato chips and an ice cold Fresca, or why they're suddenly at the drive-through window ordering a double order of fries, jumbo soda, Quarter Pounder, and a couple of chocolate chip cookies for dessert. From their perspective, it simply sounds *soooo* delicious! They also know only too well just how good this type of food makes them feel! At least temporarily.

No matter how hard you try, *dieting NEVER works!*

While you consume this food, your level of comfort skyrockets! *Ahhhh,* suddenly you feel so good, so relaxed. But BEWARE! At the very same time, your fat cells are gorging! They were triggered open by the spike in insulin caused by this food. Your billions of fat cells are now open wide and feeding! And they will remain open and ready to store new fat from any food source, *no matter how healthy it is*, for about two hours after the meal. Your body will also not release any stored fat during this time.

As your serotonin levels begin to drop (and they most certainly will), so will the feeling of emotional comfort you just derived from these foods. Your energy will plummet. Your mood will do likewise. You'll become aggravated. Quick to anger. Stressed. Anxious. Your brain will then begin the cycle all over again, creating noise, i.e., *cravings* for the types of foods and/or beverages that it knows will once again trigger the production of this won-derful, mood-altering brain chemical. This cycle is repeated over and over and over again. And this is exactly <u>why</u> we have so many new cases of diabetes in both adults and, sadly, even young children. Just take a look around. No matter the age or race, everyone seems to be overweight—if not obese. Those who are in shape are becoming a rarity, few and far between.

We must also never forget the feelings, the *emotions* that are attached to these weight loss struggles. The feelings of guilt, shame, the total loss of self-respect when you fail at another diet. These deep-seated and complicated emotions further exacerbate the rate of diet failure. You feel even more out of control. Your mood sinks deeper. You feel worthless, hopeless, and alone. No matter how hard you try, *dieting never works!*

But <u>why</u> is it so hard to lose weight, to control the cravings? Are you that weak? Do you not have any willpower whatsoever? You struggle. You cry. Desperate for relief, you eat some candy. With each bite of chocolate, your mood becomes lighter. Bite, after delicious bite, you almost feel normal. Not surprisingly, you eat the entire box. *Ooooh, my!* Relief has finally come! As comforting as it is, you know it's merely a temporary fix. That's okay. You'll take it. For now, it calms your mind. The vicious cycle you know only too well will, however, repeat within a few short hours. You say to yourself: "To hell with it! Tomorrow is another day. I'll start my diet then!" Or you may say, "Hey, I can eat all I want and then just throw it up!" With that, you rush to pick up the phone. "Hello, Pizza King....." (Note: Binging and purging are both symptoms of low serotonin.)

Emotional eating...

Is this why I eat when I'm upset?
The underlying causes of emotional eating can truly be limitless. But if you are at least able to maintain healthy levels of serotonin, you will be far stronger, *far better prepared emotionally and mentally,* to deal with these emotional issues. And when this happens, it will subsequently help alleviate the often overwhelming sense of anxiety, depression, etc., that initially fueled your cravings for junk food—and equally deepened your sense of worthlessness. Until you understand this critical link between serotonin and insulin, this vicious cycle of mood swings, depression, and "emotional eating" will control you. And because serotonin is so easily depleted—causing, at the very least, anxiety, binge eating, and yes, *highly emotional behavior*—your brain will continually compel you toward the foods it has long known will elevate it. And, trust me, your willpower is no match for your brain when it wants to maintain this major neurotransmitter! Since high GI carbs are one of the quickest and easiest ways to elevate it, your brain will start the noise, i.e., cravings, for these. You helplessly succumb to the cravings, only to experience once again that overpowering sense of failure. FACT: To control the emotional eating episodes, you must maintain healthy serotonin levels. Once this is achieved, you'll be astonished by how you will no longer seek food to comfort yourself. The emotional eating will be controlled. I promise you.

I finally get it! I really do! But how will I know if I'm eating too much sugar?
To reiterate, the weight you carry around your midsection is the first sign of insulin resistance. It is the first indication that you're consuming more sugar/high GI carbs than your body can utilize. Funny, as their personal trainer and nutritionist, my clients have often tried to convince me they're eating healthy. Sorry. Little do they know that all I have to do is look at their stomach to make this judgment for myself. Their waistline is, again, the most efficient way for me to analyze their diet.

As much as some may honestly try to lose the excess weight, statistics don't lie: 98% of all diets fail. They fail because of cravings. This is because so many things in our day-to-day life deplete serotonin. Maintaining your serotonin is absolutely crucial to controlling cravings. Controlling cravings is absolutely crucial to stabilizing insulin levels. Until this is achieved, obesity and type 2 diabetes will continue to rise at alarming rates.

I've failed at far too many diets, and suffered with those exact emotions described above. But based on what you're teaching me, I hope to never endure that sense of failure or guilt ever again!

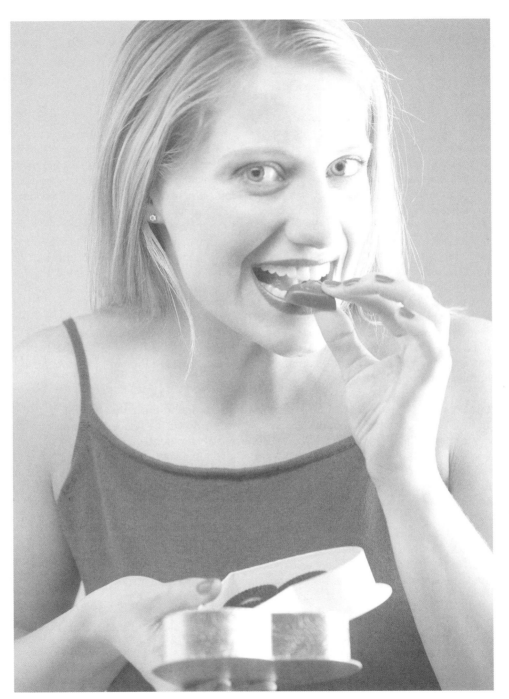

11

SUGAR
&
ITS SWEET, ADDICTIVE NATURE

How did sugar even come into our diet?
The junk-food industry got its start back in the late 1800s. Sugar intake was pretty low to start, averaging a mere 12 pounds a year per person. Suddenly, by 1928, the consumption of sugar was over 10 times that amount! As of 2004, Americans on average consumed over 100 pounds of refined sugar per year, per person!

No disrespect intended, but don't believe that you're not one of these people. I say this because I'm not talking about the kind of sugar you take out of a sugar bowl or even the little packets of sugar. I'm speaking of the sugar that is hidden in over 90% of all processed food! Sugar is *disguised* under various names in thousands of products! High-sugar products are extremely successful in the marketplace, and they're some of the cheapest fillers in processed food. Sugar is everywhere, from fruit juice, soda, crackers, bread, soups, desserts, baby food, processed foods, and canned food. Of course, all those fat-free/low-fat foods are LOADED with sugar! The list is endless. So please read the nutritional labels with the greatest of care.

Not only does sugar not have any nutritional value, but it is tremendously harmful to your health. Sugar is a poison to our bodies. It's highly addictive, and there are hundreds of clinical studies that prove just how harmful its affects can be. Sugar damages the immune system, promotes vitamin and mineral deficiencies, not to mention it drains our body's energy. And sugar ages us faster than ever!

Personally, I have never experienced anything as addictive or harmful for the mind and body as sugar. Perfect scenario: My close friend Billy always likes to give me a box of decadent truffles for Christmas. And while I don't have any cravings for sweets, I plead with him each year to *pleeeease* not give them to me, as even I, at certain times, can be seduced into eating them.

Now there are those who can enjoy one—and that's it. But not me. Once I take that first glorious bite, my mind is immediately triggered by the sugar, and it keeps forcing me to eat more. I have even gone as far as to put them in the freezer so it wouldn't be as easy to eat them. Yeah, right! *Who was I kidding?!* Instead, I would find myself taking one, slowly nibbling on it, and then simply letting it melt in the warmth of my mouth. *Ooooooh, baby!* Talk about sinful! Hmmm! But, as delicious as it may have tasted, the problem was that, only minutes after eating it my brain would create that noise, that ever-nagging little voice, that voice we now know is a craving. And as hard as I tried to ignore it, it would keep at me, whispering over and over again, "Pssssttt hey—those truffles are in the freezer just waiting to be eaten! Have one more! Come on! That's all. *Just...one...more!*" So I'd have another. And another. And then—one more. Talk about addictive! Once again, I say: I have never experienced anything as addictive as sugar! Since then, if Billy gifts me with those chocolate delights, I take only one, savor its sweetness, and then I quickly, and with great precision, whip the rest of them down the hillside!

Beyond the addictive aspect, sugar damages the body by causing hypoglycemic reaction (low blood sugar). Sugar is actually more toxic than alcohol. It was once written in a Harvard health journal that if "Sugar was just now coming out, the FDA would classify it as a drug." It should at least come with WARNING labels!

Didn't they add some silly sugar tax a couple years ago to help prevent obesity?
With regard to the two-cent "sugar tax" placed on soda/juice/candy, with intentions of diminishing obesity in children, I found this absurd. Do they really believe that an additional two cents tagged onto these items will deter kids from buying them? Of course not. The thought process behind this tax increase is, in itself, childish, as well as, useless. First of all, the FDA should heavily fine the companies who manufacture these foods and beverages, as it's not a secret that these companies will do whatever it takes to keep the consumer buying their particular products. And the best way to insure that the consumer keeps coming back for more is to get them *addicted* to their products.

The FDA and FTC (Federal Trade Commission) should go after those companies with a vengeance, particularly those who *knowingly* practice deceitful/fraudulent marketing tactics. But instead of going after the source, they disturbingly allow these huge money machines to keep putting out this junk food, getting a vast majority addicted, which most certainly contributes to the alarming rate of obesity, heart disease, cancer, depression, etc. And then, on top of that, they want to further tax these food items? *This is wrong!* It is not the government's place to try to control what we eat, through taxation or otherwise, especially considering they knew these foods were unhealthy and addictive to begin with. A tax will not solve anything. A disturbing pattern: Cigarettes—knowing full well they were addictive and deadly—but allowing them to be marketed. Then charging those who used them higher taxes. A perfect marketing plan, as the government knows these people are long addicted, and will therefore pay whatever the asking price. Never forget: They also realize the exorbitant amount of profit involved in treating the diseases associated with smoking and obesity. There are far too many people, who make far too much money, to ever put an end to selling these types of harmful products, or their deceitful marketing practices. As of the Vioxx scandal in 2004, the FDA is most assuredly one of those making billions off this deception!

I want to share a rather enlightening comment made by Ricky Williams, the NFL football payer who unexpectedly resigned in December 2004. Mike Wallace was interviewing him on *60 Minutes*. Mr. Wallace, with his usual flair, asked Ricky if he was using any other "more dangerous drugs" than his admitted marijuana. Ricky looked intently at Mr. Wallace, pondered his question, and responded with extreme clarity, "Do I use anything *more dangerous*? Hmm, yes, I suppose I do." (Camera quickly cut to Mr. Wallace with this look of astonishment!) Ricky continued by saying, "Yes, I occasionally eat sugar, as in sweets." Mr. Wallace was dumbfounded by this comment, but I thought it was *absolutely brilliant!* Good for you, Ricky! I admire you for following your heart when it concerned your career—and for recognizing and calling out where the real dangerous drugs exist: in our food!

What other hidden sugars should I watch for?
The following chapter lists the numerous names under which sugar can be disguised. Although I want you to take the time to familiarize yourself with these various names, so you can avoid them, it will be nearly impossible to avoid sugar or artificial sweeteners all of the time. Just do your best to eliminate them as much as possible.

Besides the highly addictive nature of sugar, it has also been known to:

- Fuel cancer cells • Cause hormonal imbalance • Contribute to diabetes
- Cause depression and insomnia • Lead to drinking problems, even alcoholism
- Contribute to osteoporosis, worsen PMS and increase risk for yeast infection
- Promote excessive food consumption in obese people • Cause epileptic seizures
- Promote the death of our cells • Increase harmful production of cholesterol
- Deplete vitamins and minerals • Cause hypoglycemia • Decrease growth hormone
- Cause premature aging • Age our skin by damaging collagen structure
- Slow down the ability of the adrenal glands to function properly
- Cause tooth decay, headaches, migraines, arthritis, and heart disease
- Decrease insulin sensitivity, thereby greatly contributing to obesity
- Increase the systolic blood pressure • Suppress the immune system
- Increase risk of high blood pressure • Cause drowsiness and decrease energy
- Alter the proper absorption of protein • Impair the structure of DNA
- Severely reduce learning ability in children • Contribute to Alzheimer's
- Cause hyperactivity, anxiety, difficulty concentrating, and moodiness
- Promote an increase in triglycerides • Cause a spike in adrenaline

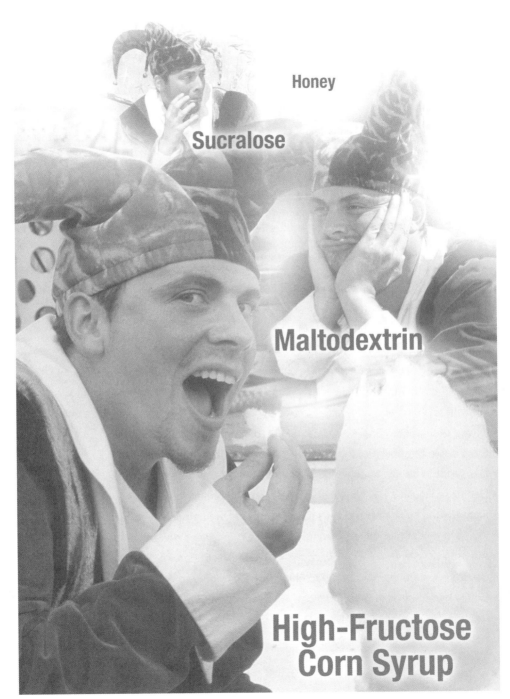

Honey

Sucralose

Maltodextrin

High-Fructose
Corn Syrup

12

THE MANY FACES OF SUGAR

With all this talk of sugar, it's important that you know the many different names under which sugar, sugar substitutes, and artificial sweeteners are masquerading. Hopefully, this list will help you make better choices when selecting your groceries. Please keep these various names in mind as you read nutritional panels, and then do your best to avoid them.

Types of sugar:

Beet sugar	Brown sugar	Cane sugar
Corn sugar	Confectioner's sugar	Corn syrup
Granulated sugar	HFCS	Honey
Invert sugar	Isomalt	Maltodextrin
Maple sugar	Maple syrup	Molasses
Raw sugar	Sorghum	Turbinado sugar

Words that end with "ose" are also a form of sugar:

Dextrose	Fructose	Galactose
Glucose	Lactose	Levulose
Maltose	Sucrose	

Words ending in "ol" are yet another form of sugar, known as sugar alcohols:

Maltitol	Mannitol	Sorbitol
Xylitol (*one of the healthiest choices)		

Artificial sweeteners:

Acesulfame-K	Aspartame	Cyclamate
Neotame	Saccharine	Sucralose

Brand names containing artificial sweeteners:

Equal/Equal-Measure	NutraSweet	Splenda
Spoonful	Sweet N' Low	Sweet One

Bottom Line...

If you truly want good health—

AVOID SUGAR AND ITS MANY SUBSTITUTES!

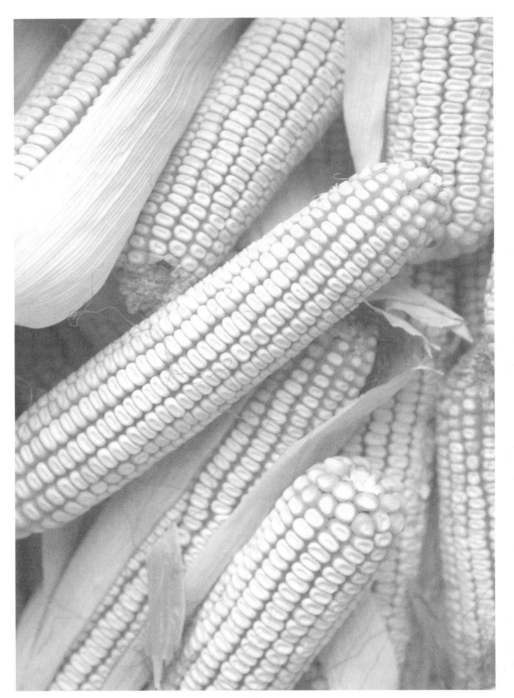

13

WARNING:
HIGH-FRUCTOSE CORN SYRUP

I see high-fructose corn syrup everywhere, but what is it?
High-fructose corn syrup, also known as HFCS, is made from cornstarch. It's a thick liquid that contains two basic sugar building blocks: 55% fructose blended with 45% glucose. HFCS is produced by processing cornstarch to yield glucose, and then processing the glucose to produce a high percentage of fructose. It's basically white cornstarch turned into a crystal clear syrup.

The process for making this sweetener out of corn was developed in the 1970s. The demand for it grew rapidly—from less than three million tons in 1980 to almost 8 million tons in 1995! Consumption of HFCS rose 1,000% between 1970 and 1990. As of 2004, Americans consumed far more HFCS than sugar. The average consumer would be surprised to learn that the larger percentage of sweeteners used in processed food comes from corn, <u>not</u> sugar cane or beets. Sweeteners made from corn account for over 55% of the sweetener market. *Annual sales are over $4 billion!* According to the U.S. Department of Agriculture, consumption of various sweeteners had risen in the United States from an estimated 113 pounds per person in 1966 to 147 pounds in 2001. As for HFCS, we consumed almost 63 pounds per person!

What's the advantage over cane sugar?
There are several advantages of using HFCS. Corn is much cheaper and twice as sweet as refined sugar. As a liquid, HFCS is also easier to blend into various food products, beverages, etc. Food manufacturers prefer it over refined sugar, as they can use less, yet get the same wonderful sweet taste as cane sugar.

Where is HFCS found?
HFCS is laced into literally thousands of food products, including chewing gum, fruit-flavored drinks, cookies, jams, soft drinks, baked goods, fast food, bread, cereal, sauces, bacon, crackers, candy bars, chips, etc. It's basically used in all processed food. Worst of all, it's even found in health products like protein and nutrition bars, as well as, purported natural fruit drinks and sodas.

How do I know if a product contains this syrup blend?
You need to read the nutritional panel, specifically the ingredients section.

Why don't you recommend it?
There are hundreds of studies that show just how unhealthy HFCS is for the body and mind. For starters, it's processed differently in the body than glucose. Glucose causes the pancreas to release insulin. Studies suggest, however, that HFCS does not trigger the release of insulin, nor does it break down like glucose. And even more alarming is that the liver converts HFCS far more readily into lipids than it does with glucose. And lipids are the chemical building blocks of trigylcerides.

Oh, I am so confused!
Sorry. I know it can be rather hard to follow. Let me simplify it: The body processes HFCS differently than it does old-fashioned cane or beet sugar. It also forces the liver to put more fat in the bloodstream. The end result: Our bodies are basically tricked into wanting to *eat more,* while at the same time we are *storing more* body fat. HFCS also depletes vitamins and minerals, and accelerates the aging process at the *cellular* level.

Now I get it. I also realize, with this toxic ingredient in so much of our food, why we're all so damn fat, always hungry, bitchy, and looking older by the minute!
Please don't get discouraged. Simply make sure you read food labels and avoid HFCS, corn syrup, and fructose.

I assume these sweeteners will also deplete my serotonin?
Most definitely. These sweeteners will perpetuate cravings and encourage weight gain, mood swings, insomnia, binge eating, depression, heart disease, and so forth.

I'm sorry, but I'm still a little confused. I thought fructose was from fruit, which is healthy, right?
Fructose naturally occurs in both fruit and corn. The fructose I'm talking about here, is made from corn. And high-fructose corn syrup is fructose that has been highly concentrated. Fructose has been aggressively touted for years as a natural sugar. This marketing deception has gone over quite well, considering we've been led to believe since childhood that all fructose comes from "fruit." Hence, it must be healthy. But hold on a minute! Once again, this particular fructose that is being used in our foods is not from fruit. It's a *refined* sugar—and harmful to our health. Fructose, corn syrup, and HFCS are large-scale *commercialized* sweeteners. Eating fruit in its natural form is far different from eating processed food containing fructose, corn syrup, or HFCS.

Understood. I'll make sure to read food (and beverage) labels to avoid buying anything containing fructose, corn syrup, and especially HFCS. Now, can you please tell me once again what triglycerides are?
Triglycerides are the chemical form in which most fat exists in food, as well as in the body and blood plasma. Calories eaten, but not used immediately by the body, are converted into triglycerides and transported to fat cells to be stored. Hormones regulate the release

of triglycerides from fat tissue so they meet the body's specific needs for energy between meals. Elevated triglycerides contribute to heart disease.

Controversial sweetener is banned!

Allow me to close this chapter with a very encouraging news story. As of July 2004, Earth Fare, a North Carolina chain of health food supermarkets, has banned all products made with HFCS! Over a third of all their sodas and energy bars will have to be removed—some of them best-sellers! Their plan is to remove all products containing HFCS by the end of 2004. This is one of the best stories I've read in a very long time! I applaud Earth Fare for following their mission of "Good Heath," no matter the effect to their profit margins. Most other vendors blindly turn their heads to the numerous health risks associated with HFCS, following instead the almighty dollar. This bold stand by Earth Fare also shows just how much they really do care for their customers. As consumers, we should expect the thousands of other retail stores and manufacturers to have the same sense of ethical consciousness.

The Natural Foods Merchandiser, reported that as of December 2004, Newman's Own has also started to remove HFCS from all their products. Again, great news! Hopefully, this trend will continue.

14

ASPARTAME—A DEADLY TOXIN!
Making us fat, depressed, & deathly ill!

To the millions of women (and men) who think they're doing the right thing by drinking diet sodas in lieu of regular sodas, PLEASE STOP! I'm sorry to inform you, but these diet sodas are actually <u>encouraging</u> fat gain, cravings, binge eating, mood swings, anxiety, depression, ADD, water retention, and much more!

How's that?
First of all, did you know that diet sodas and most diet foods actually *encourage* the storage of body fat? *Why?* Because they're loaded with aspartame, an artificial sweetener. Aspartame is marketed under such names as NutraSweet, Spoonful, and Equal. It is a DEADLY CHEMICAL POISON, disguised as an artificial sweetener! Phenylalanine makes up 50% of aspartame. Phenylalanine is neurotoxic! (Meaning: It damages the nervous system, causing headaches, dizziness, nausea, etc.) Phenylalanine goes directly into the brain, and, at the very least, it depletes serotonin. Phenylalanine can damage neurons in the brain to the point of cellular death. If that isn't enough to scare you away from diet sodas (or diet products in general), diet sodas most often contain caffeine, which will spike insulin levels, thereby further depleting serotonin. And you know by now the many serious health risks associated with low serotonin.

Are you serious? Where is aspartame used?
Aspartame is the most commonly used artificial sweetener. The average American consumes over 148 pounds of artificial sweetener each year, and most of it's aspartame.

How can this be? I don't use the stuff that often!
You don't necessarily have to use it from a sugar packet. Like HFCS, aspartame is equally prevalent in numerous foods (diet or otherwise), ranging from sodas, cereals, breath mints, chewing gum, candy, protein bars, protein powders, wine coolers, coffee creamers, tea beverages, multi-vitamins, almost all sugar-free and lite products, coffee drinks, juice drinks, yogurt, even Alka-Seltzer! If you have products with aspartame in them, throw them away—and do not buy anything ever again that contains this deadly sweetener!

Are you saying my diet soda encourages my food to be stored as fat?
This is exactly what I'm saying. And because every diet soda contains aspartame, women especially need to pay very close attention to this. Little do they realize, as they go about

their day, having an otherwise very healthy lunch of fresh salmon, spinach salad, along with an ice cold diet soda, that the diet soda with its aspartame, will actually encourage their food, *no matter how healthy*, to be stored as fat. But after what you just read, weight gain is one of your least concerns! (Karen and Janene, I'm absolutely thrilled to know that you've both stopped drinking diet sodas based on my many warnings!)

Oh, my! This is awful! All this time I thought I was doing the right thing!
Yes, you and millions of others. To reiterate, your serotonin will be depleted by the aspartame (and the caffeine), which will perpetuate sugar cravings, weight gain, binge eating, mood swings, bloating, depression, ADD, insomnia, decreased sex drive, etc.

Isn't aspartame considered safe?
No! Studies have linked aspartame to *Sudden Death Syndrome*. It's also shown to cause brain tumors, cancer, seizures, depression, impotence, sexual problems, headaches, migraines, bloating, confusion, chronic fatigue, increased heart rate, edema, menstrual problems, hair loss, chest pains, asthma, vertigo, panic attacks, phobias, memory and vision loss. At the very least, aspartame depletes serotonin, thereby perpetuating cravings, stimulating appetite, encouraging weight gain and depression!

All of this from an artificial sweetener?
Yes, and there are many more alarming and documented side effects. But don't take my word for it. As with everything I write about, I encourage you to do your own research. See for yourself. Make your own decisions. And believe it or not, it gets worse. Aspartame contains three chemicals: aspartic acid (40% of aspartame), phenylalanine (50% of aspartame), and methanol (10% of aspartame). And while both aspartic acid and phenylalanine come with their own serious health risks, methanol is known as wood alcohol, or *methyl alcohol!* Toxic levels of methanol mimics both MS (multiple sclerosis) and lupus, while causing brain swelling, blindness, and inflammation of the pancreas and heart muscle. Even more frightening is that, based on the Trocho Study done in 1998, aspartame converts to formaldehyde in those who ingest it. And many of the symptoms reported by victims of aspartame toxicity are undeniably those associated with the poisonous and cumulative effects of formaldehyde!

Why the hell doesn't the FDA pull it from the market?
Why? Money. Greed. Simple as that. Though the FDA has received well over 10,000 aspartame-related complaints, more than all other complaints combined, shockingly it doesn't believe there is any concern, since the substance is used in such small doses. Regardless, the cumulative effects of aspartame are what you should be concerned with! And yet the FDA still considers it "safe." Many believe otherwise. Avoid aspartame at all cost!

This explains why I always feel so bloated and aggravated after I drink my diet soda. Would I be better off drinking regular sodas?
No, not at all. Regular sodas are nothing more than liquid candy. They're loaded with

sugar, caffeine, and chemicals. All of which deplete serotonin. There are, of course, caffeine-free sodas, but they still contain sugar. And once again, if you drink sugar-free, you end up with aspartame.

How do you feel about saccharin and neotame?
Saccharin has been linked to cancer. At the very least, it will deplete serotonin, trigger cravings, weight gain, etc. Neotame, the newest artificial sweetener, is merely a more potent/deadly version of aspartame. Avoid both of these!

One of the latest sugar substitutes is Splenda. What are your thoughts on it?
Splenda, the brand name for the non-nutritive sweetener sucralose, is a low-calorie sweetener. Of all the sweeteners, sucralose, discovered in 1976, is the only one made from table sugar. Because it's made from sugar, McNeil Nutritionals, the makers of Splenda, claim it tastes like sugar. Studies show it's about 600 times sweeter than sugar and can be used safely in place of sugar to eliminate or reduce calories in a wide variety of products.

How is it made?
It's created by chemically altering sucrose (table/white sugar). In the five-step patented process, three chlorine molecules are added to a sucrose i.e., sugar molecule. This type of sugar molecule, however, does not occur in nature. Thus, your body cannot properly metabolize it. As a result of this "unique" biochemical make-up, McNeil makes it's claim that Splenda is not digested or metabolized by the body, making it have zero calories. But don't be fooled by this claim. The *only* reason it's a zero calorie product is because your body can't metabolize it!

So, I guess the real question: Is Splenda safe?
Ah, yes, the *real* question! "Is it safe?" No, it is not! Only six human clinical trials have been conducted on Splenda, i.e., sucralose. Out of those six minimal trials, only two were finished and published before the FDA approved sucralose for the marketplace, i.e., human consumption. Even more alarming is that the two published trials only used 36 human subjects, with only 23 actually given sucralose for testing. It gets even worse. The trial testing lasted only four days—and the studies primary focus was sucralose and its relation to tooth decay, *not human tolerance!* Furthermore, none of these studies included children or pregnant women!

Nevertheless, according to the far too few studies that have been done, the FDA currently considers it GRAS (Generally Recognized as Safe). As a result, in 1998 they gave it full release to be used in hundreds of foods and beverages. Trust me, this is based on the astronomical *profits* that will come from this latest sweetener, not because it's safe! As with anything, it takes years of being on the market before a full scope of potential health risks can truly be known. Thus far, pre-approval research showed that sucralose caused shrunken thymus glands (up to 40%) and enlarged liver and kidneys. Based on its chemical structure, it's also possible that after years or decades of use, it may contribute to serious chronic immunological or neurological disorders. My opinion is that anything that is altered chemically is not safe.

Personally, being a woman who doubts most everything, I needed to test Splenda myself. I used one packet in a cup of decaf tea. Within an hour, I found myself with a rash on my neck—and more frightening yet—my vision was dramatically affected! I saw those little back dots and waves of light for nearly 30 minutes afterward ingesting it. Fluke? I seriously doubt it. My body simply being too sensitive? Well, that is a good thing, especially when it comes to poisons! Based on what I've researched, along with what I've experienced firsthand, I will never (knowingly) use Splenda/sucralose again.

Splenda replacing aspartame!

Spring 2005: PepsiCo is launching Pepsi One, a diet drink sweetened with Splenda. Their classic Diet Pepsi sweetened with aspartame will still be available. Coca-Cola will also be offering a new diet coke sweetened with Splenda. Likewise, their classic Diet Coke sweetened with aspartame will still be available, as well. To reiterate, sodas are often loaded with caffeine. If they're caffeine-free, they still contain highly questionable and toxic ingredients. I suggest you avoid sodas whether they're diet or regular, or sweetened with Splenda or aspartame.

If not table sugar, aspartame, HFCS, or Splenda, what should I use?

Good question, as it's all a bit confusing. Personally, I would rather use something that is from an herb or a fruit than something that has been chemically altered. While I do my best to avoid all sugars and artificial sweeteners, sometimes it's nearly impossible. Nonetheless, just making yourself aware of the many hidden sugars and sweeteners will help you tremendously in reaching your weight-loss goals. My four all-natural choices would be:

Mother Nature's favorite sweeteners:

Stevia: *Stevia Rebaudiana* is an herb in the chrysanthemum family. Stevia is a non-caloric herb, an all-natural sweetener, 300 times sweeter than sugar, and it doesn't affect blood sugar levels. It's been used safely for centuries without side effects. Stevia is extremely sweet, so you need to use very little. There are those who complain of its long aftertaste. I suggest you try using less. Stevia is my personal favorite. I believe it should be freely offered in all restaurants, as we deserve a healthier choice. Until that day comes, I carry my own in my purse.

Wisdom Natural Brands, the manufacturers of SweetLeaf Stevia brand, has created a wonderful new line of stevia products called Stevia Clear. These liquid stevia-based products are 100% natural and come in some exciting flavors, including vanilla cream, apricot nectar, chocolate raspberry, English toffee, etc. You can add them to flavor your water, decaf coffee, tea, protein drinks, yogurt, etc. Great concept! But beware of similar products, as they often contain ethyl alcohol.

Xylitol:
Xylitol (also known as birch sugar), is another favorite of mine. It's a naturally-occurring sweet compound found in fruits and vegetables. Unlike table sugar or artificial sweeteners, xylitol boasts a wide range of health benefits. More importantly, studies suggest it causes little change in blood sugar and insulin levels. (Ranks 7 on the GI.) Therefore, it's safe for diabetics—and, thus, perfect for those who want to add a little sweetness—while keeping the excess weight off. Xylitol is almost as sweet as sucrose, tastes good, and unlike stevia, has no after-taste. It also has 40% less calories than sugar, with a caloric value of approximately 2 calories per gram.

Lou Han Guo: Luo Han Guo is a very sweet fruit found in China. Extracts of this fruit are marketed as a sweetener. It is a wonderful, healthy alternative to sugar and artificial sweeteners. It's up to 250 times sweeter than sugar. More importantly, it offers a pleasant, sweet taste without elevating blood sugar levels.

Ki-Sweet: Ki-Sweet is all-natural, made from 100% natural kiwi fruit. It does not contain any additives or preservatives. It's low-glycemic, considered safe for diabetics, hypoglycemics, pregnant or lactating mothers, and children, as it does not significantly affect blood sugar or insulin levels. It's without calories, as well as being fat-free. It's 10 times sweeter than sugar, with no aftertaste or bitterness. In its raw concentrated form, Ki-Sweet is 200 times sweeter than sugar.

Please never forget: It's also possible to enjoy your food and beverages without using any sugar or artificial sweeteners. Allow yourself time to adjust to the wonderful flavors found *naturally* in food.

15

OBESITY...
an alarming epidemic!

First of all, when is a person considered "obese" versus being overweight?
A person would be considered obese when they are 20% above their ideal weight for age, height, and bone structure.

Isn't obesity becoming an epidemic?
Obesity is already an epidemic, and it's out of control. Globally, there are more than one billion overweight adults, at least 300 million of them are obese. As for the United States, and reported by the CDC (Center for Disease Control), obesity rose 33% in the last decade with an *astounding 65%* of our population now considered overweight! 65%?! It's almost hard to fathom! If this trend of obesity continues, experts say 95% of all Americans will be obese by the year 2040! Needless to say, adults need do whatever it takes to break this cycle for themselves and their children. And it's not just the visual aspect of being overweight that's so terribly distressing, but mainly the many illnesses and diseases that are caused by eating poorly.

According to the National Center of Health Statistics:
A break down of approximately 127 million adults are overweight, 60 million are obese, and 9 million are severely obese. Obesity in children has caused an epidemic of type 2 diabetes. Estimated annual U.S. healthcare costs due to overweight/obesity are over $117 billion, $10 billion more than all forms of cancer. Obesity is now the second leading cause of preventable death, surpassed only by smoking. Each year an estimated 300,000 Americans die from disease caused by being overweight. As of 2000, there were 400,000 obesity-related deaths. It's now shy just 15,000 of becoming the #1 preventable death! I simply must ask: *How did it ever come to this?* Well, I think we all know the answer now.

NEWS FLASH!! April 2005: Our government is suddenly claiming the death toll from obesity is only 112,000 <u>not</u> 400,000. *Why the drastic change?* This is due to the relentless pressure by the lobbyists for the food industry. Shockingly, this same report is also claiming, and I quote, "People who are modestly overweight, but not obese, have a lower risk of death than people of normal weight." *Really?* Where are the studies to support these highly questionable claims? This is absolutely insane! Does no one question their motives? This retraction—and self-serving health claim—are both based entirely on the food industry trying to make sure we keep eating their poisoned food! And this will insure we stay fat, addicted, and riddled with disease! This action proves, yet again, it is about greed and profits—and all at the consumer's expense! Not to mention, this kind of commentary coming from our own damn government will give those who are overweight, a license to keep on eating, without guilt, care, or concern. I can't even begin to express how disgusted I am with our federal government!

I can't believe they could be so far off. It makes me seriously question their intentions. You mentioned the food companies getting us addicted, but how do they achieve this?

Getting the consumer addicted to their products can be easily accomplished, either by adding sugar on the front end, using ingredients that have naturally occurring sugar, or by using high GI carbs that *turn into* sugar once consumed. To further confuse the consumer, they cleverly hide all kinds of sugar in their products under many different names, names that most people will not recognize as sugar. And if that isn't enough, food manufacturers also add certain chemicals that can cause addiction. It's very simple—these companies only make money if you continue to buy their products. Hence, they will do whatever it takes to keep you coming back for more, regardless of how these foods affect your health. Again, it's all about profits. Period. *And then our government wonders why we are all so fat—and getting sicker by the minute?*

Didn't someone file a "fat suit?"

Yes, in July 2002, a gentleman filed a major lawsuit against the fast-food industry, claiming fast food is addictive, which subsequently led to his two heart attacks. The suit charged the biggest names in the industry for basically not informing him, the public, that their foods were inordinately unhealthy—and addictive. While I believe such companies should offer healthier food choices, it's up to us as individuals to know what we're eating. Although we are forever enticed through TV ads, billboards, $1 specials, playgrounds, toys, even ATMs for stress-free purchase, no one forced this man to eat this food. *On the other hand*, this type of food is highly addictive and always in our face! These companies spend billions of dollars on seductive ad campaigns, targeting primarily the younger generation. Their marketing approach is precise: "Get 'em hooked while they're young!" Therefore, the fast-food industry should be held liable to a certain degree. Better yet, maybe this lawsuit will bring about some positive changes to this industry. In the meantime, think for yourself and make better food choices. Maintaining your serotonin will control your cravings for junk food.

Update: Since this lawsuit was filed, there have thankfully been many changes in the fast-food industry. Burger King is now offering a veggie burger. Several other chains are offering salads, fruit plates, even quality bottled water. This is a perfect example of how one person can make a difference. So please, never be afraid to stand up for what you believe in. If you still believe eating fast food is without health risks, I insist you watch the highly acclaimed documentary "SUPER SIZE ME" by filmmaker Morgan Spurlock. This man risked his very life to show the public just how toxic fast food is. Beyond how terribly sick this food made him, you'll see how it equally affected him mentally and emotionally—happy one minute, depressed the next. This is directly related to insulin being spiked by the high GI carbs, which then increases the production of serotonin. (This is why these foods are often favorite comfort foods.) Unfortunately, the serotonin will soon plummet. Followed by craving more of the same. The same old, terribly unhealthy cycle.

Any concerns with the healthier options offered by fast-food restaurants?

Even though they're offering so-called healthier options, these foods still contain damaged fats and carcinogens—along with plenty of hidden sugars and addictive chemicals! After all, how else will these restaurants keep you coming back for more? Once again, it is all about profits. You really should AVOID fast food at all cost! If there is absolutely no other option (which there always will be), I suggest the salads, minus the croutons. For those who want something other than a salad, I suggest either a chicken breast or a burger wrapped in lettuce, both without the bun. Better yet, have a veggie burger. Avoid coffee, sodas, and juice. Instead drink bottled water. Avoid salad dressings and condiments, as they're high in sugar and chemicals. Lemon, olive oil, and vinegar make a wonderful dressing. As for their fruit plates, you need to be sure to eat the fruit along with a healthy fat and protein. Better yet, eat the fruit as dessert. (You don't want to eat if first, as it will spike your insulin.) And I sincerely hope it isn't necessary to say that you should not be eating the hash browns, muffins, pancakes, bagels, onion rings, french fries, french toast, breakfast burritos, McNuggets, tacos, taco salads, fried chicken, egg rolls, rice bowls, cookies, frozen parfaits, McFlurries, milk shakes, or deep-fried cherry pies?

October 2005: The latest buzz with regard to the fast food industry: The Cheeseburger bill. It basically states that no one can turn around and sue the fast food industry for making them sick. Look, if you didn't know it before, you do now. These companies don't give a damn about you, their loyal customer, even if their food KILLS YOU! So, forget about having to sue them. Instead, *forget they exist!* Do not give them your business. Period!

In closing this chapter, I want to applaud the many schools across the country for having the courage to take a stand against childhood obesity. These school systems are removing soda and candy machines, eliminating processed and refined foods, and replacing them with freshly prepared REAL food. And, in a very short time, the teachers are already noticing a remarkable difference in the students' energy level, attention span, and overall attitude. Little do they know, but this is only the beginning! Parents and teachers alike would be astonished to see just how quickly their kids would slim down and no longer suffer from ADD, mood swings, etc., once they're off this addictive, deadly, junk food! And can you possibly imagine how many pharmaceutical drugs would no longer be needed to treat the many professed "diseases" kids, teens, and adults are suffering from due to this food! People would be absolutely astonished at how healthy they could get—and how absolutely great they could feel!

And, finally, success in fat loss, is far more than just a number on a scale. It's about achieving excellent health of both body and mind, as well as truly liking yourself, inside and out. I want you to be (modestly) confident in all that you are!

16

FAT CELLS GETTIN' FATTER!

You mentioned fat cells. You said we have *how* many?
An adult who is at normal weight has approximately 20–27 billion fat cells. An adult who is overweight can have fat cells that range in numbers from 75 billion to over 300 billion! Most people believe fat cells are predetermined at birth. Though the actual number of fat cells grows primarily through late childhood into early puberty, you most assuredly can produce more later. Fat cells also increase far more rapidly in obese children than in thin children. The amount of fat someone has, is a reflection of both the number and the size of their fat cells. And, I'm sorry to say, but due to various factors, women have more.

Oooh no! Can I ever get rid of them?
Not exactly. We all know, especially women, just how damn easy it is to fill up our fat cells. Fat cells can shrink, but they don't ever just disappear. Liposuction can remove some of your fat cells, but unless you're able to control your cravings, you will never maintain the fat loss. You will eventually, as with all your diets in the past, succumb to the cravings and put the weight back on, plus some. You must also be willing to make other necessary changes. Your new, healthy lifestyle must include not only healthy foods and habits, but it must also include regular exercise. If not, the fat cells will again grow in number and continue to enlarge.

Do overweight people have a harder time shrinking their fat cells?
Overweight people have an extra hard time losing excess body fat, because not only do they have more fat cells (about three times as many), their fat cells are now about 1/3 bigger than those at their normal weight. So, yes, those people who are overweight have more fat cells, which can be more difficult to shrink.

It seems absolutely hopeless! What can I do?
The more fat cells a person has, the harder it will be to lose weight. But that's *not* to say that you can't lose it, with effort and long-term commitment. This is why you need to start making a serious effort <u>today</u> to lose the excess body fat. You must also teach your children good, healthy eating and lifestyle habits—starting today. They might not like it at first, but they will, without a doubt, thank you later.

What are fat cells used for?
Fat cells are used by the body to store excess calories. Calories are energy, used by the body for future use. The energy that your body uses today may be coming from a meal

you ate weeks prior. Just remember, the excess calories that your body does not utilize for energy is promoted to fat storage. All the more reason you need to build lean muscle, as muscle is a metabolically active tissue. (8 times more active than fat.) It requires a precise number of calories daily to maintain itself. More muscle = more calories burned.

Okay, but why do I feel fat from my ankles up after a high-carb meal?
Some of the bloating comes from those carbs triggering your insulin, which then leads to a higher level of sodium. In addition, a high-carb meal, of course, also opens your fat cells, causing them to store new fat. Ironically, this reminds me of my own struggles from many years ago. Please allow me to share:

Childhood memories...

I was one of 7 children, raised in the Midwest with pretty typical eating habits: Finish what's on your plate, eat three square meals, with my stepmother always freshly preparing anything from ham, pot roast, pork chops, meatloaf, chicken, etc. These dishes were accompanied by a variety of veggies, potatoes, salads, and desserts. There was also my father's Saturday morning breakfast of eggs, bacon, and cinnamon toast and the Friday evening yippee-the-parents-are-going-out-quick-fix-meals—everything from hot dogs, sizzle steaks, fish sticks, Sloppy Joe's, tater tots, mac' and cheese, pot pies, french fries, and an abundance of s'mores! In and around all of those traditional foods, we still managed to eat copious amounts of sugar-coated cereal, pancakes, Pop-tarts, Wonder Bread sandwiches, potato chips, Snowballs, Ding-Dongs, and Twinkies! And I'll never forget how my younger brother Tommy and I would race our bikes down to the lakefront store nearly every day, eager to spend our weekly allowance. We'd take our tiny, but overflowing brown paper bags filled with nickel candy, washing each sweet delight down with delicious sugar-laden ice cold pops—and then proceed to look for trouble.

Lucky for me, I was a tomboy, never sitting still. I'm sure I burned up the excessive overload of sugar by chasing the boys, then running *from* the boys, playing red-rover, duck-duck-goose, hide-and-seek, kick-the-can, and racing my brother's motorcycles. Then there was tag football, shootin' hoops, horseback riding, water skiing, swimming, and the many athletic sports I played through school. As kids we never stopped! Like cattle, my stepmother would literally have to ring a huge bell to get us to come home.

Later on, though, as a young woman, I came to believe I wasn't meant to eat. I came to this startling conclusion because I had long given up the candy and the many other things we were told were unhealthy. (Even way back then, it was all about low-fat.) But I still began to gain weight. I had always been so athletic and lean, but things seemed to be changing. I was not happy! All I'd have was a toasted bagel with some orange juice and only moments later, I felt like a blow fish! I felt so fat, but why? I had eaten so little, yet my pants were suddenly tight! I felt bloated! Aggravated. Bitchy. Tired. *Why, though?* I couldn't understand *how* I could feel so fat (and moody)! After all, I only had a bagel and a lousy glass of fruit juice! I mean, come on, a bagel had NO fat! And the juice was from fruit, which was all-natural. Again, NO fat! So how could I be gaining weight? To make matters worse, I was hungry all the time, never felt satiated, and the only foods I craved were more of the same. Ah, I was miserable and awfully frustrated!

Oh! That sounds *just* like me!

I felt it was important to share the above story, as I'm sure there are many adults, teens, and even children who can relate to this exact scenario. The truth of the matter is, I was eating the so-called "recommended diet" provided by the AMA and the FDA. Both my bagel and juice fell perfectly within their guidelines of low-fat dieting. They were indeed low-fat, but unfortunately, extremely high in sugar and high GI carbs! Based on what you've just learned here, you now know precisely *why* my body and mind reacted the way they did. Moreover, why their recommended low-fat dieting did NOT work! In fact, low-fat dieting is one of the biggest direct contributors to our current rate of obesity.

Obviously, this was long before I ever began my research. But, as you can see, even two decades ago, I was learning to listen to my body. By doing so, I began to understand, on my own, what foods my body thrived on. I discovered that when I ate fruit, and more so when I drank fruit juice, I could actually feel the sugar rush through my system. It made me feel terribly hyped! Caffeine, whether it came from sodas or coffee, also made me feel far too anxious, followed by mood swings and a severe drop in energy. Cereal, chips, and bagels were all very comforting, but I never felt full, at least for very long. I also felt bloated after eating those foods. Eventually, I began to avoid them and instead leaned toward cheese, eggs, chicken, and...diet sodas. Yes, diet sodas. I was still learning. I hate to think of all the aspartame I've consumed!

The junk food I ate as a child is not terribly different from what the kids eat today, but we always had a base of healthy food, followed by the less than desirable treats. The biggest differences: We ate mostly home-cooked meals, rarely if ever eating fast food, and we were always physically active! Not only have schools stopped scheduling Physical Education (which I find absolutely astounding!), but the kids don't motivate themselves to play. Parents need to make them turn off the TV, computer, video games, and get their not-so little butts MOVING! Sedentary lifestyles are a <u>major</u> contributor to obesity in children, teens, and adults. And this is precisely why we're suddenly seeing so many new cases of type 2 diabetes. In addition to balancing your serotonin, this is a perfect example of where a dramatic change in *lifestyle* is desperately needed.

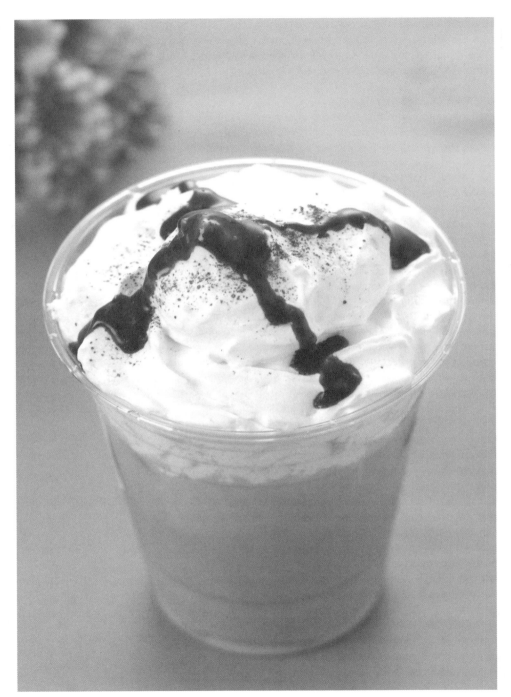

17

STIMULANTS NOT NEEDED
But freedom of choice is a MUST!

Why don't you recommend stimulants for fat loss?

Products that use stimulants to speed up your metabolism are harmful and unhealthy. (This includes the latest Brazilian diet pills. The reports coming out claim that, among other ingredients, the morning dose contains speed. The evening dose contains Prozac and Valium. Stay clear of these! This is not a healthy way to lose weight!) Stimulants put excessive stress on your adrenal glands and heart. For those millions of people who are told they need to be on lifelong thyroid medication, the excessive stress brought on by stimulants is most often a contributing factor. Although you may lose pounds according to the scale, most often it's from lean muscle mass and water, not fat. Moreover, once you go off these stimulant-based diet products and begin to eat normally, you will most likely gain all the weight back, plus some. This relates directly to the old "lose 10/gain back 20" scenario. With each new attempt to diet, it will be even harder to lose the fat. What you've done instead is risk your health, drastically reduce your lean muscle mass, change your total body composition, thereby *increasing* your fat stores. While it may seem you're losing fat quicker with stimulants, it's a false and unhealthy fix, not a long-term solution. Furthermore, you have not learned "how or why" the body stores fat, or why you crave high GI foods. Don't forget that all stimulants spike insulin levels, which *encourages* the storage of body fat. They can also increase weight gain due to salt and water retention.

Different type of stimulants would include?

Stimulant sources are endless and can vary from prescription/nonprescription drugs, OTC (Over-the-Counter) meds, to ephedra, caffeine, sugar, high GI carbs, nicotine, sexual enhancing herbs, alcohol, soda, your child's chocolate milk, and your frappuccino.

And stimulants deplete serotonin, right?

Stimulants do indeed deplete serotonin, causing depression, insomnia, agitation, and continued carbohydrate cravings. They also cause the body to produce a harmful form of cholesterol which can lead to heart disease, high blood pressure, stroke, type 2 diabetes, etc. Bottom line: You can't use stimulants, whether they come in the form of coffee, sodas, high GI carbs, chocolate, recreational drugs, ephedra, alcohol, nicotine, etc., if you want to achieve a healthy body and mind. It requires commitment, consistency, and knowing long-term weight loss is about a *healthy lifestyle,* not a quick fix with stimulants. (I go into much greater detail about caffeine in the next chapter. Please, read it carefully, as I explain how the latest coffee craze is directly related to weight gain, depression, suicidal thoughts, binge eating, rage, ADD, ADHD, etc.)

How do you feel about ephedra?
In addition to the health concerns just mentioned, I would <u>never</u> suggest ephedra to my clients, nor did I ever use it myself, as I know only too well its many serious side effects. Personally, I am overly sensitive to stimulants. I also hate that feeling of being amped, on edge, or unable to sleep. Thus, I do whatever it takes to avoid all stimulants. That would include ephedrine, caffeine, yohimbe, guarana, etc. Ironically, my first supplier of raw ingredients feverishly tried to convince me that because I refused to use ephedra (or any other stimulant), I was "missing the boat and failing to realize the 'real needs' in the fat-loss market." When I explained my research, he was condescending, claiming I was being foolish and making a huge mistake as a product developer/owner. He then accused me of trying to change the world. I humbly replied, "Yes, I suppose I am."

His next attempt to force my hand was to remind me that Wal-Mart's best-seller out of thousands of products was Metabolife, an ephedra-based fat-loss product. Again, I told him I didn't care. More importantly, I'd be nothing more than a pathetic hypocrite if I used it, as it was against everything I knew to be healthy, for fat loss or otherwise. I explained to him that while people may lose weight with stimulants, it was unhealthy, and they would more than likely gain all the weight back after they went off those products, as they had not learned why they crave all those insulin-producing foods. His quick reply was, "Perfect! You just sell them another product!" Sorry. This approach is not at all who I am, or how I work. I'm not some self-righteous woman either, but it's unfortunately terribly common in our industry. All one has to do is read the ingredients (and deceptive claims) on any given product, to realize that far too many companies do not give a damn about their customers. Instead, it's only about profit margins. This is also a perfect example of standing up for what you believe in, learning to think for yourself, and never letting yourself be manipulated by guilt or money.

Wasn't ephedra pulled from the market?
Yes, as of February 2004, the FDA banned all ephedra-based supplements. It was the first dietary supplement ever banned. I chose not to use it because of its many side effects: increased heart rate, blood pressure, and at the very least, depleting serotonin. Regardless, as with anything, if you choose to abuse it, it can cause serious side effects such as stroke, or even death. Examples: Drink too much alcohol and you could die. Eat too much sugar and you could go into a coma. Even drinking too much water can kill you. Far too many Americans believe that if one is good, two or maybe three are even better. This is neither accurate nor a healthy choice. This is what so often leads to such unfortunate news stories. The records show 155 deaths, along with numerous heart attacks and strokes, were related to ephedra. Many of these reports indicated, though, that other critical factors played a role. Nonetheless, the FDA quickly condemned this herb as "deadly" and pulled it from the market. With all due respect to those who suffered any such loss,

this is absolutely *nothing* compared to the number of people who die *every damn day* because of pharmaceutical drugs! And let's not forget the tens of thousands of people who don't die—but instead suffer serious liver, kidney, or heart damage from these same drugs! How about those who die each and every year just from OTC meds such as aspirin? That would be an astounding 9,000! (Please read chapter 27 for more staggering pharmaceutical drug statistics.)

Update: A company from Utah sued the FDA over this unlawful ban. I'm thrilled to report that, as of April 2005, the FDA was found guilty as charged. Ephedra will once again be available. Whether I believe it's a healthy choice or not, it is a huge victory for all of us. Nevertheless, pulling ephedra from the market went far beyond any so-called health risks. The FDA's motive here was about frightening the consumer into believing that supplements are dangerous and deadly. The FDA's motive had <u>nothing</u> to do with being concerned for our health, rather it was, once again, about keeping the drug companies in control, while eliminating any alternative choices! This action was about one thing and one thing only: MONEY! If we aren't careful, if we don't start paying closer attention, if the FDA, FTC, and AMA have their way, they'll make all supplements, including a simple vitamin, available only by prescription! This is already proposed by the AMA.

Hold on a minute! There's more! This is merely a fraction of what's going on around us. Our government is slowly—but most assuredly—stripping us of our rights. Whether it's censoring our music, TV, sexual partners, dress code, or marriage partners, our government suddenly feels they have the almighty right to censor all that we are. But who are they to tell us what to watch, listen to, and eat? Who are they to tell us who we can have sex with or fall in love with and marry? Who are they to tell us how to live our lives? What is considered immoral to one, is not to another. So who are they to force their religious beliefs on us? Our country was built upon, among many things, FREEDOM OF CHOICE! But those currently in power are raping us of all those rights!

Hypocrisy at its finest: Watching a movie, I was astounded to see that, while they censored the words "ass, damn, and hell," blurred out both a joint that a boy was smoking and a man flipping someone off, they instead, allowed me, the viewer, to see men getting their throats slit and, more gruesome yet, showed a man carrying two severed heads as he casually smoked a cigarette! Excuse me, people, *but who the hell is at the controls here?!* They censor foul language, one little joint, and the finger, but show such brutality? And why is it okay to show a cigarette, a known deadly and addictive product that has killed billions? We all know the answer to that: PROFITS! But if they expect us to believe they're doing this to "protect the children," then cigarettes (and alcohol) should definitely be on their hit list! BTW: Their next targets are sexy cheerleaders, cable TV, and satellite radio. And then what? A woman's right to choose? *Where does it end?* This all frightens me. You should be equally concerned. Do not sit in silence. We must all be willing to defend our rights before it's too late!

18

DIRECT LINK...
DEPRESSION & OUR DIET—
sugar, high GI carbs, caffeine, nicotine, etc.

Is depression caused by low serotonin?
Whatever the *underlying* cause, depression is due to the depletion of serotonin, the major neurotransmitter among all brain chemicals. Each year depression strikes over an astounding 17 million adults, teens, and children in the U.S. Over 12 million diagnosed are women. The numbers are at alarming, epidemic proportions! Remember, serotonin is depleted by many things. A few primary factors are the over-consumption of processed and refined foods, sodas, caffeine, nicotine, high GI carbohydrates, sugar, HFCS, and artificial sweeteners. Regrettably, Americans consume these in *excessive* amounts.

Obviously, our diet plays a major role in our mood, yes?
Absolutely, it does! I'm shocked that no one in the medical industry ever questions the direct link between diet and depression. Never have I heard anyone say that, when they went to see their doctor for depression, their doctor asked, inquired, and/or expressed concern about their "diet." It simply does not happen. It's far easier, not to mention financially more rewarding, to prescribe yet another drug. Instead of our doctors, AMA, FDA, or FTC promoting wellness and preventive methods of treatment and educating people about how to eat a healthy, nutritious diet, combined with efficacious herbal supplementation to *naturally* alleviate depression, they'd rather prescribe DRUGS—be it Prozac or another deadly antidepressant. European countries have used herbal remedies to treat depression for centuries, and with tremendous success.

It's shocking how the U.S. pharmaceutical industry has been glorifying their many antidepressant drugs. For example, a certain TV commercial that used to run: *"Do you have a special event coming up? A family affair? A celebration? Call your doctor today to see if you're eligible for Prozac Weekly!"* This advertisement was terribly alarming. It seductively played more like a beer commercial! More disturbing yet is that they found it acceptable to treat depression, to offer happiness, for only a week at a time!

In lieu of the medical community making the necessary effort to find out the underlying causes of depression, they'd rather sell a drug to *mask* the symptoms. Remember, these pharmaceutical drugs are just that, D-R-U-G-S, all of which will lead to serious side effects. People need to realize they can help take control of their mental health by supporting healthy levels of serotonin, *naturally*. If you question the deadly side effects of these drugs, drugs that big pharma actually manipulated their clinical findings, I urge you to read *The Shooting Drugs, Prozac Exposed* by Donna Smart. It documents hundreds of terrifying cases of those who went on psychotic rampages brutally murdering their families, strangers, then committing suicide—all while on antidepressants! (Columbine is merely one example!) It also documents the depth to which the drug companies will go to protect the future sales of their DEADLY drugs, i.e., bribery, threats, falsifying records, etc. *You MUST read this book before taking any antidepressant!*

If this discussion isn't enough to concern you, I once met a psychiatrist in passing. I was sincerely intrigued by his work. But when I questioned if he ever discussed how his patients' diets played a critical role in their mental health, he looked at me with a cold blank stare and said, "*Why* would I do that? Their diet has <u>nothing</u> to do with their depression!" *Excuse me?* This doctor wasn't just a family practitioner from whom you might expect such a limited understanding. He was a licensed and practicing psychiatrist! Another prime example of why you must be willing to educate yourself.

FACT: Less than 2% of all doctors are trained in nutrition! Hence, you <u>must</u> educate yourself. Research. Research. And research some more. Protect yourself and your family. Plus, commit to a healthier lifestyle starting today! And seek out a health expert who will help treat the depression <u>minus</u> the drugs. Whatever choice you make, weigh the benefits and the many risks.

Alarming statistic: The fastest-growing market for antidepressants is *preschool children*. To imagine these children being drugged, at an age when their young minds are developing most, is horrendous! *Why is this being allowed?* The drug companies will stop at nothing! Do not be fooled by their self-serving diagnosis! Research on your own! Get a second, even third opinion. Use a PDR (Prescription Drug Reference) to substantiate side effects, which will be numerous—and life-threatening! No disrespect intended, but I cannot believe parents would allow this without questioning such a harmful prescription. (This also pertains to the drugs doctors are prescribing for ADD, ADHD, etc.)

What do you suggest parents do?
Before you or anyone else (and especially your children) start taking these antidepressants, you must immediately take a closer look at what you and yours are eating and drinking. Based on what you've learned thus far, you now know that, in fact, diet does play a MAJOR and CRITICAL role in your mental and emotional health. So, please, take a fresh look at all the foods and beverages (as well as nicotine and alcohol) you and your family consume on any given day. Then make the much-needed changes. More than likely, it will not be easy weaning off the highly processed junk food, as your brain will continue to tempt you with the foods that it knows have always triggered the production of serotonin. SESs are developed specifically to help people control these cravings.

I've noticed my mother is rather depressed. What can I do for her?
Due to age, often failing health, and the far too many medications that most seniors are on, combined with a diet that is terribly high in sugar, caffeine, alcohol, etc., their mental health is often dramatically affected. Statistics prove one of the biggest health concerns with seniors is depression. From my own personal experience, I've been blessed throughout my life to befriend many amazing elderly people. Whether I met them as neighbors, at my gym, or simply by going to visit local retirement or nursing homes, I've always had an incredible attraction to those much older than myself. There is such an honesty there, no pretense, no bull shit, no ulterior motives, just pure, raw thoughts and emotions shared between two human beings. Through these friendships, I've witnessed the kinds of meals they eat—either those they prepared themselves or were served in the homes. From morning till night, they also eagerly consume an endless array of sugar and caffeine, from iced teas and coffee, sodas, juice, candy, etc. Add to that the often questionable meals they eat and the far too many senseless pharmaceutical drugs they take, which, of course, also deplete serotonin, and well, I'm sure the next time you, their loving and devoted child go to visit them, you'll know exactly *why* they're so depressed.

But what can I do?
Please take what you've learned here and help them. Be there for them. Spend time with them. If they live in a home, do not assume these homes have your parents' best interest at heart. You need to be their advocate. Visit them and visit them often. Make sure they're eating healthy. Don't let their doctor overload them with senseless drugs. Take them for walks. Have lunch with them. Read to them. Stimulate their minds and emotions. Be part of their life. Don't let them feel forgotten. And while you may not be able to care for them full time, at least do whatever it takes to make sure the time they do have left is lived with a clear and emotionally fulfilled mind. The time you spend with them, and with the many other residents who will literally beg you to get them out of there, will surely make you cry or, at the very least, make you wish you could do more for them. I also sincerely hope it will further inspire you to live a much healthier life. (Note: Being able to maintain healthy levels of serotonin with an SES can be surpassingly beneficial, and more importantly, without side effects. In addition to helping control cravings, SESs can also enhance mood, sleep patterns, energy, etc. These products can indeed offer you and your aging parents many positive health benefits.)

My mother is on way too many drugs. She also has 3 or 4 cups of coffee before noon, plus several iced teas. By the way, isn't caffeine a drug?
Yes, all the more reason to be concerned. Caffeine is the #1 socially accepted, *legalized* DRUG! Caffeine also happens to be highly addictive. Caffeine, along with the sweet taste of added sugar, is the reason why sodas are consumed by our youth (and adults, too) at a startling rate of 54 gallons per person, per year! This doesn't include the caffeine you can get from your local coffee café. While I most certainly respect Starbucks business savvy, people seem to forget that caffeine is a <u>drug,</u> and it plays a major role in their inability to lose excess fat, stabilize their mood, lower cholesterol, etc.

There are nearly 9,000 Starbucks locations worldwide. In 2003, they did $4.1 billion in sales. Statistics show that over 25 million customers visit Starbucks every week, with people going on an average of 18 times per month. Besides the excessive amount of caffeine, at a <u>minimum</u> of $3, plus tip, this caffeine habit alone adds up to no less than $60 per month, $720 per year. And unless you're wearing blinders, how can anyone possibly resist their sinfully decadent pastries that *SCREAM* to be eaten! Sweets were never my weakness, but when they're in your face like that *teasing you...and...tempting you,* well, no wonder most people succumb to this manipulative sugar-tease! (Thankfully, I remain in complete control because my serotonin is balanced.) Nevertheless, 18 times a month you enjoy a latte (plain, nonfat, large latte = 30g carbs/sugar!), with maybe a sesame bagel (440 calories, 630mg sodium, 92g carbs/sugar!), or maybe a chocolate cream cheese muffin (450 calories, 420mg sodium, 53g carbs/sugar!). Add this to your other not-so-healthy daily habits. Now, can you start to see why so many people are stressed out, on edge, depressed, suffering from insomnia, shocking cholesterol panels, sexually unavailable, and quickly gaining weight?

Caffeine, the #1 socially accepted, legalized DRUG!

But I enjoy a cup of coffee with my friends!
I'm sure you do. So do I, as it's a wonderful way to socialize or to take a quiet moment for yourself. I'm not saying you can't enjoy a cup of coffee, just please consider drinking *decaffeinated*. You also need to be aware of all the sugar in those flavored syrup blends, as well as the milk, nonfat or otherwise. And do not add sugar or artificial sweeteners.

I can't believe you actually go to Starbucks. Is this healthy?
Starbucks or otherwise, life is <u>not</u> about living like a monk. I go *maybe* once a month. More importantly, I have either a decaf green tea or a small decaf latte with a splash of vanilla. But, as of late, even this basic latte is becoming too much sugar for my body. (For the record: to claim "decaf," 97% of the caffeine has to be removed. That leaves approximately 3mg, compared to the whopping 100–150mg in 6 oz. of regular coffee.) I'd have to say that the vanilla flavoring is my most sinful treat. I also prefer to use the product with sugar versus those with aspartame, HFCS, or Splenda. And I use organic soy milk versus low-fat cow's milk. Other than in my latte, I rarely drink soy, as it makes me feel so bloated. Instead, when at home, I use lite coconut milk.

Why don't you use low-fat milk?
I'm so glad you asked this, because I hear so many people ordering their lattes, frappuccinos or cappuccinos, and it's *always* with nonfat milk. Unfortunately, the fear of dietary fat still runs rampant. You're actually better off using milk *with* the fat, as the dietary fat actually helps lower the blood sugar response from the sugar naturally found in milk. Yes, you heard me right. The fat is a good thing, as it helps lower the glycemic response. Skim, 2%, 1%, low-fat, or nonfat milk still contain plenty of lactose (milk sugar), but without any fat, this milk will affect blood sugar levels much more dramatically.

You're right, it makes perfect sense. But what are your concerns with soy?

Soy and its many food products were touted as the best thing out there, but lately studies are showing otherwise. Soy food products made from soy protein powders, soy protein isolates, textured soy proteins, as well as soy milk, have been shown to contain both natural and added chemicals. These chemicals are proving to be harmful to the body. *Why?* For starters, non-fermented soy products contain phytic acid, which contains anti-nutritive properties. Phytic acid binds with certain nutrients, including iron, to inhibit their absorption. The best fermented soy foods to eat include natto, miso, tempeh, and tofu. (I must admit this is all a bit too much. First, soy is great—then it's bad for us. Look, if you can find fermented soy, buy it. But if you can't, buy the regular soy. Either way, soy milk is still far healthier than cow's milk.)

And your concerns with cow's milk are?

First of all, cow's milk is intended for *baby calves*. There are numerous studies that clearly demonstrate just how unhealthy cow's milk is for humans. All the while, the NDC (National Dairy Council) spends millions of dollars on clever ad campaigns. "Got milk?" is there most successful by far. However, I find one of their recent ads, an ad that shows men eagerly scrambling to buy as much milk as possible, because they're claiming milk "may" help reduce symptoms of PMS, is misinformed—and insulting to women.

"Got milk?" *GAIN WEIGHT!*

I'm ecstatic to report that their latest campaign, a campaign that has cost over $200 million since 2003, has prompted lawsuits against the biggest names, i.e., Dannon, Kraft, General Mills, etc. The ad claims, "Drinking 24 oz. of milk per day 'may' help people lose weight, particularly belly fat." *Reeally?* "Got studies?" Oh, of course they do, but guess who funded the studies? The NDC! Hence, their deceptive claims. Michael Zemel, professor of nutrition/medicine at the University of TN, received $1.7 million in research grants since 1998 to secure statistics that would support their campaign. Obviously he was unsuccessful. Thus, the lawsuits. Not only will milk NOT help people lose weight, but because it's a liquid carb—and people most often only drink fat-free milk—it will actually *encourage* weight gain! Can you say moo? (BTW: Where is the FDA, the FTC? Hmm? Why have they allowed these ads to run so long without holding the NDC accountable for their fraudulent claims? Yet another example of the disreputable, illegal—and harmful relationship between big business and our government!)

Furthermore, cow's milk contains many harmful components. Proteins in cow's milk are different from human milk proteins. It causes problems with digestion, impaired absorption of other nutrients, intolerance, and autoimmune reactions. Few of the proteins meant for a calf are found naturally in human mother's milk, and <u>none</u> are found in any natural adult human food. In addition, cow hormones are not meant for humans. Over time, cows have been selectively bred to create high levels of these exact hormones, those that help cows to grow the fastest and produce the greatest amount of milk. There is also a high concentration of pesticides and pollutants in cow's milk. The high amount of drugs now given to cows makes this all the more serious.

I thought milk was required for building strong bones?
This is precisely what the NDC has perpetuated for decades. It is not factual, though. The high protein content of milk actually causes a net loss of calcium in the body. Studies that were even paid for by the NDC have shown that the excessive protein in milk *lowers* blood calcium levels, causing the body to actually draw on calcium from the bones. The advertising propaganda put forth by the NDC with regard to drinking milk to prevent osteoporosis is sadly inaccurate. Milk can actually encourage this medical condition. I realize most of you will not believe this, so I kindly ask that you research this further on your own. The studies are clear.

Wow! More deceit, more frustration! What do you suggest?
Be aware of the health risks, but then make the best choices possible. Personally, I eat plenty of nonstarchy vegetables and assorted fresh cheeses, organic whenever possible. And again, I only use organic soy milk on the very rare occasion that I enjoy a latte. Also, please don't forget that dairy cows are forced to endure such awful lives, as well as being slaughtered as soon as they are no longer able to produce milk. Their innocent lives are filled with abuse—and then cut terribly short! And lastly, by drinking cow's milk, you inadvertently support the veal industry. I certainly want no more part of that torture! So please, please, please, drink organic soy milk rather than cow's milk!

What if I make my coffee at home and use a flavored coffee creamer?
I'm sure you already know the answer. Anything that tastes that sweet cannot possibly be good. There are many varieties of these oh, so richly delicious creamers, and not one is a healthy choice. *Why?* Because they're loaded with sugar. This is why you need to read the nutritional panel. The first ingredient: water. The second: sugar or corn syrup solids. The serving size is 1 tbsp, and it equals 5g of sugar! If that isn't enough, is anyone really going to pour in only 1 tiny little tbsp? I think not. (Thank you, Keven, for inspiring me to write about this, especially because you actually listened to my advice.)

Here's another wonderful example of how such little things can make a difference in your health. Keven hits the weights hard 5 days a week, and he's very conscious of what he eats. But since he cut out the creamer and caffeine, and with absolutely no other changes in his diet, he lost a quick 5 pounds. He says he's never felt so lean. And this weight loss was not from muscle mass, but rather from water weight that was caused by the caffeine and creamers spiking his insulin, which was causing his body to retain water and store fat. Remember, less insulin equals less fat stored, more fat burned—and less water retention. All of this adds up to a much leaner, more defined and healthier body.

Once again, it is about choices and picking your *occasional* treat. But stop and ask yourself: Considering these creamers are nothing more than sugar water, then added to caffeine, both of which will spike your insulin, deplete your serotonin, put your body into a fat-storing mode for hours, cause bloating and mood swings, and even further perpetuate carb cravings and fat gain, why, then, would you want to use them?

Confession: Long before Starbucks, I bought those sinfully delicious creamers to top off my equally decadent flavored decaf coffee to enjoy at home. *Ooooh, both were so good!* I knew the creamers were pretty much pure sugar, but I figured, because it was my one and only treat, I was entitled. *Wasn't I?* I mean, come on, how bad could they be? Well, I can assure you I don't feel this way any longer. Ironically, even after I became fully aware of the dangers of the ingredients, both in the creamers and soothing cup of Joe, my brain kept quietly, but continually forcing me toward that sweet delight. It wasn't until I started developing SESs that I finally got rid of the craving for this syrupy drink. And while I could, like many others, simply keep on enjoying this warm sugar concoction, even though the craving was long gone, I could no longer ignore the numerous health risks associated with sugar, corn syrup, etc. Eliminating them from my diet is simply one more way that to help keep my body as lean as possible, my moods stable, and my energy constant.

Point taken. I'll leave the creamer out. Should I stop drinking coffee altogether?
In a perfect world, yes. At the same time, I would never tell you or anyone else what to do. Nonetheless, I would hope that you'd consider drinking water-processed decaf. My only intention is to educate you. It is then your decision, as to what you will do with this information. This brings me to an interesting observation: I'm probably like a lot of women who don't really care about the caffeine. It's more the habit, the tradition of making coffee first thing in the morning. The grinding of fresh coffee beans. The intoxicating aroma as it permeates the house. Maybe meeting the girls out to socialize and then—taking that first glorious sip. Ahhhh, it triggers such a wonderful sensation! Well, here's the good news: You can still enjoy all of that *without* the health risks associated with caffeine!

Furthermore, ladies, for those who have men in their life who think they need caffeine to start their day, I suggest you start weaning them off it with decaf. Day by day—cut it back, until it is only pure decaf. Let it be your little secret. Most will never miss it. Trust me. This also goes for those women (and teens) who think they need caffeine to get their day going. No one should "need" caffeine, ever. If you do, you'd better be asking *why*? Don't forget all the things caffeine does to your body and mind. Can you really tell me this is a healthy choice? (SESs will definitely help control cravings for caffeine.)

I guess I should also be concerned about my kids drinking all those coffee drinks?
You should be very concerned. I'm astounded at how many teens, even young children, I see so often buying those highly caffeinated-chocolate-dripping-overflowing-whipped-cream drinks. *Are the parents not aware that caffeine is a drug?* If not, please take notes now. The chocolate is another stimulant source. A double whammy. Add the milk with all that lactose—and the whipped cream. *Getting the picture?* And considering the latest craze is for high school, even middle school kids, to grab a flavored latte (averages 320

calories, 39g carbs/sugar!) double espresso, or mocha mint frappuccino (390 calories, with a staggering 74g carbs/sugar!) before and after school, the health issues with our youth will only get worse! I'm further dismayed that no one in the health industry is concerned by this fashionable trend. But now add the aforementioned concerns to the typical teenage diet of fast food and endless sodas, and well, it's no wonder our youth are so damn depressed, emotionally out of control, unable to concentrate, filled with rage, gaining fat at an alarming rate, and—suicidal. Parents need to realize that caffeine, *no matter the source* (coffee, iced tea, chocolate, sodas, Red Bull-type energy drinks, etc.) deplete serotonin, causing cravings, eating disorders, weight gain, depression, agitation, anxiety, ADD, and, yes, even suicidal thoughts.

Oh, you're absolutely right. Is this why ADD/ADHD are so prevalent?
Yes, more often than not. Remember, when serotonin levels are depleted, among many things, our ability to concentrate is greatly affected. But instead of the medical industry wanting to find out the underlying cause of your serotonin depletion, they'd much rather prescribe a pharmaceutical drug. This is because the doctors don't make money by telling you to go home and reevaluate your eating habits and lifestyle. Instead, they eagerly prescribe a drug, which will, in turn, create new side effects, which will create yet another illness, for which they will again eagerly prescribe yet another drug. It is a vicious and continuous cycle driven solely by greed.

What about the latest adult ADD?
Same thing. This is, sadly, nothing more than the drug companies looking to expand their drug sales. After all, there are only so many children they can get on their drugs for ADD/ADHD. But by creating this new disease called "Adult ADD," they open the door to earn billions more. In reality, it is a *condition* that is due to low serotonin. And low serotonin is due to poor diet and lifestyle habits. Once again, it's important to realize that I have personally lived most of what I speak: mood swings, cravings, bloating, fat gain, etc. This is no different. Please allow me to share my personal experience with adult ADD: I've been taking SESs for nearly six years. Except when I'm testing formulas, I'm never without it. Only recently, while I was trying to finish this book, did I actually experience the symptoms of what the medical industry has recently labeled "adult ADD." Please allow me to share:

I wrote most of this book in about 11 months. Because it's my passion, there was very little effort—it simply flowed. So much, in fact, that at times I would get up and review my work from the day before and not remember half the chapters that I had written. I'm not kidding. It was as if someone else had written them. (That someone else was definitely a Higher Power working through me.) Nevertheless, it was effortless. However, after I was off product for about a week, I was suddenly no longer able to concentrate. It was like a TV channel that kept switching. As hard as I tried, I couldn't stay focused. Thoughts were there one minute, gone the next. Hell, I couldn't even focus long enough to write one lousy sentence, let alone a chapter! I was stunned! Frustrated! I needed to finish my book, but it was hopeless, as I was unable to hold a thought long enough. I also found it all very telling. Suddenly, I knew exactly what all those commercials about ADD, adult or otherwise, were talking about. But I also knew that by merely boosting and maintaining my serotonin, *minus any drugs*, my mind would once again be in total control, sharp, focused, and creative. And that is precisely what happened. Back on product and within only three doses, I wrote four new chapters in one afternoon. More importantly, it was, once again, effortless. My mind was sharp, focused, creatively driven, and long-lasting. What a huge difference!

That's amazing. Both my children were diagnosed with ADD, and recently, my sister was diagnosed with adult ADD. Considering their horrendous diets, mine included, I'm quite sure this is the underlying cause. A healthier diet is an absolute must. Now, as if I don't already know the answer, what are your thoughts on cigarettes?
In addition to nicotine being a stimulant, it's a horrendously addictive and deadly product! Besides increasing your risks for heart disease, stroke, lung cancer, and sudden death, it will deplete serotonin—which will lead to numerous other health issues. Adults should not smoke, nor should our youth. Here's another flashback: Candy cigarettes. Ahhh, remember those? Back in the 1960s, they had names and packages that were nearly identical to the real thing. They were long, white candy sticks with tiny red tips. They were the ultimate in cool! Or so we thought. As a child, we used to love to pretend to be smoking. *How sick is that?* Only now, as I write this chapter, do I suddenly realize the dreadful marketing scheme that was behind these candy cigarettes. There's compelling evidence that the candy makers actually worked with the cigarette companies to attract young smokers! Little did we know, as children, what their motives were. Unfortunately, neither did most parents.

Isn't there a lot of peer pressure for kids?
Of course. Studies show that much younger kids are feeling the peer pressure to drink, smoke, take X (ecstasy), and have sex. Whether it's the "friends with benefits" type of sex or a serious relationship, it's way too much pressure and responsibility at that age. Sex and all the emotions, health risks, etc., are tough enough to deal with when you're an adult, let alone a teenager, and most certainly not at 10 and 12! And if you think for one second that I don't understand the insatiable desire to explore, be it sexually or with things that alter one's mind, well, I can assure you, *you would be wrong!* Very wrong.

In high school, I, along with my few close friends, drank alcohol, smoked dope, even occasionally snorted blow, ate shrooms, and dropped acid. As a rebel—and as a teenager struggling emotionally—I wanted to experiment. But I did these drugs *freely,* not because of peer pressure. To a greater extent, I was trying to escape the reality of my home life. Furthermore, I was also, and still am, a very sexual being. Uninhibited. Eager to explore. (More importantly, highly selective and protection was, and is, a must.) But, up until about age 14, I was perfectly content with just racin' around on motorcycles, shootin' hoops, and playin' football with the boys. Shortly thereafter, however, things began to change. Boys, or should I say men no less than 5–10 years older, were suddenly my entire focus. So, you see, I, too, understand and appreciate the need, the *desire* to quench one's sexual thirst.

"Friends with benefits!"

The biggest difference between my generation and what's going on now is that whether or not we engaged in oral, vaginal, or anal sex, we didn't lie to ourselves; we knew it was S-E-X, and we didn't pretend to be virgins. Moreover, we became sexually active because we thought we were "in love." Yet the young girls today freely admit they're using their bodies, *their sexual abilities*, to just be more popular with the boys. And not just with one or two guys but many—from orgies, rainbow parties, to tossing salad, etc. Well, here's a rude awakening, girls: This is NOT the kind of popularity or reputation you want! Furthermore, why would you ever let a boy use you like this? This is such a pathetic game, a game in which you're being made fools of! In case you're not aware, your value as a female is NOT measured by your body parts! You do NOT need to give a boy a handjob, blowjob, or any other sexual favor to be an appreciated, admired, and lovable human being! You are worth so much more than this! Take your power back! Rise above this selfish trend, and let the pretty boys do their own dirty work!

To those girls who will most certainly seek the sexual thrill, at least I hope that when you do explore, you'll engage in this emotionally, mentally, and physically risky behavior with your eyes wide open and making damn sure the boys are *STRAPPED UP* before they put it down! Getting pregnant will seem like *nothing* compared to being infected with HIV! And anal sex drastically increases this deadly risk! Don't forget, condoms fail far too often. (Equally, the boys, though few there may be, should not feel pressured into having sex.)

Most teens, including myself, also know the pain of losing a parent through divorce or another tragedy. This pain, this sense of loss, can be devastating. Now, combine that with the above, along with the normal hormonal changes that any teenager will experience, and, well, I hope you're starting to realize why they're so depressed, and why it's so absolutely critical for them to eat healthy and properly maintain their serotonin levels. But please help them eat a healthier diet before you put them on any pharmaceutical drugs!

What things should I cut out?
Cut out any and all sodas, fruit drinks, iced tea, and any other caffeinated beverages. This includes the many new, hip energy drinks that are loaded with sugar, caffeine, and numerous other stimulants. Avoid alcohol, nicotine, chocolate, aspartame, high-fructose corn syrup, sugar, cereal, milk (especially fat-free/skim milk), nachos, rice cakes, fast food,

pasta, white bread, rice, potatoes, bagels, pizza, biscuits and gravy, fried food, etc. The list is endless! I think you have a good idea. Simply stated: You need to read the food labels. This alone will help you tremendously in selecting the right foods for you and your family. Just remember, you need to eat REAL food, not processed or refined food. I know this will seem overwhelming at first, but your health and the health of your children depend on it. These are all healthy habits that you need to make part of your life starting NOW!

To reiterate, healthy levels of serotonin will help control the cravings for the foods that spike insulin. And because insulin is what causes the body to store fat, the less insulin spiking, the less fat stored. These same unhealthy foods, however, also cause depression. Please understand that once you boost and maintain your serotonin, your mind will become quiet—the cravings will stop. You will no longer have the desire for those types of foods or beverages. It will happen effortlessly. You will finally be free of those insatiable cravings and so-called food addictions. Your mood will also become much more stable. You'll feel less anxious, less stressed, slower to anger. You'll be more focused and feel so much happier. You'll feel in control of your life once again.

I'm concerned about my son. What are the statistics on teens and depression?

I was stunned to discover that suicide is the third leading cause of death for teens! Each year, approximately 20% of all high school students think about committing suicide. 10% try. To reiterate, the antidepressants doctors are prescribing to these teens are actually causing *more* suicidal thoughts, even suicide itself! There is currently an investigation into these drugs. The drugs thought to be effective in treating children with major depression are themselves now being investigated as a possible cause of suicidal behavior! Numerous lawsuits have been filed against the makers of these drugs.

Update: August 2004, the medical industry came out in an attempt to defend their drugs and these latest charges. They're claiming that "because these kids are now able to 'talk about' their depression means that the drugs are, in fact, working. They see it as a positive sign that these kids are actually getting better." *Excuse me?* While I am not a medical doctor, I seriously doubt this rationalization. So should you. But hold on a second—let's be fair here. In the *farthest stretch* of one's imagination, let's say it's true. How, then, do they explain that during the clinical trials on these various antidepressant drugs, dozens of patients were not only experiencing suicidal thoughts, but several actually committed suicide? Huh? How in the hell do they rationalize that? They can't! Period. Chillingly, the FDA allows these DEADLY drugs to be marketed! *But why?* How can a drug be sold that causes the exact same deadly side effects that it's intended to be eliminating? *Where is the outrage by the parents and our government?* This all leaves me absolutely speechless!

Latest update: As reported by CNN, February 2005, the FDA has suddenly backed off its warning that antidepressants such as Zoloft, Paxil, and Prozac can cause suicidal actions among children and teens taking those drugs. Instead, the FDA, in a revised warning, changed the wording to state only that the drugs "increased the 'risk' of suicidal thinking and behavior in short-term studies of adolescents and children." Limiting their warning to a mere "risk," rather than admitting the drugs actually can *cause* suicidal behavior in younger patients, is a major and exceedingly disturbing retreat for the FDA! And do you want to know *why* the FDA backed down? Here is yet another contemptible example of the FDA being bought off by the pharmaceutical industry. The record is clear: They backed off after several months of lobbying by the pharmaceutical industry. *HELLO?!! Doesn't anyone find this alarming, let alone illegal?* God, I should hope so! The FDA, FTC, and the pharmaceutical industry need to be investigated before even more people die at their greedy, lying, manipulative hands!

I agree! Along with a healthier diet, aren't there safer ways to treat depression?
Elevating serotonin does <u>not</u> have to include risking your life with pharmaceutical drugs! This is what I'm desperately trying to share with you. The following supplements have impressive clinical studies supporting their ability to safely/effectively enhance serotonin.

<u>5-HTP versus antidepressants:</u>
Clinical studies indicate that 5-HTP is one of the safest, most effective methods of elevating serotonin. Unlike MAOIs (Monoamine Oxidase Inhibitors) such as Nardil, Parnate, etc., 5-HTP does not interfere with the activity of the enzyme that breaks down serotonin. And unlike SSRIs (Selective Serotonin Reuptake Inhibitors) such as Prozac, Zoloft, Paxil, etc., 5-HTP does not block reuptake of serotonin. 5-HTP is an amino acid. It does not interfere with the body's natural process of serotonin release, absorption, or elimination. It's safe, natural, affordable, non-habit-forming, exceptionally effective *without* side effects, works much faster than drugs, and no prescription is required.

<u>SAMe versus antidepressants:</u>
SAMe, an amino acid, naturally occurs in the cells of our body. SAMe is essential to at least 35 biochemical processes in the body, including maintaining the structure of cell membranes and safely balancing neurotransmitters such as serotonin and dopamine. Studies have shown SAMe to be extremely effective in safely alleviating depression.

<u>Vinpocetine versus antidepressants:</u>
Vinpocetine, an extract from the Periwinkle plant, has tremendous studies supporting its ability to safely increase serotonin. It's known as a cerebral enhancer and neuroprotector.

<u>Noni versus antidepressants:</u>
A tropical fruit, the highest serotonin-binding plant of the Rubiaceae family. Though it's limited in clinical studies to support its various claims, it's still another safe option to help elevate serotonin. Just be aware of the amount of fruit juice/sugar in the noni products.

With all this talk of depression, I feel the need to share my own personal story, as it may help you, or your teen. I feel it's paramount that you know that I speak not just as a researcher, but also as someone who has experienced what I write about.

A very personal reflection...

Obviously, by now, you know that I'm not pretending to be some sort of angel or puritan. Nor did I <u>ever</u> do anything based on peer pressure. That being said, throughout my late teens and into my early thirties, I loved going out, most often alone, and the edgier the place, the better. For me, that included going to clubs, dancing, drinking alcohol, and a few other party favors. But I still did my best to eat healthy and exercise five days a week. I was fortunate to maintain my physique while enjoying a few less than desirable habits. For me, it was all about balance and moderation, with an occasional escape from reality. Nevertheless, as time went on, alcohol no longer gave me the same pleasure it once did. I wasn't going out nearly as often as years prior, but when I did, I drank more than I should, I started to have blackouts, hangovers were pure hell, and even after the hangovers finally subsided, my mood would be altered for days. Hence, I cut back even more. But, still I found myself feeling emotionally weak, not my usual strong, carefree self. My tears fell quicker and more frequently. I also craved carbs, anything from subs, cereal, pretzels and pasta, foods that I would normally *never* care for, were suddenly my only desire. (Considering I was years away from discovering this research, my only concern at that time was finding out why I felt so sad after a few lousy cocktails.)

I wrote my mood swings off to simply being hormonal, financial stress, boyfriend issues—all those things people at my age worried about. Although I'm blessed with the most wonderful friends, I've always been content in my time alone. It was at those sad times that I would find solace in working out—and writing poetry. Not rhyming type of poetry, rather free-flowing-let-your-mind-run-wild kind of poetry. I <u>had</u> to write; it was my *only* way of releasing all that I felt. I never felt suicidal, but I definitely felt lost. Hopeless. Desperately alone in the world. And that is a terrible place to be. (On a very personal note, I also feared that I had possibly followed in my mother's footsteps. She had, sadly, been diagnosed with mental illness many years prior.)

Ever since I was 15, writing had been my chosen therapy. Robert (AKA Coach) Grimes, my high school creative writing teacher, was truly an amazing man—a man who inspired me in many ways—but he also insisted I keep a journal, a journal that was a safe haven for me to pour forth all that I was feeling. Right or wrong, I would never be judged. It was through this writing process (along with his genuine compassion) that I was able to mentally and emotionally survive those tormented teenage years. Ironically, years later, I discovered that my writing was once again the venue I chose to express my grief, my darkest fears, my overwhelming sense of foreboding that would unexpectedly envelope me. Writing allowed me to do this privately, without shame or judgment. And then, come the next morning, I felt fine. And life went on. Happily. Until I drank again. (I still have those writings. It's rather sad to see just how dark my mood was. As for my high school journals, my stepmother found them and was horrified by what she read. I can't recall exactly what I wrote, but whatever pain she felt reading them couldn't *possibly* compare to the pain I felt when writing them. To my grave disappointment, she threw them away.) With regard to my drinking,

I continued on this unhealthy path for years to come. To be honest, I assumed it was just who I was. Too emotional. Too sensitive. The fact of the matter was, my mental state of mind had *nothing* to do with my mother's illness or with my being too emotional. These mood swings were rather directly linked to the alcohol.

Why didn't you stop?
Why? Good question. I suppose I didn't really want to stop. I loved going out. As a single woman with a very adventurous spirit, I enjoyed meeting new people, and going to night-clubs and intimate wine bars was the way I preferred to socialize. However, and more importantly, it was actually that quiet, but oh, so powerful little voice within, that voice we now know as a craving, that kept me coming back for more. No matter how bad I felt, it all seemed worth it. Little did I know it was just another craving. After all, alcohol is primarily sugar, and it's recognized by the body as sugar. This craving is absolutely no different from the cravings you get for bread, candy, chips, or soda.

Are you serious?
Yes. Alcohol is made from either grain or fruit, both of which are carbohydrates. Alcohol is a combination of alcohol and sugar. Alcohol will hence, have the same effect on brain chemistry as the high GI carbs we've discussed. You drink it. Insulin is spiked. Insulin leads to serotonin elevation. Between the alcohol and the shift in brain chemistry, you start to feel good. Really good. And whoever stops at one drink? Regardless, the next day, you're undeniably serotonin deficient. Your brain then shifts to other cravings for the foods that will once again trigger the release of this blissful, mood-altering brain chemical. This is exactly why after a night of partying you'll find yourself craving things like bagels, fries, pizza, chips, sodas, caffeine, maybe even another drink. It is your brain merely trying once again to stimulate the production of serotonin. It is a cycle. Once you're aware of this cycle, this pattern of cravings, whether it's for alcohol or junk food, you'll hopefully be able to take control of these bad habits.

And your depressive moods?
While alcohol first triggers the production of serotonin, it also depletes it. After a night of partying, my serotonin would plummet. This caused not only food cravings, but also mood swings. Some days, these mood swings plummeted to depression. *"Depression?"* What the hell did I know about depression? I just felt blue. Or so I believed. It is only now, after I've spent numerous years researching serotonin and its essential role in our physical, mental, and emotional health, that I can reflect and honestly understand what was hap-pening to me. By sharing this story, *the direct relation to alcohol and depression,* I sincerely hope it helps save you, your spouse, and your teenager from this senseless, self-inflicted emotional trauma.

How did you eventually stop?
I had no choice but to start listening to my body, as it was certainly letting me know that alcohol was not good for me, in many ways. Over the years, I had drastically cut back. And

since I began this journey, even one drink a month became too much for me. After about 7 months of being on an SES, it amazingly squelched all desire for alcohol. Where I used to have my Thursday night urge to go out, craving a dirty martini in some soulful Ebony underground club, I now have no desire to drink. Best of all, I don't miss it. I feel absolutely wonderful without it. My moods are much more stable. I no longer suffer from those dark days. I haven't felt the need to write poetry in over 10 years. And god knows I've stopped wasting time nursing hangovers. Maintaining my serotonin has given me far more than a lean body—it has literally saved my life by keeping me from abusing my body and mind any further with this intoxicating yet potentially dangerous drug.

But how does this happen?

Serotonin helps control carbohydrate/sugar cravings. And alcohol is, once again, made from either grain or fruit, both carbohydrates. Don't forget that most people like to mix their preferred alcohol with some sort of soda, fruit juice, etc., which adds even more sugar, plus caffeine. All of these will further deplete serotonin. So you see, my desire for alcohol was the same as someone craving a chocolate bar or a bowl of cereal. The brain exhibits low serotonin in many different ways, and it will continually make you want the things it knows will elevate this brain chemical. Without a doubt, my brain knew that alcohol would elevate my serotonin.

It's not like I drink that much. Are you saying I should quit altogether?

I'm not telling you or anyone else to quit drinking. I am merely conveying information about the effects alcohol has on your health, on your life. It's up to you how you choose to use the information. Over the years of training clients, I've had many who expect me to give them a perfect body while they ignore all the things I teach them regarding diet, alcohol, caffeine, and many other health concerns. While I'm more than confident in my abilities as a trainer, I am not a magician. I need their help once they leave the gym. You need to realize that if you're really serious about losing excess body fat, lowering blood pressure, reducing cholesterol, and so forth, alcohol is something you most definitely need to limit. Alcohol is a leading contributor to high blood pressure. Alcohol triggers insulin, thereby causing the production of harmful cholesterol. High levels of insulin also fuel cancer cells. Alcohol depletes serotonin, which leads to numerous health issues including PMS, ADD, rage, insomnia, low sex drive, body pain, carb/sugar cravings, weight gain, depression, and anxiety. Many of those who drink, also don't realize that their body has to first burn off the alcohol *before* it will start to burn their stored fat. Alcohol is nothing more than useless calories and a momentary break from reality. While I admit we all certainly need a break from reality now and then, you need to look at the bigger picture and see the effects alcohol has on your life. I've personally seen a huge change in my body (and emotions) since I stopped drinking. (An SES will help control these cravings, but if someone doesn't make the effort, no amount of working out or product will help them. You have to be willing. You have to make the effort to get the body you desire. And please don't use your age as an excuse. Age is the not determing factor when it comes to achieving your fitness goals.)

101

What do you suggest?
Start by getting on a quality SES. I also respectfully insist that, for the first 30 days of this new healthy lifestyle, you avoid all alcohol for the reasons just mentioned. If, after those 30 days, you want a drink, please limit drinking to the weekend. Studies suggest dry red wine, Scotch, or vodka—minus any tonic, soda, juice, or sugary mix—are acceptable in moderation. Personally, I prefer that you stick to red wine, with no hard liquor. Better yet, avoid all alcohol during the initial stage of reduction. Allow yourself to really get into a healthy workout regimen and eating program. Give yourself a month of feeling what it's like to just focus on being healthy. Your body composition will start to change. Toxins will begin to flush out of your system. Your mind will become clearer, more focused. Your emotions will be far more stable. You will start to feel a difference in all aspects of your life. You will be astonished at just how good you can really feel without all the poisons that come from alcohol, processed food, and sugar.

My personal guarantee: If you devote one full, unadulterated month to this healthy lifestyle, I guarantee you will not want to go back to your old habits. You will feel *sooo* much happier, healthier, stronger—and more self-confident—and all of this combined will motivate you to continue on this path. The sense of pride you will feel for having accomplished this lifelong goal is enough to inspire you to take it even further, much further. You will be amazed at what you can create with your body! But know this, your goal is simple: Do not let yourself get overwhelmed by looking too far down the proverbial road. Instead, I want you to focus on one month at a time. Each passing month will bring even more exciting changes in both your body and mind. Once again motivating you to take it further. Your success will equally inspire others around you!

It's much less stressful to look at it one month at a time. I can easily commit to that. But isn't there pressure to drink when you go out on a date or with friends?
First of all, I rarely date. When I do, the man respects my decision, especially after I tell him why I no longer drink. As for my friends, likewise. Please understand that I'm fine with those who drink. We make our own choices. It's simply my choice now not to. The reward: I'm a sober, safe driver, no risk of DUIs or harming another. (I'm also much better prepared to drive defensively.) Come the next day, I wake up bright and early with no headache, no hangover, no regrets, sexual or otherwise. I'm ready to work out, run my dogs, go to the stables, anything to enjoy the day. And I must be honest, sex has never been better since I quit drinking. I think many of us are used to being intimate with the help of some sort of mind-altering substance, alcohol being the most common, that we forget where such intense passion can truly take our bodies—and minds. (With the right lover, of course.) Furthermore, avoiding alcohol makes it a lot easier to maintain a lean, healthy body since I don't trigger cravings. My moods are also much more stable. I'm less emotional, less stressed, and less anxious.

I'm ready to quit drinking after that! What about the elderly and drinking?
This is a serious issue. Researchers are now calling this phenomenon "Late-Onset

Alcoholism." In one clinical study, 41% of the people age 65 and over who were enrolled in an alcohol treatment program, reported that their alcohol problems began after age 60. Most seniors who do have an alcohol problem are unable or unwilling to recognize it. Others simply can't recognize it because of cognitive impairment caused by the alcohol.

I worry that my mother drinks too much. But what can I do?

I know this is a very sensitive and personal matter. Nonetheless, my suggestion is to first talk to her, compassionately. Tell her your concerns. If she is open, then start with her diet. Use the information you've learned here and put it to work. Next, get her on an SES. This will help her control the alcohol cravings. You must understand that both changing her diet and using any such product will require time, effort, and tremendous patience before you start to see a shift in her behavior. (Caffeine is also a concern, as it's depleting her serotonin, thereby perpetuating her cravings for sugar, i.e., alcohol.) If your mother chooses to ignore you, you'll at least know that you made an honest and loving attempt to help her. And while you may have nothing but good intentions, we each have to live our own life. Your mother has the right to do with her life as she wishes, just as you do with yours. If she chooses to drink, in excess or otherwise, it's her choice. It won't be easy to watch, but it's not your life. Be there for her, but without contributing to her drinking lifestyle. Your teenage son, however, is a different story. He is your son and living under your care. You need to do whatever it takes to help him.

Once again I'm amazed at this information. I certainly relate to the senseless hangovers, as well as the depression. My son is often depressed after a night out with his friends. I'll do everything I can to help him improve his health through a healthy diet <u>before</u> I put him on any drugs.

I'm sure you can understand my extreme frustration when I see the endless drug commercials marketing their antidepressants. With regard to teens, considering their horrendous high-sugar diets, along with drinking, smoking, takin' X, hormone shifts, and the stress of just being that age, it's no wonder they're depressed, even suicidal. Their serotonin is frighteningly depleted! But you have choices. Please keep those many choices in mind before you put your family or yourself on any pharmaceutical drugs.

BTW: For those parents who aren't aware, ecstasy works primarily by releasing serotonin. Some teens are hip enough to take 5-HTP to help avoid the depression that most often follows after partying. Now, if you could only get them to take the 5-HTP <u>minus</u> the X, you'd see so many wonderful changes in them. Personally, I question the many so-called risks of taking X, as I think the real danger comes from the hazardous drugs and chemical compounds that X is often cut with. But, even if the risks are real, why then, are alcohol and cigarettes—two products that have *long been proven* to be addictive and deadly—legal and so heavily promoted? Easy answer: Big business. Bigger profits.

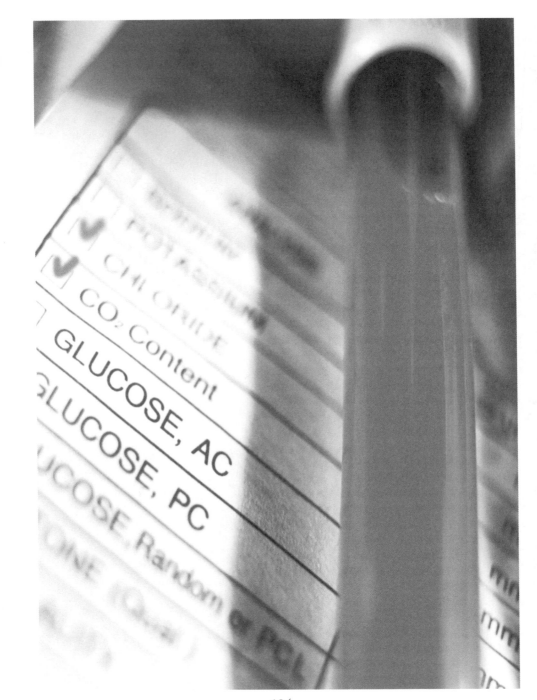

19

INSULIN & HOW IT AFFECTS CHOLESTEROL
The key to helping cure heart disease

We hear all these warnings about high cholesterol, but I'm not even sure what it is. Cholesterol is a type of fat. It is a soft, waxy, fat-like substance found in the bloodstream and in all of our cells. And, in case you didn't know it, *we need cholesterol.* It's an important part of a healthy body. Cholesterol not only helps produce cell membranes, it also provides structure within cell membranes and keeps those cells permeable. Several of our major hormones (cortisol, testosterone, estradiol, and progesterone), are all made from cholesterol. Cholesterol provides a type of insulation around nerves. This helps electrical impulses move freely. Neurotransmitters are dependent on cholesterol. Cholesterol is, therefore, necessary for proper brain function. Furthermore, cholesterol and other fats are water insoluble, i.e., they cannot dissolve in the bloodstream. Thus, they have to be transported to and from the cells by special carriers. These cholesterol-carrying proteins are called lipoproteins. There are three types:

VLDL = Very low-density lipoprotein. This is the "bad" cholesterol. VLDL contains high amounts of triglycerides, with very little protein. VLDL deposits cholesterol on the walls of arteries, increasing risks for heart disease. It makes up 10–15% of total cholesterol. (The lower the number the better.) Recommendations for triglycerides: <150 mg/dL.

LDL = Low-density lipoprotein. This is also a "bad" cholesterol. It's a combination of fat and protein. Too much LDL can clog your arteries. Again, this increases your risk of heart attack and stroke. It makes up 60–70% of total cholesterol. (The lower the number the better.)

HDL = High-density lipoprotein. This is the "good" cholesterol. Most HDL is made by the liver. HDL carries cholesterol away from the arteries and back to the liver, where it is then removed from the body. Studies show that high blood levels of HDL can reduce your risk of heart attack. Thus, lowering your risks of heart disease. It makes up 20–30% of total cholesterol. (The higher the number the better. 60+ is protective against heart disease.)

As you can see, each lipoprotein has its own unique function in the body. Therefore, the "total" cholesterol number is not an accurate way to asses one's overall risks for heart disease. The best way to achieve healthy levels of these lipoproteins, thereby reducing your risks, is by living a healthy lifestyle. This healthy lifestyle will help increase HDLs, while at the same time *decreasing* VLDLs and LDLs.

How does one get cholesterol?
Your body i.e., your liver, either makes it, or it can come from the foods you eat.

You're saying we actually need to eat cholesterol?
Yes. Contrary to what most experts will tell you, you need to eat healthy foods rich in cholesterol to shut down your body's internal clock and keep it from producing its own. If you deprive your body of this vital nutrient, your body will be forced to produce its own. To avoid this health risk, you need to eat foods (at every meal) that contain cholesterol. If you don't, your body will make cholesterol from carbohydrates. And this is not a healthy type of cholesterol. Excellent dietary sources of cholesterol-laden foods are red meat, shellfish, milk, butter, poultry, fish, cheese, and eggs. Other than the meat and milk, I enjoy plenty of these foods, making sure I eat one with every meal.

Eggs? I thought eggs were bad for us?
This scare tactic was perpetuated over 30 years ago by the cereal industry. Eggs are a perfect protein, a healthy source of cholesterol—and one of the most perfect foods.

Wow! Another fear campaign. A very successful one at that!
Yes, that campaign was unfortunately terribly effective. But eggs are truly one of the healthiest foods there are. They're low in calories, carbs, sodium, and an excellent source of protein, dietary fat, and cholesterol. In addition, eggs contain a wonderful abundance of vitamins and minerals: And so I ask: *With all these many benefits, how can eggs possibly be bad for us?*

I agree. I've eaten eggs all my life and my cholesterol is fine. Plus, I feel great after I eat them. By the way, what is a perfect protein?
I'm glad to know you've been eating eggs. Please continue to do so. As for what makes a perfect protein, allow me to explain: Egg whites contain the purest form of protein found in whole foods. Experts use eggs as the standard when comparing other whole food proteins. Without getting too technical, they measure how efficiently a protein is used for growth. And the higher the value, the better the protein is absorbed by the body. Eggs are at around 93, with milk at 84, fish at 76, and beef at 64. Personally, I happily eat about a dozen eggs a week in many various ways.

What is the connection between insulin and cholesterol?
Anything that triggers insulin increases the production of cholesterol. This list includes sugar, stress, alcohol, prescription and nonprescription drugs, over-the-counter meds, poor diet, cigarettes, lack of healthy fats and proteins, caffeine, ma huang, all stimulants, processed and refined foods, a sedentary lifestyle, excessive, and high GI carb intake equals high insulin levels, which creates the most harmful form of cholesterol. This is what increases your risks for heart disease, heart attacks, and stroke.

Doesn't an SES also help control insulin levels?
Exactly! An SES will help you greatly reduce your intake of the types of foods that trigger insulin. But the key to a healthy cholesterol panel is to live a healthy *lifestyle*. It is <u>not</u> just about a number. You need to do what it takes to stabilize your insulin.

The latest controversy regarding cholesterol: Recent studies suggest that the current method of determining actual health risks associated with cholesterol are now themselves being questioned. Recent reports show people are actually having *more* strokes and *more* heart attacks when their cholesterol levels are <u>exactly</u> where the AMA and FDA claim they "should" be. <u>FACT</u>: A majority of people with so-called high cholesterol *never* suffer heart attacks. <u>FACT</u>: More than 60% of all heart attacks and strokes occur in people with *normal* cholesterol panels.

How do you feel about the latest change in guidelines for "total" cholesterol?
When the medical industry, i.e., the *drug companies*, changed the cholesterol guidelines from 220 to 200mg/dL (recently even as low as 180), the number of people who were suddenly "sick or at risk" tripled! Literally overnight, 104 million Americans were scared into believing they had to be on these drugs! This alone increased cholesterol drug sales by over an astounding 32%, earning the drug companies over $12.5 billion!

If that wasn't enough, in July 2004 the NCEP (National Cholesterol Education Program) suggested that the new guidelines for LDL be lowered from 130 to 100mg/dL or less. Those considered high risk should aim for <70. This suggestion was based on clinical studies performed by who else, *the drug companies!* Not to mention, the NCEP works hand in hand with the FDA! My first reaction to this latest change was, "When will it ever end? This means the drug companies basically want <u>every</u> <u>single</u> <u>adult</u> on their lifelong, cholesterol-lowering drugs!" This will create *billions* in new revenue for these pharmaceutical companies! Lowering their guidelines will have an astronomical effect on millions of people who will be scared into believing they must be on these drugs! There are currently 40 million people on some sort of cholesterol-lowering drug. This new guideline will push the number to over *100 million!* I guarantee you that most people will, unfortunately, *never* even question this. I find this outrageous! This tactic is once again based on nothing but the GREED of the pharmaceutical drug lords!

What are these drugs designed to do?
These drugs, called statins, are HMG-CoA reductase inhibitors. They were designed to inhibit the production of cholesterol, primarily to help lower TC (Total Cholesterol) and LDL cholesterol levels. The proposed goal of these statin drugs: To help prevent coronary heart disease. However, this is far from reality! These statin drugs, like most other pharmaceutical drugs, are NOT what the medical industry claims! Furthermore, based on the latest guidelines set by the medical industry themselves, serious consideration should be given to this report: "Nine statins, commonly used at a dose to lower TC to <160mg/dL, are associated with higher cancer rates."

Cancer? I'm afraid to ask, but are there any other side effects?
Yes, of course, there are literally dozens of other serious health risks to consider. Researchers from the U.S. National Institutes of Health found that the use of cholesterol-lowering drugs during the first trimester of pregnancy is associated with limb deformities and severe central nervous system defects. These medical findings were published in a research letter in the *New England Journal of Medicine*. It disclosed that 20 of 52 babies exposed to these drugs in the womb were born with malformations. And 1 to 3% of the prescriptions for these medications are for women in their childbearing years. Lipitor, Zocor, Pravachol, Crestor, Lescol, Mevacor, and Baycol were all linked to these studies.

Anything else to watch for?
Plenty! Other side effects reported range from constipation, myopathy, polyneuropathy, myalgia, liver and kidney damage, amnesia, and congestive heart failure. *All of this for drugs that do NOT work!* In August 2002, CNN reported that statin drugs were known to cause nerve damage in one in every 2,200 patients. For those over 50 and on the drugs for over two years, the chances of nerve damage were 26 times higher than for the normal population. That puts over 6,000 people at risk for nerve damage each year! (My own father is suffering from this statin (Zocor) side effect. When he complained to his doctor, he said it was not related, worse yet, he insisted he stay on it! Sadly, my dad, like millions of others, are scared into believing they have to be on these drugs!) With regard to the brain and central nervous system side effects, a separate study showed that 100% of the participants, after *only* six months on the statin drugs, suffered measurable declines in cognition! To avoid these deadly drugs you need to take a much closer look at your diet and lifestyle, then make the necessary changes starting today!

With over 20 million people on Lipitor alone, it was crucial to include some of its many serious, not to mention, underlined side effects. Shockingly, most of these side effects were documented during the clinical trials. But yet the FDA considers it safe: "*Abdominal, back, and chest pain, abnormal heartbeat, changes in eyesight, constipation, decreased sex drive, depression, diarrhea, dizziness, dry eyes/skin, fatigue, flu symptoms, fluid reten-tion, gas, hair loss, headache, heartburn, indigestion, inflammation of sinus/nasal pas-sages, itching, joint pain, leg cramps, liver damage, muscle aching/weakness, nerve dam-age, purple/red spots on skin, rash, rectal hemorrhage, sore throat, tingling of extremities, unstable emotions, urinary problems, vomiting, weakness, weight gain, and weight loss.*" (Let's not forget stroke, heart attack, and death!)

Statin update: As of May 2005, the medical industry is claiming that statins cut the risk of developing various cancers by 50%. *Talk about pushing drug sales to an all-time high!* Well, BEWARE! Considering the studies generating most of the positive press are funded by the companies that actually make these drugs, I seriously doubt this claim! Furthermore, if statins really are the "miracle drugs" that the drug industry would like us to believe they are, *why* then are more people than ever before dying of heart failure? *Why?* I'll tell you why. While these statin drugs are doing *nothing* to help prevent heart attacks, they are instead, *and at the very least*, dangerously affecting your liver's ability to make CoQ10 (coenzyme Q10), a substance found in most tissues in the body and in many foods. It's an antioxidant and used by the body to produce energy for cells. Without CoQ10, the cells in your muscles can't produce enough energy. Subsequently, these muscles weaken dramatically. The *heart* just happens to be one of these muscles!

To reiterate, I suggest you make the much-needed changes in your diet and overall lifestyle. Research on your own. Educate yourself about your options. Then, for the next 90 days, avoid any and all things that trigger insulin. This includes, but is not limited to, alcohol, cigarettes, caffeine, sugar, high GI carbs, processed/refined foods, etc. It may not be easy in the beginning, but maintaining healthy serotonin levels will help control your cravings. Controlling your cravings will help stabilize your insulin. Also, start some sort of exercise program. You need to be devoted to this if you really want to make these changes. It's possible to turn your health around by simply making better, healthier choices. Don't cheat yourself or your loved ones. After 90 days, go back to your doctor and ask her (or him) to run the *appropriate* test—the test that will determine whether or not your "arteries" are clogged. After all, this is what causes heart disease. Please understand that you can reverse many of these health problems without having to risk your life by using drugs. Not only do these drugs merely mask symptoms, they inevitably come with serious, if not, life-threatening side effects! These drugs, will, undoubtedly cause new diseases/illnesses in your body! Is it worth it? The answer is obvious to me.

I'm willing to research on my own, but where do I find this type of information?
You can find most anything you want online. Go to Google. Start searching. The information made available is unlimited. That being said, don't believe everything you read. Check sources, look for ulterior motives, dig deep, and use your common sense. Once again, I recommend you immediately read *"The Schwarzbein Principle,"* an extraordinary book written by Diana Schwarzbein, MD. She's one of the most respected medical experts. Her studies in this precise area are truly impressive. Two other excellent sources for finding the latest medical information would be *Life Extension* magazine and *Alternatives*, a monthly newsletter written by Dr. David Williams. Both dare to speak the truth, no matter how ugly, no matter how risky—be it against the FDA, AMA, FTC, CDC, drug companies, etc. (Note: While I certainly value the articles in these health subscriptions, I do not buy and/or endorse their products. Unfortunately, when I read something that seems scientifically brilliant, it greatly diminishes the validity when I turn the page only to find their products being sold. I'm not saying their products don't have value. Just don't be unwillingly seduced into buying them.)

FINAL WARNING: Heart disease, heart attacks, strokes, etc., are not caused by high cholesterol! They are, though, caused by plaqueing of the arteries which is caused by high insulin levels. Therefore, it's critical that you avoid anything that causes your insulin levels to rise, especially long-term! SESs can help stabilize your insulin levels by helping you live that much-needed healthier lifestyle.

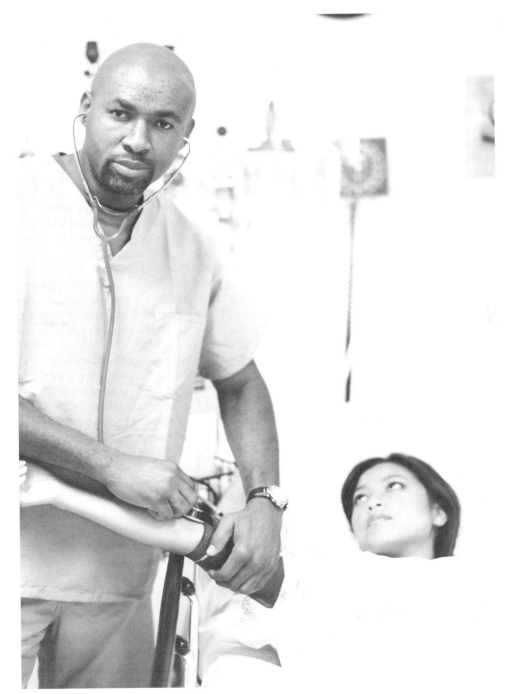

20

INSULIN & HOW IT AFFECTS BLOOD PRESSURE

How do high insulin levels affect blood pressure?
First, allow me to say that those with high blood pressure have a much higher risk of getting heart disease. High blood pressure can be caused by several factors, but my focus is on those related to "high insulin" levels. High insulin levels can affect blood pressure in two ways:

1) Insulin promotes an abnormal increase of salt retention. And while the kidneys are responsible for regulating sodium levels in the blood, this salt increase leads to water retention. This higher fluid levels equals higher blood pressure.

2) Insulin excites the nervous system. This increases the amount of blood being pumped out with every contraction of the heart. Not only will this cause high blood pressure, but it will also lead to stiffer, less pliable artery walls. This can lead to heart damage, a heart attack, even sudden death.

What exactly is sodium?
Sodium is a mineral that the body requires, but in small amounts. Read your food/drink labels and watch for the name "sodium chloride." (Sodium chloride is another name for table salt.)

Does table salt contribute to high blood pressure?
Yes, it can, so do not add salt to your food. You should be getting plenty of sodium through a healthy, balanced diet. Please understand, though, you do not have to actually add salt to your food to be eating way too much salt. Once again, read the nutritional panels to see how much sodium is in the food you eat. Foods to watch out for are all processed foods, soups (canned and freshly made), snack foods, crackers, condiments (mustard, ketchup, dressings, relish, soy sauce, etc.) smoked, salted, pickled, canned fish, meats, and vegetables, pickles, sauerkraut, processed cheese (includes cottage cheese), tomato juice, etc.

How much sodium do I need each day?
The body needs, at minimum, 500 milligrams of sodium daily. However, most experts agree that sodium intake should be around 2,400mg per day (milligrams not grams!) for

healthy adults. Unfortunately, most Americans consume far more sodium than this, often consuming 2,300 to 7,000mg per day! This is way too much—and asking for serious trouble! In addition to high blood pressure, a build-up of sodium in the body can cause thirst, water retention, and shortness of breath. This can greatly increase your risk of a stroke or heart attack. (BTW: One teaspoon of salt = 2,000mg of sodium.)

Furthermore, studies show that certain people are more sensitive to sodium. For example: African Americans, Hispanics, and obese individuals are especially sensitive to salt and would, therefore, need to monitor their salt/sodium intake much closer. So please, be very aware of the amount of sodium you take in each day. The most effective way to do this is by reading food labels.

What is considered to be a normal and healthy blood pressure?
Excellent question, considering that after the drug companies saw such a profitable response when they lowered cholesterol guidelines, they wasted no time in doing the same thing with blood pressure guidelines. Where once you had always been told you were healthy, *with normal blood pressure*, suddenly you were at serious risk for a stroke or heart attack! Please! Doesn't anyone question their motives here? Why doesn't anyone demand explanations for this drastic and terribly convenient change?

To truly determine your blood pressure, it should be taken on at least three separate occasions. Take it when you're rested and calm—not in the busy, stressful part of your day. Blood pressure can also vary 5 to 30 points within mere minutes. The top number can be anywhere from 90–240, and the bottom number can be anywhere from 60–140. Blood pressure is measured in millimeters of mercury, which is written down as: mmHg. The following is a range from optimal to high:

Optimal BP: Less than 120/over less than 80
Pre-hypertension: 120–130/over 80–89
High–normal BP: 130–139/over 89
High BP: 140+/over 90+

What do the numbers actually represent?
There are two components of a blood pressure reading. Example: 115 over 65. The top number, 115, is the systolic pressure. This is the blood pressure in the arteries when the heart is pumping blood. The bottom number, 65, is the diastolic pressure. It represents the pressure in the arteries when the heart is resting and filling with blood.

One more time, please.
The systolic pressure shows the pressure in your arteries when your heart is forcing blood through them. The diastolic pressure shows the pressure in your arteries when your heart relaxes.

Medical update: Many doctors are now rethinking these guidelines. Nonetheless, I urge you to let your physician check and monitor your blood pressure. (In between my check-ups, I periodically check mine using BP machines found in various pharmacies.)

What are the symptoms of high blood pressure?

Another excellent question, because high blood pressure is considered the #1 SILENT KILLER! It is considered extremely dangerous because it has absolutely NO symptoms! High blood pressure is a far more deadly health risk than so-called "high cholesterol." People with high blood pressure may occasionally complain of headaches, shortness of breath, or nosebleeds. This is not always the case, though. Regular health checkups are the best way to make sure you don't have high blood pressure.

What are the risk factors for high blood pressure?

Risk factors for high blood pressure include family history, race, age, being 20% above ideal body weight, smoking, more than 2 or 3 drinks per day, foods high in sodium, stress (more so for those who hold anger in), diabetes, and kidney disease.

How many people are afflicted with high blood pressure?

High blood pressure affects about one in four adults. This totals about 50 million people! As frightening as this may sound, this is at least one cardiovascular risk factor you can help control. If you are overweight, have high blood pressure, high cholesterol, or you are insulin-resistant, you should immediately start restricting sodium, sugar, and high GI carbs. An SES will help you do this by controlling the insatiable cravings.

How will an SES help control insulin levels?

An SES will help control the cravings for the countless high GI foods and beverages that spike insulin levels. However, take notes here: High GI carbs are found in most processed/snack foods, i.e., pretzels, chips, crackers, etc. These same foods are often excessively high in sodium. A double whammy, as high sodium also leads to high insulin levels. An SES will, though, by controlling your cravings for junk food, inadvertently control your intake of these high sodium foods.

An SES will, as well, help you avoid alcohol, caffeine, and nicotine. Each of these lead to high insulin levels. An SES will help reduce stress and anxiety. Both equally lead to high insulin levels. An SES, will, in essence, help you live a much healthier lifestyle (which includes regular exercise). Insulin levels will subsequently become much more stable. Once again, do whatever it takes to avoid spiking your insulin, especially over an extended period of time.

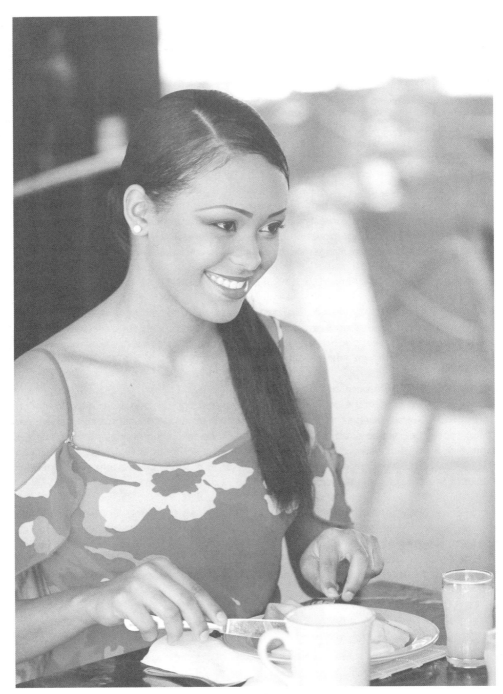

21

EATING HEALTHY
WITHOUT EVER FEELING DEPRIVED!

Are you saying you never feel deprived?
That's exactly what I'm saying. To reiterate, life is <u>not</u> about living like a monk. Life is to be enjoyed in many delightful ways. Food just happens to be a small part of that. And while food can be absolutely divine, especially during the holidays, with family, sharing an intimate evening with someone special, or just a quiet meal alone, food stimulates a lot more than just our appetite. It also creates wonderful memories. Above all, though, food is fuel for our body. It is necessary for survival. Just please don't obsess about it.

So, do I eat healthy all the time? 99% of the time, I eat remarkably healthy, and what's more amazing, considering how stressed my life is, I can do so without any effort. I may occasionally want something I wouldn't necessarily recommend to my clients, but there isn't any effort to eating healthy, and I never have any sense of feeling hungry or deprived <u>if</u> I maintain my serotonin. Again, S-E-R-O-T-O-N-I-N is the key. I'm able to eat plenty of delicious foods, combining healthy fats and proteins with complex (low GI) carbohydrates, while maintaining a lean, strong, and healthy physique.

The fact of the matter is, we are all creatures of habit. To achieve optimum health, we must learn (and be willing) to exchange the bad habits for healthier ones; that includes not skipping meals. I realize that, after 25 years of being told "not to eat fat," there will be an adjustment. But, believe me, eating good quality fat does NOT make you fat. It is eating the *wrong* type of carbs (along with eating damaged fats that are found in junk/processed/fast food) that has caused the alarming rate of obesity in this country.

Okay, so what should I eat if not low-cal, low-fat, or low-carb?
Eat balanced, nutritious meals. Combine food groups, eating a quality protein, healthy fat, with a complex/low GI carb. Don't eat processed or refined foods. Eat real food. Stop counting calories and fat grams; instead watch your carbohydrate/sugar intake. Cut out sugar, HFCS, artificial sweeteners, sodas, diet or otherwise. Avoid caffeine, nicotine, ephedrine, guarna, and all other stimulants. Limit your consumption of alcohol. Eat less, more often. Eating a small meal every three hours will keep your metabolism going strong. Remember: Low-calorie dieting puts your body into a starvation mode, in addition to changing your total body composition. And less lean muscle mass = <u>more</u> fat stores!

As for skipping meals, what if I don't have time for breakfast?
Make the time. If you want to achieve lifelong health, you cannot skip meals. When your car is running low on fuel, do you just keep on driving because you're short on time? Of course not. "I don't have the time" is a far too common excuse when it concerns both skipping breakfast and working out. It is precisely these habits people <u>must</u> be willing to change if they ever hope to achieve lifelong health. If you want your body and mind to perform at their best, you must provide them with the proper, most *efficient* fuel, and do so at regular intervals. Eat 3 primary, yet smaller meals, along with 2 to 3 snacks. This means you're fueling your body basically every 3 hours. And then stop eating (especially carbs) 3 hours before bedtime.

Eat less, more often!

What do you mean by smaller meals?
The goal here is *never* to eat low-calorie. But, based on what most Americans eat at one sitting, I think it's safe to say that, in theory, I want you to eat smaller portions versus stuffing yourself. You'll be eating less at each sitting, while eating more frequently.

What is the most effective way to safely increase my metabolism?
The safest, most effective way to increase your metabolism, and thereby lose weight, is by EATING! And breakfast is one of the most important meals! *Why?* Because it literally <u>breaks</u> <u>your</u> <u>fast</u>, which means you to need to "eat" to get your metabolism going. Having lean muscle mass—and eating smaller meals more often—are the two best ways to keep your metabolism in high gear. So, as soon as you get up, EAT! I eat 5 to 6 times throughout the day (3 main meals with 2–3 snacks). Grazing, as I call it, has always been my preferred way to eat. Also, try to eat your daily meals as close to the same time as possible. This consistency will further help boost your metabolism.

But how do I really know what I'm eating?
When you grocery shop, you must make a new habit of reading the nutritional panels. However, you need to really understand what you're reading so you can subsequently, make better food choices. Take an interest. Be concerned. Expect more from the foods you buy. (For more details, please read chapter 34, "How to Read a Nutritional Panel.")

What about meal replacement shakes and bars?
Beware of the diet products and programs that consist of drinking only a shake or eating a bar as two of your main meals. All one has to do is read the nutritional labels to realize these products are often loaded with sugar. They are not nutritionally sound and will perpetuate your sugar/carb carvings. Furthermore, does anyone really eat these meal replacement bars *in lieu* of a meal? Most often, not. Instead, they eat them in addition to their regular meals, which equals way too many calories. And if you were to only eat them as a primary meal, they would fall under the "low-calorie dieting" category. While you may lose a few pounds by forfeiting a real meal for a meal replacement bar or drink, especially

if you forfeited two meals, the pounds lost will be water weight and will occur only because you drastically cut back your caloric intake to bare minimum. This is low-calorie dieting at its worst. You'll lose weight at first, as your glycogen stores are depleted, but then you'll plateau. At that point, your body will go into a starvation mode. This stage, if allowed to go too long, can be very dangerous. This is not a healthy way to lose weight, nor will you be able to keep the weight off long-term.

How about a certain cereal that claims I can lose up to 6 pounds in 2 weeks?
Ahhh, operative words: *up to*. Nevertheless, this is merely another manipulative advertising blitz that will only fuel our obesity rate. Beware of this marketing ploy. For those who are not familiar, Kellogg's, the makers of Special K breakfast cereal, have been running a clever advertising campaign that claims you can "Lose 'up to' 6 pounds in 2 weeks!" *Really?* Pray tell. Well, they claim it's possible by merely replacing two of your main meals by eating two bowls of Special K, along with 2/3 cup of skim milk, plus fruit. They also recommend you eat your third meal (and beverages) as you normally would, along with choosing snacks from fresh fruit, veggies, or one of their very own breakfast bars. Oh, how convenient!

Sorry to say, but this is another instance of incredibly poor nutritional advice, and, at the very least, it's misleading marketing. I was further taken aback when I read the list of ingredients: Sugar is third, and HFCS is fifth! Sugar is expected, *but HFCS in a breakfast cereal?* They can't be serious? Even I am stunned to see where they hide this sweetener! (Post's Raisin Bran cereal is not much better. They claim you can "Lose 10 pounds" in pretty much the exact same manner. Their 4th ingredient is sugar, with corn syrup being fifth.)

Kellogg's has since stopped running that particular ad, but I'd like to know why the FDA and FTC allow this type of deceptive advertising to go on for so long? They know damn well this is nothing but self-serving advertising, not to mention an unhealthy way to lose weight. Based on what you've learned here, would you care to tell me why these proposed diet plans wouldn't work?

Is it because they're basically low-calorie with way too many high GI carbs?
Exactly! I'm so proud of you! Yes, it's not only low-cal with nothing but high GI carbs (the cereal itself with the added sugar and HFCS, plus the skim milk and fruit), but Kellogg's also recommends you eat "normally" for your third meal, along with *whatever* beverages you want. Whoa! Knowing how most Americans eat and drink, that is most certainly asking for trouble. On top of being low-calorie, this diet of high GI carbs will spike your insulin and deplete serotonin, perpetuating cravings, water gain, mood swings, all the many things that come from low serotonin. But, hey, most consumers won't care, because they will feel great while they're on this cereal diet since cereal is a very common comfort food. Just remember, that feeling of emotional comfort is only temporary.

And I suppose if I were to lose some weight, it wouldn't last. Right?

Yes, more than likely, you'll lose a couple of pounds. But it will only be temporarily, as this weight loss is false at best, and due only because you'll be consuming a lot fewer calories. With each "cereal meal" containing as little as 200 calories, including the skim milk and fruit, this is extremely low-calorie. The little weight you lose will be from water and muscle, NOT body fat. The bigger problem is that when you start to eat normally again, you'll gain the weight back, plus 5–10% more. This type of dieting and highly questionable marketing practices has been, and still is, contributing greatly to our obesity epidemic. You must remember: DIETS DON'T WORK!

It's obvious very few give a damn about the consumer. It seems most only care about selling their product. No wonder we're getting so fat! Nothin' but lies!

This low-calorie dieting is certainly old school thinking. But it serves the manufacturers quite nicely in their product promotion. With this type of marketing allowed, it's no wonder people no longer know what to eat. It's no wonder they're fed up. It's no wonder Americans are getting heavier by the minute. This is precisely why I'm writing this book: To educate you, to help you make sense of it all. (Be sure to read my next chapter, "Marketing Scams That Are Making Us Fatter Than Ever!")

I will definitely read it. Now, if I shouldn't drink sodas, what can I drink?

Drink plenty of water—and on a consistent basis. Here are several reasons why: About 60% of body weight is water. The body's water supply is involved in almost every bodily function, including absorption, circulation, digestion, and excretion. Water is the key transporter of nutrients throughout the body. Water is vital for the proper functioning of the body and mental well-being. Water is a natural appetite suppressant and it hydrates your skin. Water is needed to help flush metabolized fat out of the body and regulate body temperature. When you think you're hungry, more often than not, you're just thirsty. Drink water before you get thirsty. Over 75% of all people are constantly dehydrated. 2% dehydration = thirst. 4% = dry mouth. 10% = heat stroke and even death!

Water, at room temperature, is one the best sources of hydration. However, when you exercise, especially if you're involved in a physically demanding sport such as basketball, football, tennis, hiking, jogging, weight training, etc., you'll definitely sweat more, which means you'll lose electrolytes, i.e., sodium, potassium, and chloride. These electrolytes must be replaced to keep the electrolyte concentrations within the body constant. The best way to replace electrolytes is by drinking sports drinks, as they contain various levels of fluid, electrolytes, and carbohydrates. They also contain sugar to provide extra energy. But unless you're an athlete involved in strenuous exercise, beware of how much sugar (and sodium) you're taking in. (Gatorade seems to be the preferred sports drink of most athletes.)

Bottled Water Alert: Bottled water is a six-billion-dollar-a-year industry. Unfortunately, just as with countless other markets, the water industry has its share of less than honorable companies selling their goods. Recent studies show that over 31% of the 52 brands tested were contaminated with bacteria. The low-grade plastic that's most often used is also of serious concern, as it can easily leach toxins such as carcinogens and methyl chloride into the water, and, drinker. So, choose your bottled water wisely. Better yet, consider buying a quality distiller for your home. You can then be guaranteed a much cleaner, healthier water. Plus, it will save you quite a bit of money over the years.

What do you do for quality water?
When I'm out, I buy bottled water. For home use, I double filter. I put a filter on my faucet, and then I run that water through a pitcher with an additional filter. While I am concerned about the quality of water I drink, I also don't want to be completely neurotic. In addition, to insure I drink enough water throughout the day, I use a creatively designed sports bottle that holds just over 2 liters (67.6 oz.) of water. I also drink it at room temp.

I like both of those ideas. I get tired of buying all that bottled water. Plus, I'm sure I don't drink nearly enough. That particular bottle, will help me keep track of how much I drink. But don't you agree that water gets rather boring?
Absolutely. This is why I recommend my clients take quality water and squeeze in a touch of fresh fruit: grapefruit, strawberries, raspberries, lemon, or lime. Adding sliced cucumbers can be equally refreshing. Sometimes I add decaf green tea with stevia. If this is too much trouble, there are several kinds of bottled water that come with a slight hint of fruit flavor. They offer many unique combinations of flavors, and hopefully they're using quality water. Just make sure you select the water that is <u>without</u> the sugar and high levels of sodium. And beware of bottled water that claims it's sugar-free, as it is often artificially sweetened with aspartame! AVOID this deadly sweetener! Again, if something is sweet, you need to ask *why!* Read the ingredient section carefully.

If I should avoid coffee, what then?
If you are truly healthy, which means at the very least—your serotonin is properly maintained, you should not have any desire for coffee. But, if you insist on having it, please drink organic, water-processed *decaffeinated* coffee, as caffeine comes with far too many health risks. Better yet, in lieu of drinking decaf coffee, consider decaf green tea, hot or cold. Green tea has proven to have many wonderful health benefits. It contains powerful antioxidants called catechins (a class of polyphenols) that destroy potentially damaging free radicals in the body. EGCG (Epigallocatechin Gallates) are also found in green tea and are proven to promote normal blood sugar levels, enhancing insulin activity. They are also a clinically proven thermogenic. (And no, the studies clearly show that you do <u>not</u> need the caffeine to reap the thermogenic benefits of green tea.) And because restaurants don't carry "decaf iced tea," order a hot decaf tea, with a pitcher of ice on the side. Again, you need to be creative in your thinking.

22

MARKETING SCAMS THAT ARE MAKING US FATTER THAN EVER!
(Not to mention sick as hell!)

What marketing scams are you talking about?
By far the worst and most despicable marketing scam perpetrated by the food industry is the harsh reality that all processed/junk food is intentionally poisoned by the food manufacturers. They add assorted harmful chemicals, chemicals that the FDA and FTC don't require to be accounted for on the food labels.

Harmful chemicals? **Why would they do this?**
The purpose behind the deliberate and precise manufacturing of these foods is multi-dimensional. First, it's to get us addicted. *Why?* To keep us buying their products. Their next intention is to get us fat—and sick. *Why?* To enrich the medical and pharmaceutical industry. These chemicals, though, are not the only culprits here. The exorbitant amounts of sugar, HFCS, aspartame, etc., that are also added to these foods will equally cause addiction, obesity, depression, heart disease, and many other serious health issues.

This is all dreadfully alarming! It seems the food companies make us sick with their poisoned food while the drug companies make us even sicker with their drugs! I'm finally starting to see the bigger picture here. It really is all about greed and with absolutely no regard for the consumer's health or well-being.
It is hard to accept that it truly comes down to corporate greed, which equals profits, huge profits! All the more reason to avoid processed, refined, canned, fast food, etc., and instead eat only "real" food as often as possible.

Are there other marketing scams I should beware of?
Oooooh, too many to mention! They're endless! Beyond the ruthless reality of what the processed food industry is really about, all one has to do is walk down any grocery store aisle and see just how many scams are intentionally put over on the consumer every day. I actually can't believe there are so many fat-free/low-fat products still on store shelves. And in case you're not aware of this, while most snack foods aren't generally a healthy choice, it's NOT the fat in these foods that is making us fat. It is, however, the highly refined and processed, high GI carbs that these foods are "made from" that is making us fat—and depressed. And, as I stated earlier, these foods may not have fat, but they are LOADED with all types of sugar! And if they're not jammed with sugar, they contain olestra, an indigestible fat substitute that has over 15,000 complaints, due to side effects

reported—ranging from gas, diarrhea, bloody stools, to cramps so severe that people had to be rushed to the emergency room. Once again, please avoid any and all fat-free/low-fat foods! (If the food has fat, watch out for trans fats.)

How awful! I hate to ask what's next?

Well, after the terribly unsuccessful low-fat movement promoted by the FDA and AMA, the next marketing scam launched by the food manufacturers (and eagerly allowed by the FDA, AMA, and FTC) was the low-carb movement, followed swiftly by the net carb/impact carb campaign. Trust me, this is a *multi-billion-dollar marketing blitz* that will frighteningly exacerbate our current rate of obesity! At the same time, it will make those involved even richer!

With the FDA and FTC finally cracking down on more accurate labeling claims, I believe this whole net/impact carbs scheme resulted from this. This is nothing more than another pathetic marketing scam to confuse the unsuspecting and ever-trusting consumer. Just as the fat-free/low-fat foods gave millions of consumers a free ticket to eat those foods in abundance, so will this marketing tactic. The manufacturers would love you to believe this is "carb-friendly" food. All one has to do is read the label to realize this is not true. While some carbs do indeed break down more slowly, affecting blood sugar levels less dramatically, a carb...is a carb...is a carb. At the end of the day, all that matters is how many carbs you've consumed. And—are you active enough to burn up all those carbs?

Moreover, with deception running rampant in marketing and elsewhere, I would *never* believe any of these claims. It's nothing but a ploy. You need to read the label carefully. First and foremost, read the list of ingredients. This will give you a much better idea of what is actually in the product. Then count all carbohydrates, not just their claims of so-called net carbs/impact carbs. Then determine whether or not you want to eat this type of product, and if you can afford to eat it. These are NOT free foods! (Note: Warning letters were *finally* sent to food manufacturers indicating that the phrase "low-carb" is not an FDA authorized term and should not be used.)

Then why is it on most carb products?

Good question, considering it's been used for several years. I think this is another reason why wannabe-carb-friendly food manufacturers transitioned their labels to claim "net carbs/impact carbs."

Why is all this marketing deception allowed?

It's allowed because the food industry is not properly regulated by the FDA or FTC. I also believe that it's another example of "big business" at work. The sugar industry, no matter what form it takes, is ENORMOUS! A lot of people make an extraordinary amount of money from these transactions! It is again only about profits!

Another area to watch out for is the recent candy/chocolate industry packaging their many assorted sweets with "sugar-free" labels. You must be wondering *why* something so deliciously sweet can be sugar-free, aren't you? Well, if you haven't, it's time to start. Remember, if something is sweet, ask <u>why</u>! Those labels proudly screaming sugar-free are not quite accurate. Those products contain a sweetener called maltitol. But because this particular type of sweetener supposedly has a minimal effect on blood sugar levels, the FDA does not consider it a sugar. Consequently, food manufacturers are allowed to make this claim.

How will I know what makes these foods sweet?
I want you to first read the label to see how many sugar alcohols and "other carbs" the product is claiming. Please understand that these are simply an attempt to disguise the sugar. Trust me, nothing that sweet is ever sugar-free, or good for you. Next, look in the ingredient section. This is where you'll find what actually sweetens the product.

What is maltitol?
Maltitol is an alternative sweetener known as sugar alcohols. There are those who claim it's a healthy choice for people with diabetes because it has so little effect on blood glucose and insulin levels. But I, along with many others, disagree. Even if that claim were true, if you plan on indulging yourself with these so-called sugar-free sweets, you might want to have a diaper close by.

A what? A diaper? What are you talking about?
Maltitol is well known for causing bloating, gas, and diarrhea. Ooooh, my goodness! Now doesn't that sound healthy, let alone physically charming. From my personal experience, although I didn't feel the typical sugar buzz after eating one of these sugar-free bars that are instead loaded with maltitol, it did, though, make me crave more of the same. Worst of all, my stomach cramped painfully for hours soon after. It played such extreme havoc on my tummy that I refused to even throw this food down the hill, fearing I'd hurt the unsuspecting little animals that might eat it. Instead, I threw it in the trash.

I can't begin to tell you how sorry I feel for most consumers, with all that the food manufacturers relentlessly throw at them. I'm sure the intentions of most people are to eat healthy, with an occasional treat. And yet, with this type of marketing deception allowed, it's no damn wonder the poor consumer is getting fatter and fatter, even though they're eating nothing but the recommended fat-free, sugar-free, carb-free foods!

I agree. This is why I bought your book. I'm hoping you can help me make better sense of all of this. That being said, what else do I need to watch out for?
If I could walk down any given grocery store aisle with you, I'd show you literally hundreds of similar marketing scams. I'd have to say, however, that the protein and nutrition bars are one of the next biggest scams perpetrated on the consumer. *Why?* Because long before

these bars became so popular, the only people who were eating them were athletes, people who really cared about what they put in their bodies, people who required extra protein. But now these bars are *nothing* but over-hyped, over-priced candy bars!

Oh, no, protein bars? Are you serious? I thought they were so healthy!
This is what the manufacturers would love for you to believe. But these are nothing more than highly processed foods. And are you aware that most of these bars are loaded with sugar, often hidden under several different names other than "sugar?" (Not to mention most health bars are equally high in calories and hydrogenated oils.)

A different name from sugar? Such as?
Those names can range from glycerine, HFCS, corn syrup, fructose, molasses, honey, maltitol, etc. And some have over 25g of sugar in a 2 oz. bar!

But what if the bar claims it's sugar-free?
First, I would highly doubt that claim. Then I'd read the label more closely and look for artificial sweeteners such as aspartame, Splenda/sucralose, neotame, etc. You do not want to eat these. Next, you need to remember that whatever the amount of carbs in the bar, *and they are usually exorbitant amounts*, they will break down into sugar once consumed. And you realize by now what sugar does to insulin levels and how it causes the body to crave more sugar, store fat, etc. Considering how competitive this market is, you need to do more than just read the nutritional labels. Their alleged claims of the amount of sugars within do not distinguish between refined and naturally occurring sugars. You have to read the ingredient list to get more accurate information. The FDA requires all ingredients be listed in order of the quantity used. If you see refined sugars anywhere but the very bottom of the list, this bar would not be a good choice.

Which sugars should I watch for?
All of them. Once again, those sugars can range from glycerin, high-fructose corn syrup, corn syrup, fructose, chocolate, to brown rice syrup, sucrose, maltodextrin, dextrose, maltitol syrup, cane sugar, chocolate liquor, etc. (Chapter 12, "The Many Faces of Sugar," lists many of the names under which sugar is disguised.)

Still doubting me? Okay. But please read on: In 2002, due to the extremely lucrative yet fiercely competitive market, an independent lab revealed that many of the largest protein and health bar manufacturers were caught lying about the actual ingredients in their products. Out of 30 bars tested, an astounding 60% failed to meet their labeling claims! Only 12 bars passed on all criteria.

Are you serious? What were they lying about?
Although they lied about amounts of protein, the most prevalent problem, as well as the most disturbing to me, as the relatively trusting consumer, was not declaring precise and

total amounts of actual carbs. And I am NOT talking about small indiscernible amounts either! I was shocked to see that *half* of all the bars tested *exceeded* their claimed levels of carbs often by staggering amounts! One bar that claimed to be "low-carb" with only 2g of carbs actually had 22g of carbs!

This can't be!

Sorry. Yes, it can. And there's more, I'm afraid. Eight of the top-selling bars also exceeded their *sugar* claims. These protein/health bars on average exceeded their sugar claims by a whopping 8g! That equals 2 tbsp of sugar! Add the additional carbs, with the additional sugar count and what do you have? A Snickers bar with a 300% markup! As bad as this is, it is exactly why I focus on the claim of "total carbs" versus just the sugar claim. *Why?* Because all those lovely carbs they're claiming will *turn into sugar* either way. Yes, some carbs may burn slower, but all carbs are recognized as sugar by the body. And while these companies should be honest, and, if not, then be held liable, I also realize that this particular industry can only survive if it's somehow able to disguise the sugar within.

Caught lying!

This is horrendous! No wonder I'm always craving a lousy protein bar! They're nothing but sugar! This also keeps me from losing weight! This should be illegal!

You're right. This is unacceptable. I find this type of marketing deception absolutely unconscionable! Those behind this deceit should be thrown in jail. Instead, the FDA simply comes in, warns them, possibly fines them, tells them to make the appropriate changes, and then allows them to continue doing business. It's one thing to make an honest mistake; it is entirely another matter to *knowingly* deceive the buying public, especially when it concerns things we are putting into our bodies. And don't believe for one second that these companies are innocent. They know all the tricks when it comes to getting consumers addicted to their products! Once addicted, we are their lifelong customer. No questions asked. So you see, a fine is merely a small part of the marketing game. (Of course, I know that throwing these people in jail is not an option, but the harsh reality is that monetary punishment for these huge companies will *not* deter them from future marketing scams.)

If that isn't disturbing enough, in or around 2001, Atkins Nutritionals was also found guilty of deceptive product labeling on their diet/nutritional bars. The FDA sent out warning letters to them and 16 other companies, informing them that "their bars were misbranded, adulterated, and in violation of the Federal Food, Drug and Cosmetic Act." In addition, in August 2001, Tim Bryson of Alabama filed a class action lawsuit against Atkins Nutritionals for "intentionally misleading with regard to the characterization of the actual number of carbohydrates." Bryson's group won, with a settlement of $100,000. Now I have to ask: If we can't believe the company and/or the man who was the biggest advocate for low-carb eating, *whom can we believe?* The protein bar market is a $1.5 billion market, with Atkins Nutritionals alone having sold more than $30 million worth of bars in the past year. Sadly, it always comes down to profits. Again, buyer beware. I tell my clients they need to look at protein bars as nothing more than expensive candy bars. In fact, I suggest that if they desire this kind of occasional treat, I'd rather have them eat a PayDay candy bar.

A PayDay? Please! You must be joking!

No, not really. For starters, at least with a PayDay you'll know exactly what you're eating. There's no reason for the manufacturer to lie. It is what it is. Plus, all those peanuts will help lower the GI, as they're a good source of fat and high in protein. Funny, I've actually compared a PayDay's nutritional panel to several of the leading protein bars, and the PayDay is often a healthier choice. Personally, I have boycotted protein bars. Not only are they not real food, but their manufacturers have cheated us, lied to us, and all with the greedy intention to get us addicted to their glorified candy bars!

Here's a great example of why you need to "listen" to your body: I woke up one night and thought to myself, "Hmm, a protein bar sure sounds good! *Excuse me? A protein bar?!* It's one o'clock in the morning! Why am I craving a protein bar?" This craving stunned me, particularly because the bars I was eating claimed a mere 2g of carbs, with zero sugar. I hurried into my kitchen to read the label. Though, it of course, claimed only 2g carbs, I knew right then and there these bars were <u>not</u> what they pretended to be. I knew my mind was making me crave this bar for one reason only: SUGAR! It was only a few short months later that I read that all-telling article describing the extent of the deception found in the protein bar industry.

Sugar addiction—like any other DRUG habit!

Why do these companies lie to us and cheat us?

Why? Profits. Huge profits. Don't be fooled, either. These companies know *exactly* what they're doing. So what if they have to pay a $10,000, $100,000, or even $1,000,000 fine. When you're making tens of millions, this is what these major conglomerates call CDB (Cost of Doing Business). In the meantime, their deception is cleverly getting us <u>addicted</u> to their products.

Most consumers buy a protein bar (or any product) that they see heavily advertised. They generally don't even bother to read the nutritional panel. They often blindly trust what the ads and packaging claim. Even if some do take the initiative to read the nutrition facts to make sure these bars are a healthy choice, they won't read them time and time again. So if the consumer's favorite bar happened to be one of those caught lying, and subsequently, had to start claiming the much higher amounts of carbs and sugar, this trusting consumer would never know this. This is because, by then, this consumer is long addicted to these sugar-laden bars and will continue to keep buying them with the greatest of confidence.

Addicted?

Yes. <u>Sugar</u> <u>is</u> <u>ADDICTIVE</u>! The more bars we eat, the more bars we will crave. *Don't believe me?* I knew a man who used to have a $300-a-month protein bar habit! And trust me, this sugar addiction is like any other drug habit.

Food for thought: I feel it is important to include the first few and most crucial ingredients found in two very popular protein bars. The first is PowerBar. I selected this particular bar because it was the forerunner of this booming industry. All the more reason why I was so shocked to read its ingredients. I chose to feature Slim-Fast, as it's the bar that most women gravitate toward, because of the multi-million-dollar advertising campaign Slim-Fast runs each year to promote their weight-loss products. I was equally shocked.

PowerBar/Original/Cookies & Cream Flavor:
Ingredients: High Fructose Corn Syrup with Grape and Pear Juice Concentrate, Oat Bran, Maltodextrin, Milk Protein Isolate, Cookie Bits (Rice Flour, Sugar, Canola Oil, Alkalized Cocoa, Rice Starch, Sodium Bicarbonate, Salt), Brown Rice Flour, Almond Butter, Glycerin, Natural Flavors, Soy Protein Isolate, and so on.

I'm constantly amazed to see what food manufacturers put into our food, but I am further dismayed when it comes to supposedly *healthy* food choices such as protein bars. PowerBar's 1st ingredient is HFCS, the worst sugar there is! Plus, it has a staggering 45g of total carbs! 20g of which are sugar and 23g of "other carbs!" And, after all that, it only has 9g of protein. Based on the primary ingredients, this is a *candy* bar, NOT a protein bar.

Slim-Fast Bar:
Ingredients: High-Fructose Corn Syrup, Milk Chocolate Flavored Coating (Sugar, Partially Hydrogenated Palm Kernel, Palm Oils, Partially Defatted Peanut Flour, Graham Cracker Cookie Pieces, Cocoa Processed with Alkali, Nonfat Milk Whey, Soy Lecithin, Salt, Artificial Flavor), High Maltose Corn Syrup, Soy Protein Isolate, and so on.

I was stunned to see HFCS (and corn syrup) in Slim-Fast's various bars (and their other products). HFCS is also their 1st ingredient, followed by nothing but more sugar and hydrogenated oils! And whey, which is the actual protein, is the 10th ingredient! So the real question is: Do these bars sound like real food, let alone healthy? I think not. My final warning: The better a bar tastes, the more sugar it will contain—and the worse it is for you.

How do you suggest I get my protein?
In lieu of these *processed* protein sources, please find a healthier source. Get your daily protein from real foods such as organic chicken, eggs, duck, lamb, turkey, fermented soy products, fresh cheese, salmon, tuna, mahi-mahi, shellfish, and quality protein powders. But first, please read the following chapter with an open mind for far healthier, kinder, and cruelty-free suggestions. While I sincerely appreciate that this is a very sensitive and personal subject, I hope you will at least be willing to consider other options.

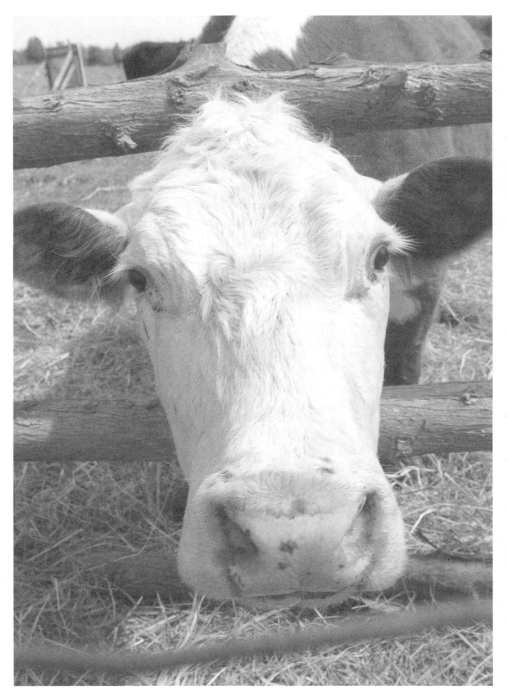

128

23

FROM PETTING ZOO TO DINNER TABLE
When did it go so terribly wrong?

Remember when our parents would eagerly take us to the petting zoo? As children, we were so amazed by these wonderful, loving creatures. We would feed them their favorite treats, reaching out with hope to simply touch them, feel their soft fur, to rub their pink little bellies. And ooooh my, if the little lamb or calf licked us, we would scream with such absolute delight! Ah, the pure joy of petting these many beautiful animals was *sooo exciting!* And this is why I <u>must</u> ask: *When did it go so terribly wrong? When did we go from wanting to love, adore, and care for these innocent animals to EATING THEM? How did it ever become acceptable to serve these animals at our dinner table?*

While I certainly respect the fact that we are each entitled to our own choices, I feel the desperate need to convey my very personal thoughts, concerns, and torment: Are you aware that more than <u>25 BILLION</u> of these once-cherished animals are slaughtered every year in the U.S. for food? Raising animals on factory farms is not only devastating to the land and to the earth, but eating animals (especially red meat) is bad for our health, leading directly to many diseases and illnesses, including heart disease, heart attacks, strokes, diabetes, cancer, and obesity. The astronomical amount of food it takes to raise these millions of farm animals every year could, instead, be put toward ending world hunger. And don't forget that factory farming is responsible for *unfathomable* cruelty and senseless suffering for the animals involved!

First of all, would you eat your dog? Your cat? Your horse? Of course not! So, why do people eat pigs, which are known to be smarter than dogs, and equally as affectionate? And why do people eat cows, which are nothing but gentle, timid creatures? And how could anyone *ever* eat a calf? The calf's only crime in life is to have been born a male. Hence, the severely short and tortured life of a veal calf. The same goes for every other animal, fowl, fish, etc., that we serve on our plates. All innocent creatures. Therefore, who gave us the right to end their lives, simply for our dining pleasure?

Shameful confession...

Personally, for over twenty years I have chosen not to eat most meat. Even though I felt I was doing my best for the rights of these animals, for my health, and Mother Earth, I am ashamed to say I continued to eat, somewhat guilt-free, chicken and turkey. And maybe because I was brought up in the Midwest, where the privately owned, small family farms were run dramatically different from the factory farms I speak of here, but I *genuinely* wasn't aware of any problems with eating eggs, butter, and cheese, as no animal was "killed" in this process. While I recognized chickens and turkeys gave their life for me to enjoy their flesh, it somehow seemed less tragic to eat them than it was to eat a cow, pig, or helpless little calf. I also thought these animals were at least treated *humanely* until the time of their death. Hence, I made it okay to eat them. But I am now tormented by this as well — and dreadfully ashamed.

Why are you suddenly tormented?

Recently, I met Paul. Through our brief encounter, we discovered we were on the same path regarding health. He recommended I read *The Food Revolution* by John Robbins, heir to the "Baskin and Robbins" fortune. He told me it would be one of the most enlightening, and equally disturbing, books I would ever read. Oh, how right he was!

Now, I've long been aware of the horrific life veal calves live, as well as pigs and cows. But never was I aware of how chickens and turkeys are tormented in life, and at death. Based on what I read in Robbins' book, and then doing some additional research, I am repulsed and *infuriated* by what these animals, and all other farm animals, are forced to endure at the hands of "MANKIND!" Moreover, our government doesn't do a damn thing to stop this cruelty! *But why is this allowed?* Cruelty is cruelty. Right? Be it to dogs, cats, children, or the elderly, there are laws to prevent such atrocities! Then please tell me why there aren't laws to protect innocent farm animals, as well?

I feel a frantic need to confess that I was shamefully ignorant when it concerned what farm animals in general go through in their short lives. I guess I wanted to *believe* these animals were at least treated humanely until the time of their death. *But this is not so!* The torture of these helpless animals is truly beyond words! And for those who may not care about how these animals are treated, you should then, at the very least, be concerned about what these farm animals are forced to eat. *And why should this concern you?* Because what these animals eat is then eaten by YOU — when you eat them! The ultimate food chain. And the ole' adage, "You are what you eat" was *never* more true!

What are you saying?

I'm saying that in addition to the many assorted hormones, antibiotics, drugs, etc., that these farm animals are fed to simply keep them alive in otherwise *deadly* conditions, to make them grow faster, produce more babies, eggs, milk, and so forth, their feed also contains everything from downed, diseased, cancerous, unwanted farm animals, to euthanized pets (yes, our beloved pets!) to road-kill, along with every unimaginable animal part! This so-called feed, which is commonly fed to farm animals, is considered an *acceptable* food source by our government!

Ohhh, my god! You've got to be kidding me!

No, but I wish I were! I've long known that 99% of all commercial dog food is made from this absolutely repulsive by-product, but I wasn't aware that the spread of such practice was so commonplace in the farming of animals that go to the marketplace—that market-place being our dinner table! And then we wonder why so many people (and our pets) are getting cancer and other life-threatening diseases? So you see, there are many other concerns here beyond just the cruelty to these farm animals. If we eat them, we are, in essence, eating our own pets and *all the other animals* that were too sick to be properly slaughtered and sent to market! We are eating everything these animals were fed. I don't know about you but, it makes me absolutely ill just thinking about it!

Our government knowingly and willingly allows this horrendous abuse to go on, and they allow this feed to be fed to the farm animals. But they also allow animals that are too sick, too damn ill to even walk to the transport truck, to be sold at auction, where these poor helpless animals are then again dragged, hauled, kicked onto the trucks in any way possible to get them to the actual slaughterhouse! If they survive that final ride, these animals are then *further* brutalized, all while they scream in such absolute terror, trying to run, *desperate* to get away—but they are too weak, too sick! The next time you'll see these helpless, diseased animals will be at your local grocery store, wrapped in cellophane, sold under desensitized names: "Bacon. Ham. Sausage links. Babyback ribs. Hot dogs. Hamburger. Steak. Prime rib. Headcheese. Sweetbread. Saltimbocca. Lamb chops."

This can't possibly be true! How could anyone allow this to go on?

Well, it is true. It is literally HELL ON EARTH for these helpless animals! In addition to refusing to eat cow or pig, and never ever eating veal—knowing now how chickens and turkeys are treated—how they're caged, driven insane, forced to cannibalism, self-mutilation, and worst of all, how they're so brutally killed, I can't possibly keep eating them! These animals were <u>not</u> put here for us to eat them, more so TORTURE them! As for most dairy products, unfortunately, by eating them I support the violence and slaughter of milking cows, and *indirectly*—the veal industry. Therefore, I must find healthier, much kinder substitutes for any products made from cow's milk.

I'm more than eager to rethink my diet, but my husband loves his steak!

Yes, most men love meat. Nevertheless, I *plead with you* to at least watch "Meet Your Meat," an exceedingly disturbing video narrated by Alex Baldwin. Download it for free at meetyourmeat.com. Watch it alone, with your husband, or grab a friend. You will be positively *mortified* by what you see! The images still haunt me months later! Then go to PETA.com (People for the Ethical Treatment of Animals) and veganoutreach.org. Each of these Web sites will show you just exactly what these farm animals go through in their far too short and tortured lives—and at their death. Also, consider reading John Robbins' book. You owe it to yourself to open your eyes to the numerous health risks involved—*and the unthinkable cruelty!* Next, try to get your required protein from assorted real foods, and preferably from plant-based protein sources NOT animal. Unlike years ago, there are unlimited choices when it comes to vegetarian foods. It may require a little more creativity, but it will be well worth it. I promise you.

I thought you said eggs were good for us?
You're exactly right, I did. This is why I must respectfully disagree with vegetarians who claim eggs, butter, and cheese are unhealthy due to their fat/cholesterol content. Sorry, but this is another example of old school nutrition. Our bodies need good dietary fat. Although I will try to get my needed fat from olives, olive oil, tofu, nuts, and avocados, I still believe eggs are crucial to good health, as they are a perfect protein, a perfect food. If I could get my eggs fresh from a local farmer, knowing the laying hens had been fed properly and had not been subjected to abuse, I would most definitely keep eating eggs.

To reiterate, we to need to eat dietary cholesterol to shut down our internal production of same. Therefore, as I begin this new journey, I have to admit that I'm struggling a bit about how to make sure I give my body and mind all that they need <u>without</u> contributing any further to the carnage of these innocent animals.

What about those who say these animals are raised precisely for food?
It's one thing to raise animals for food because we have no other options, but we <u>do</u> have options. To ignore those options, only to make these animals suffer throughout their entire young lives, to then be skinned and/or boiled alive, or dismembered while they're still conscious, is beyond comprehension! I have to ask: *Who is the animal here?* Just because we're at the top of the so-called food chain, just because we don't speak their language, just because we don't feel their pain—*doesn't make it okay!!*

However, I am not about to force my beliefs (or agony) on anyone else. We each have freedom of choice. So if, and only <u>after</u> you and yours watch the video, you still insist on eating meat and dairy, then I highly recommend you buy organic, free-range, antibiotic-hormone-cruelty-free food. It may cost a bit more, but your health is at stake here. It's also about helping put an end to the senseless abuse these animals are made to endure. Buying these foods will <u>hopefully</u>, in some way, help insure that these animals are at least treated humanely, fed properly, and when the time comes, *killed with compassion*. (WARNING: The FDA doesn't currently have regulations on what "free-range" really means. Free-range animals are not necessarily free of exploitation. They certainly aren't running free, enjoying fresh air, or the feel of cool green grass on their little feet as the packaging wants us to believe. Beware of these claims!)

I unquestionably want to do the right thing for the health of my family, while not contributing to the senseless slaughter of farm animals. But how will I know if these animals were truly free-range, without hormones or drugs—and treated humanely?
You won't, unfortunately—not until the FDA enacts stricter guidelines—and then actually enforces them. I can only suggest that you try to shop at stores that focus on healthier, farm-fresh, organically grown foods. Whole Foods, Trader Joe's, Wild Oats, Mother's

Market, and Farm-to-Market are all excellent stores to patronize, if you have one in your area. If not, ask your grocer to please start carrying vegetarian foods.

As terribly disturbing as all of this is, I believe most people are wonderfully compassionate, with no desire to hurt another living thing. We could literally be driven to tears, though, if we focused on all such brutality and misfortune in the world. And, obviously, it goes far beyond farm animals. I also realize that we each have to find our own way. I can only hope that we all do our very best to give of ourselves in whatever way we can to help others—and to STOP cruelty to both mankind and animals!

To conclude this terribly emotional chapter: Please consider becoming a vegetarian. If you aren't willing to go that far, at least cut your meat and dairy intake back to half. If everyone did this, this alone could help stop the suffering of billions of animals! Also, take a moment to write to Congress and demand laws that will protect farm animals. Boycott companies known for cruelty. Refuse to buy fur. Find a way to reach out beyond your own needs. Find a worthy cause. Donate. Don't turn your back. Speak up. Dare to defend others, both man and beast. And, please, at the very least, *eat with a conscience!*

WARNING: KFC is one of the WORST when it comes to torturing animals! From slamming live birds against walls, stomping on them when they refuse to die, to boiling them alive! 850 million chickens are viciously slaughtered each year by KFC! Update: In April 2005, KFC refused to implement kinder, more humane treatment for even one, single helpless bird! *Is this really so much to ask?* It's bad enough they give their life for us, but do they need to be tortured in the process? Absolutely not! Boycott KFC.

McDonald's, the largest purveyor of beef, was under fire for allowing, on average, one in every one hundred cows to go through the assembly line ALIVE! Which means these cows were skinned and dismembered while fully conscious! *Talk about horror!* I can't even begin to grasp the suffering involved here! PETA and other animal rights activists have fought for years to get McDonald's to address this serious issue. McDonald's finally made changes to insure their cattle are killed humanely. With regard to their chickens, unlike KFC, both McDonald's and Denny's have taken critical steps toward implementing CAK (Controlled-Atmosphere Killing), the most humane method of slaughtering chickens. PETCO and Iams are also under fire for cruelty to animals. At the very least, please boycott these and any other companies that use animals for testing or subject them to cruel and inhumane treatment.

CAUTION: The following pages contain photos that are graphic and disturbing. They are, nonetheless, necessary to help convey the brutal truth about the subject at hand. Hopefully, they are thought-provoking. Please understand, though, these images are merely a *glimpse* into what really goes on behind the scenes of transforming these sweet and completely helpless farm animals into food.

Chickens, hung by their feet, ready to be slaughtered—alive!

A veal calf, lying hopelessly in his crate, is _NEVER_ allowed to move!

A baby pig, screaming and crazed, desperate to free herself!

The transition from farm animal to food—a pig being skinned.

A downed cow, too ill to even walk, but being prepared for slaughter.

Cow parts. What more can be said?

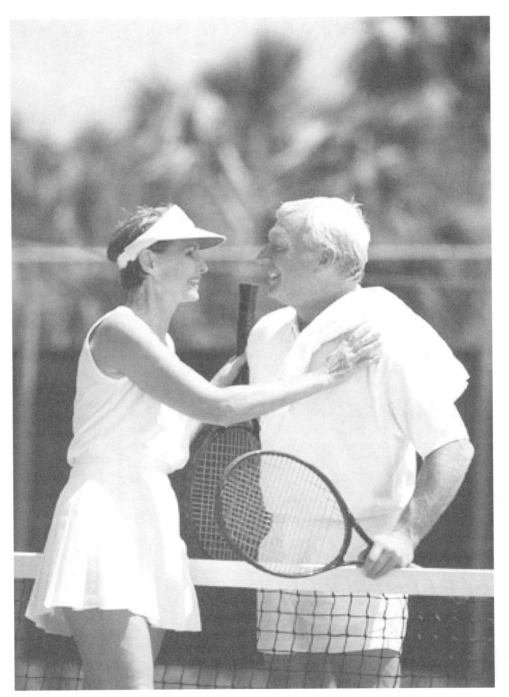

24

EXERCISE & ITS MANY GLORIOUS BENEFITS

Besides eating less meat and dairy, and eliminating sugar, processed food, and caffeine, what else do you recommend for this healthy lifestyle?
You must start some sort of exercise routine, even if it's just 45 minutes a day. (In a perfect world, it would be 60 minutes, *especially* for children!) And please don't tell me you don't have the time. Everyone has 45 minutes to devote to themselves. If you don't, you need to rethink your life. Some believe working out or having a trainer is a "luxury." It is not. If you want to be healthy and be around for your family, you must take care of *you!* God knows women are never short on time when it comes to getting their nails done, going shopping, or socializing over a decadent latte. And men, you always find the time to watch TV, golf, play video games, or hang with the fellas. So please, please, please, make the time to exercise. You will feel *soooo* much better about yourself—mentally, emotionally, and physically! There are few things in life that will return so much as regular exercise.

What do you suggest?
There are so many things you can choose from. It can be as easy as playing ball with your children, going for a brisk walk with your dog, swimming some laps, riding your bike, surfing, skiing, dancing, playing golf, taking up yoga, or working in the garden. Maybe you're healthy enough to play tennis, handball, shoot hoops, kickbox, or lift weights. The key is: Do anything to get your body moving! Do it alone, with a friend, or with your spouse. Remember, competition is great for the soul. It motivates and inspires.

Why is exercise so important?
There are so many glorious benefits from exercising. For starters, exercise is a fantastic way to naturally stimulate the production of serotonin, norepinephrine, and endorphins, all of which help alleviate depression and mood swings, while improving sleep and libido. It suppresses your appetite and lowers your risk for heart disease, osteoarthritis, osteoporosis, type 2 diabetes, and other serious health conditions. Exercise slows the signs of aging, boosts growth hormone and metabolism, as well as strengthens the cardiovascular system. Exercise builds lean muscle and strong bones. And the more lean muscle you have, the more calories/fat your body will burn—and it will burn them long after you've stopped exercising. I can't say this enough: The most effective way to maintain long-term fat loss, to achieve a lean, yet strong, healthy body with minimal fat is to build lean muscle mass. The right combination of a healthy diet and living a healthy lifestyle will further insure your success. (An SES will help you adhere to both.)

Will exercise help get rid of my cellulite?

Weight training, cardio, and a healthy diet are the best ways to get rid of cellulite. Stop wasting your time, money, and hopes on those expensive and most definitely useless creams that promise you leaner, smoother thighs and buttocks by simply slathering on their magic potions. They do not work! If you want to get rid of that lumpy and unsightly skin, *live a healthy lifestyle*. That means a diet that is devoid of sugar, artificial sweeteners, damaged fats, refined and processed foods. Focus instead on low GI carbs, good fats, quality proteins, plenty of water, and consistent exercise.

What do you do to stay in shape?

I started weight training way back in 1977 at the age of 18. I've tried many different things along the way, but have found that resistance training is what allows me to truly create the physique I want. I believe it's the most effective, most efficient way to build lean muscle, strong bones, deplete fat stores, and actually *sculpt* my body. To reiterate, weight training has proven to not only dramatically slow the signs of aging, but it has also been shown to *reverse* the aging process. (BTW: I train just as much for my mental state of mind as I do for my physical body.)

How often do you train?

I'm fortunate to maintain my physique with no more than 2 or 3 days of weight training a week, devoting approximately an hour per session. Considering I've been in and out of gyms for 28 years, I know exactly what I need to do. I know what works best for my body. I also push myself hard throughout each session. With very little rest, I get my heart rate up as well.

Is 2 to 3 days enough?

For me, yes. I prefer no less than 3 days, especially for what that does for me mentally, but I easily get by with 2 because I'm basically wanting to maintain versus lose weight. I suggest that you commit to no less than 3 days of weights per week. You'll see much quicker results and this will help keep you motivated. If you can push it to 4, even better. Both men and women can use that fourth day to focus on key problem areas.

Now I know there are those who train 5, 6, or even 7 days a week, with 2 or 3 hours per session. No, thanks. I want a life outside the gym, just as I know you will, too. Don't get me wrong, though, I'd rather see people in the gym making an effort than not at all. The more intense type of training is rarely necessary, unless you're a professional athlete, competing, or your diet is not as it should be. I just don't want this to discourage those who are starting out. Believe me, you will not have to spend every waking moment in the gym to get a strong, sleek, healthy, and sexually appealing body. On the other hand, with so few days, you'll have to make sure your workouts are focused, intense, and consistent. You'll also have to commit to a healthy diet and lifestyle, if you sincerely hope to achieve your fitness goals. One will not work without the other. And to insure you eat this healthy diet, you must make sure your serotonin is balanced.

Do you still train others?

Yes, but most of my work now is dedicated to consulting. However, when I do train others, I prefer to train my female clients in pairs. For one thing, having a partner gives them a comfort level. It also motivates them to show up on a regular basis, as they know someone else is counting on them. It's far easier to cheat yourself when the only ones you have to answer to are yourself and your trainer. Your partner will be relying on you, and vice versa. This greatly increases both your level of commitment and your dedication. Picking a good workout partner is, therefore, equally important. Find a friend who is relatively in the same shape as you are, with similar fitness goals, and who is reliable.

How often do your ladies train?

I'm proud to say that, through the many years of training, I've been able to help my clients achieve some exceptional results based on a mere 2 days a week. And that's with only one hour per session. You must realize, though, that this is *bare minimum*, it was often a selling feature to those women who either did not want to spend any more time than that in the gym, or simply couldn't afford it. Rather than lose them as clients, I chose instead to squeeze the usual minimum of 3 days into 2. (Having a partner also helps reduce the cost.) So, for a mere 2 hours of weight training per week, these women physically changed their bodies. Together, we've sculpted them new body parts.

New body parts?

While the body parts are there, of course, I simply help my clients *improve* those parts—to sculpt them and redefine them. This is why it's so important to hire a qualified trainer. Example: Many of my clients—through their dedication, along with my gentle driving force—created strong, sexy new shoulders that before simply sloped downward. Where once their arms were flabby and loose, they are now firm, tight, and so beautifully defined. Some had no fannies, and now, after lots of hard work, they actually have a bottom, one that is nicely rounded, lifted, and, more importantly, one they are proud of. *(What more motivation does a woman need than that?)*

Through my clients' hard work and perseverance, they have developed firmer, more defined arms and buttocks; stronger, sexier backs and chests; shoulders that are strong and sculpted; smaller sleeker waists; tighter abs; significant loss of body fat and much better overall body composition. On top of all that, they also achieved much healthier mental attitudes. My role as their trainer is merely to guide them, motivate them, encourage them, push them harder than they'd push themselves, and to do all of this *without* injury.

Denise, one of my recent, most dedicated clients, once told me she had some girlfriends who were raving about her new physique. Then, as some sadly will do, they tried to say that her phenomenal shape was due solely to the fact that she could "afford a trainer." Denise quickly responded by saying, "What do you think, this comes easy—without any effort on my part? Hell, *this* (as she pointed to her body) takes HARD work! And while I choose to have a trainer, my trainer is <u>not</u> the one doing the work! She's not the one doing the damn exercises. I am!" Denise was absolutely correct. It is the clients who do the work. I am merely the driving force. I was very proud of her for saying this, because no matter who the client is, their results are only as good as the amount of effort they're willing to put into it. And while Denise teasingly liked to kick and scream at most of my demands, she kicked ass in the gym!

It takes hard work!

Denise, as well as her partner Lisa, were both exceptionally committed to staying healthy. They gave 110% when they were in the gym. They rarely missed a session, and they let me do my job. Combine all these fundamental elements, and you get results. They looked unbelievable for any age, but especially since, at that time, Denise was 46 and Lisa was 51. They were truly inspiring, as well as being a tremendous walking advertisement for me. Thus, for all of those who say they're too old or it's too late, DON'T BELIEVE IT!

Considering there are far too many women who are unhappy with their bodies, it's impera- tive that I share this story: One glorious summer day, Lisa was headed to enjoy the beach with her daughter and a few of her college buddies. As they wandered down the shore, Lisa noticed they were walking quite a ways behind her. Though she felt a bit left out, she thought maybe her daughter and the others were embarrassed to be seen with her. After all, she was "the mother"—and 30 years older than they were. Only when she jokingly mentioned it later to her daughter did she find out the real reason. Lisa was told they were keeping their distance because "she looked so much better in a bikini than they did!" It was *they* who were embarrassed to be seen next to her! Lisa, being the humble woman that she is, was stunned by this admission. She was, nevertheless, flattered—and proud of her accomplishments. As well she should be. Lisa's worked out her entire life, and she, too, allowed me to kick her little butt in the gym weekly!

Now, can you imagine that at 51 years of age you could look better than a group of 20-year-olds and to do this in a BIKINI? Well, imagine it! And then believe it, because it's possible if you're willing to make the effort.

I'm impressed and further motivated. What are your goals when training yourself?
At 5'11", strong, but a lean size 4, my goal is to maintain my muscle mass and definition, keep my body fat around 12–13% while maintaining my weight between 138–142 pounds. This is where I'm most comfortable. Each of you will need to find what is right for "your" body. My goal is modest: Maintain. I currently weigh 140 with 11.8% body fat, and my LBM is 88.2%. (12% is considered "essential" body fat for women.)

How do you maintain and define your muscle mass?
I achieve this by training each body part directly once a week within 2 or 3 sessions. I do 3 different exercises per body part, no less than 3 sets each, with a range of 12–18 reps per set. I move from one set to the next. I may superset. (2 antagonistic exercises. Examples: back/chest or quads/hams.) Or I may tri-set. (3 exercises that complement each other.)

After the first set, I steadily increase the weight or I might drop-set. Either way, I always go to muscle fatigue. My routines are never the same. I prefer free weights over machines, but still combine both. I hydrate often. My workouts are intense, focused, with minimal rest. No more than an hour per session. And, I use this quiet time to do my affirmations, to empower my mind/spirit at the same time I empower my body. So, to those who fear they'll have to live in the gym to get a strong, sexy, and healthy body, you will not. You just need to find what works best for *your* body.

What do you mean by train directly?

In resistance training, you'll generally focus on 2, 3, maybe even 4 primary muscle groups per session. As you train those primary muscles, secondary muscle groups are also being worked. Example: When you train your back, your secondary muscle group would be your biceps. *Why?* Because as you do exercises designed to work the back, it requires biceps to activate those muscles. Another example: If you're training chest, the secondary muscle group is triceps. Same premise. While I focus on training each body part directly at least once a week, I'm actually working those muscles several times, but with different intensity and routines. (This is merely a brief overview. To get maximum results and to avoid injury, please hire a qualified trainer to assist you.)

Once again, the key point here is that it would not be so easy to achieve my diverse fitness goals if I were unable to control my diet. Diet plays a MAJOR role in my (and your) success in the gym. My healthy lifestyle makes everything I do in the gym go a thousand times further. And maintaining my serotonin is precisely *why* I'm so easily able to adhere to a *healthy lifestyle*. Keep in mind, maintenance is a lot easier than when you first begin. I tell my clients it's like putting money in the bank: The more you invest in your health early on, the more you get in return as the years go by. I'm reaping the many benefits of having stayed physically active throughout my adult life. But no matter when you decide to start, please do not get discouraged. You have to first *want* to make a change. Next, you have to believe in yourself. Once you realize that it's not a quick fix, that it's instead about living an overall healthy lifestyle, all things are possible. Please, take the challenge. There's no better time to start than right now!

What do you do for cardio?

I don't have a strenuous cardio routine, nor have I ever. (I admit this goes against what most experts recommend.) With such low body fat, a strong heart and exceptional blood panels, my body seems to do well without it. That having been said, I get my cardio in several other ways. When I weight train, I warm-up with about 5 minutes on a treadmill. Then I move through the session with little to no rest. And for as long as I can recall, I've eagerly devoted an hour a day, 6 to 7 days a week, to exercising and training my many beloved dogs, which, of course, would include playful sprinting and running. For the last two years, I've also helped care for a beautiful, but sadly neglected horse named Mavros. The owner basically abandoned him and never paid his board, which led to the stables unfairly putting Mav on lock down. So, six nights a week I would sneak in after hours to get him out. I'd briskly walk him around the grounds, and when I'd take him into the arena where the sand is rather deep, I'd occasionally jog with him. All of this got my heart rate up—and his, too. More importantly, I did this *alongside* Mav, <u>not</u> on his back. (Thankfully, Mav now has new owners who love him dearly! Vince and Mike are kind enough to let me still help care for him. And, because there's almost no better place I'd rather be, I happily visit the sweet boy every Sunday.)

For those who choose to do a more serious type of cardio, my recommendation would be kickboxing. In addition to the highly effective cardio aspect, it's a tremendous way to release stress and promote mental stimulation. Plus, it teaches great defense moves for women. I would, however, limit it to 3 times a week due to its intense nature. For those who aren't up for it, a brisk walk, hiking, or swimming is perfectly acceptable. Bottom line: Get out in the fresh air and get your body moving on a regular basis, and for at least 45 minutes. You must remember, each of us are different, with different metabolisms, body types, and fitness goals. My cardio routines are what work best for "my" body. You'll need to find the type of cardio, as well as the intensity required, for *your* body to either burn fat or to simply maintain your weight. I believe, though, that the key to reaching your fitness goals is by living a "healthy lifestyle." It's also a process. So, don't stress over the excess weight, as those who are thin are most definitely not always healthy.

When does my body actually start to burn fat?
Carbs, stored in the body as glycogen, are the body's preferred choice for fuel. They're readily available and quickest to burn. (I discuss this further in chapter 30.) But it takes about 20 minutes of moderate to intense aerobic exercise before your body will shift from burning carbs to a slower burning, far more efficient fuel. That fuel is body fat, i.e., free fatty acids. This is why you need to carefully monitor your cardio, more so the *intensity* of your cardio. Make it work for you, giving you the best results possible. (FYI: 1lb of body fat = 3,500 calories. To lose 1lb of fat, you must burn or reduce your calories by 3,500. Most effective method to lose body fat long-term? Build LBM and eat healthy!)

How do I stay motivated to exercise?
Boredom is one of the biggest reasons why people either don't ever start a workout program, or why they eventually quit. The key to your potential success is rather simple: *Do things that give you pleasure.* Personally, my body and mind have always thrived on training with weights. And my simplistic walk/jog/sprint routines allow me to do things that I love to do. At the same time, I'm giving these beautiful animals the love, attention, and exercise they also need to stay healthy and happy.

While I'm on the subject of reasons why people don't commit to exercise, cost is another leading excuse. To this, I kindly suggest you look over your monthly expenses and adjust them accordingly. Most women could easily afford a gym membership (along with a train-er) if they gave up their weekly manicure/pedicure and Brazilian bikini wax, hair extensions, daily lattes and bagels, and their weekend Cosmopolitans. After all, it's about choices and priorities. Now, I'm not saying that having "me time" or keeping yourself groomed isn't important. Both are, *without a doubt.* But the senseless time and money some women spend on these things, more so acrylic nails, is absurd. Trust me, I know. I wore those silly-ass nails for several years and wasted far too much time and money getting them fixed. Never mind the toxic fumes I inhaled and the harmful chemicals absorbed into my bloodstream via the nail bed.

To be honest, I found it rather fascinating to observe the type of women who frequented the nail salons. I was amazed at how overweight 90% of them were, and yet their nails were absolutely flawless. I often wondered if these women thought that this was all that mattered? Why did these women choose to ignore the rest of their body? Did they not care? If so, why not? Had they simply given up? Were they happy? Content? What about their lover, spouse, or potential new man? Did they think he only cared about long, beautifully sculpted nails? I can't help but try to respectfully analyze this: Is it because these women have total control over their nails, whereas with their diets (and subsequently their bodies), they do not? Maybe. Nonetheless, ladies, please adjust your spending so as to afford regular exercise. It's the one thing that will have a much longer-lasting, far more rewarding and powerful effect on your entire body and mind!

As for you men, you will need to do likewise. If you were to cut back on your double espressos, beers, martinis, video games, golf, and nights out with the boys, you, too, would have more than enough money to afford a gym membership, with a trainer.

You're right. It's all about priorities. I can cut back on my lattes, nail appointments, and either shave or do my own waxing. Now, how do you feel about jogging?
First of all, great attitude! Secondly, I don't recommend jogging for my clients, more so long distance—and most definitely not for my older clients. There are many other wonderful ways to get your cardio rather than the harsh impact on your joints/organs that comes with jogging. Most gyms have elliptical trainers. They offer a smooth, non-impact, and effective cardio workout. You can also ride a stationary or street bike. Swimming is another great option. Or lace up and punch a heavy bag. Or...turn up the music and MOVE!

Can I just do cardio and achieve good results?
If you want to really sculpt your body, cardio alone is not enough. I watch so many people in the gym running endlessly on the treadmills. They run literally forever, and yet, over the months—sometimes years—I never see any difference in their bodies. Besides the fact that you must eat a healthy diet to see changes, you also need *resistance* on your muscles to "sculpt" them. In addition, having LBM is one of the best ways to burn fat/calories, as muscle is remarkably active—and 24 hours a day. Compare this to when you raise your metabolism through jogging; its fat burning benefits may last only 6 hours after you're done. So, which sounds more effective to you? I know I want my body to work *with* me, not against me. Having lean muscle mass gives me numerous health benefits, long after I leave the gym.

CARDIO ALERT: Many experts are now saying that the high level of stress that most cardio exercises have on your heart is too much. Thus, the stimulation brought on by intense cardio is actually breaking the body down, rather than building it up. Case in point: How many times do we hear about the athletic 45-year-old man dying of a heart attack while he's out jogging? Once again, I've <u>never</u> done a regular, high impact cardio workout. My body does fine with weight training, daily brisk walks, along with my healthy eating habits and lifestyle. All of this, though, is greatly dependent upon me properly maintaining my serotonin. (On a personal note: With the right lover, sex can also be a wonderfully stimulating workout. I like to call it "playfully aggressive." Between the sexual arousal and the endorphins kicked into high gear—you will most certainly get your heart rate up—and hopefully for several hours.)

Ooh! I like that idea! So, what would your perfect workout program include?
It would include 8 hours of quality sleep, balanced nutrition, 5–6 smaller (but definitely adequate) meals per day, plenty of water, 3-4 days a week of weight training, with 45 minutes of mild cardio 4 days a week. Remember, cardio does not have to be that intense to reap its benefits. Just get your body moving—and ENJOY it! Finally, please devote 30 minutes a day to enrich your mind and spirit—be it through meditation, yoga, affirmations, etc.

Body, mind, AND soul! Perfect! Now, how do you keep your stomach so flat?
How? Simple. Balanced serotonin levels. This makes it *soooo* easy to control my eating habits. As I've said a dozen times, there is absolutely no effort whatsoever for me to eat healthy. I never feel cheated, deprived, or hungry. I'm sure this is completely the opposite of all the diets you've tried. Those diets not only left you hungry, but they also made you radically irritable. And who wouldn't be, when you're deprived of food. An added bonus of healthy serotonin levels is that while you're losing the weight, your mood will be better than ever. And those who have been gracious enough to notice my efforts (in particular the women), assumed that I either did not eat or that I did a ton of ab work. I hated to disappoint them, but I told them I never go hungry, I never feel deprived, and I only hit my abs directly twice a week. (*Indirectly* is another story. If you exercise with proper form, your abs are most often being worked.) Furthermore, no one could ever do enough crunches to keep their waistline lean and without that typical little (or not so little) pooch if they don't eat healthy. I don't care how intense or how many ab exercises you do, diet is crucial to achieving a lean body with *minimal* body fat, which then greatly contributes to lean muscle definition, abs and otherwise. My abs are the direct reflection of my d-i-e-t.

Didn't you say our stomach is our insulin gauge?
Yes, you're exactly right. My stomach, just like yours, is what most accurately reflects my eating habits. Go ahead. Measure yours right now. This is what you need to pay very close attention to. My waist, *my insulin gauge,* ranges from 24" to 25". It is indeed the best indicator of how healthy I'm eating. Or not. My stomach is, hence, the first place I'll see the effects of eating poorly. I then make an immediate adjustment. I recommend you do the same. It's often a very easy and effective method of controlling your weight.

144

A perfect example of our waist being our insulin gauge is easy enough to observe if you look at the many girls and young women who wear the latest fashion: skin tight, low-riding pants. Sadly, for most of those who wear them, their little tummies bulge out, rolls of fat hang over, and then, on top of that, they wear a belly jewel, which draws even more attention to their pudgy and not so flattering waistline. Not to mention, the very design of these pants completely flattens out even a nice full rounded bottom, merely adding insult to this already unsightly fashion statement. Maybe this is indeed the "style," but I can't believe these young ladies think this looks appealing. Do they not look in the mirror, to see how they look from all angles? Not only is this not attractive, but my primary concern is that these ladies are so young and already headed for serious weight problems. For starters, their waistline reflects their risk of developing diabetes. It doesn't take a genius either to know *why* they're getting so fat, so young. Rarely do I ever see one who doesn't have a large soda in hand with a bag of chips, happily munching away. (As for the boys, they're hiding their weight under all those baggy, hip-hop clothes.)

You just described my 15-year-old daughter to a T. All she eats is cereal, Hot Cheetos, bagels, and sodas! She's gained 15 pounds, she's moodier than ever, but no matter how much I try to help her, she refuses to listen. What can I do?
Once again, take what you've learned here and put it to use. People need to realize that no matter one's age, low serotonin effects most of us in one way or another. Whether it's cravings, weight gain, mood swings, depression, PMS, or ADD, I suggest you get your daughter on an SES to help control both her cravings and her mood swings. Furthermore, stop buying all those high GI carbs. *Why tempt her?* Also, try to get her motivated to start working out. Take her with you to the gym, if at all possible.

Are you saying healthy levels of serotonin will help control her angry outbursts?
Absolutely. One of the most common side effects of serotonin fluctuating drastically is fits of rage, emotional outbursts, and being quicker to anger. This comes from ingesting too much sugar, which then spikes your insulin, followed by your serotonin soaring—then plummeting. Most women know that feeling that suddenly comes from out of nowhere, yet it is all-consuming. We feel absolutely fine one moment, but the very next second, we feel our head ever so slooowly spin around. Our claws come out. Our seething words cut with precision, like that of a rusty, jagged knife. Our facial expressions alone, could kill. We are ready to literally rip the flesh off anything that moves. Most often it is our unsuspecting mate. We know our anger isn't warranted, but we can't stop it! As quickly as this angry-terribly-unattractive-outburst takes us over, it's gone. Whew! We take a deep sigh and quietly pray we will be ignored, more so *forgiven* for this irrational outburst. *But hold the laughter, gentlemen!* Before you dare judge us, you, too, are more than capable of these fits of psychotic rage. God knows I've dated more than a few men who are a perfect case study of this scenario. But man or woman—it's not a pretty sight. Knowing what I know now, I at least know where this unjustified anger comes from.

You are so right! Unfortunately, I witness this drastic mood shift not only in my daughter, but also in myself and my husband. While men so often and unfairly accuse women of being premenstrual or simply a bitch, I have often wondered what *their* excuse was. Thank you so much for explaining this!

Speaking of menstrual cycles, it's imperative that I comment on the many young women who allow their doctors to put them on the pill. If you're wondering why you feel so bloated, fat, and irritable, well, don't look any further. I know birth control is a very personal decision, but the pill comes with numerous health risks—weight gain is merely one. Stroke is yet another. Please consider another form of birth control. Then, when menopause comes knocking, please understand, ladies, that it is <u>not</u> a disease. Menopause is a *natural* stage of the aging process. It's perfectly natural to want to treat your symptoms, but beware of the pharmaceutical industry's proposed HRT (Hormone Replacement Therapy). These drugs have proved to be deadly! While the drug companies promised aging women far better health, the studies that came back proved to be extremely alarmingly! Women who were on HRTs were actually having more heart attacks, more heart disease, more strokes, more fatalities! At the very least, these women were heavier, more bloated than ever before! All you have to do is look around at most women over 50 to see the results of those purported wonder drugs.

But please! Is anyone *really* that surprised? I mean, after all, these drugs are NOT natural, they are synthetic! Premarin, *once a $3-billion-a year drug,* contains over 50 horse estrogens from pregnant mares' urine. *Horse urine?* How could anyone have ever believed this would work in a woman's body? Horse urine is not only completely foreign to the female body, but the entire medical concept is absolutely insane! As if that isn't frightening enough, the pharmaceutical companies cruelly abuse these beautiful horses for years, slaughtering their foals immediately. Then, after they've served their purpose, the mares are also killed. Please, ladies, BOYCOTT THIS DRUG! Treatment for menopause should focus on treating your symptoms. Research your options. If you need estrogen replacement, use "real" hormones. And real hormones do *not* come from horse urine! I'm speaking about *natural bioidentical hormones* such as estradiol, estriol, estrone, testosterone, and progesterone. Find a doctor and compound pharmacist who are trained in bioidentical hormone therapy.

I started getting migraines and hot flashes last year. My blood work confirmed that, at 39, I was going into early menopause. My doctor insisted I go on the pill to help balance my low levels of estrogen. In less than three weeks, I gained 10 pounds! And it was all in my stomach, like a big fat water balloon! And while I know I need to lose weight, this additional water weight has made me nearly crazy! I feel so awful! Is this what you're talking about?

If you gained this weight since the time you started taking the pill, then I'd say it's more than likely. This is another perfect example of why I say it's important to learn to think for yourself and to follow up with some research. Don't let your doctor put you on the pill, HRT, or any other medication without weighing the countless risks. And here's where you'll definitely have to listen to your body. While your doctor will run the appropriate tests, finding the right balance with the various bi-hormones takes time and patience. But don't ignore your body when things don't feel right. Talk to your physician.

Bioidentical hormone therapy versus DEADLY drugs!

Are you taking them?

Yes, minimally, for just over a year. I was 42, however, when blood tests confirmed I was in perimenopause. I was shocked! Suddenly I felt so old! Nonetheless, all my primary caregiver could offer me was HRT. No, thanks! I chose to endure the weekly migraines and occasional hot flash. By age 44, my migraines and hot flashes were far more frequent, along with joint pain—and I wasn't feeling as sexually motivated. I knew I had to do something. Thankfully by now, though, I had a new doctor, an ob/gyn, Dr. Stephanie McClellan. She's a highly educated and compassionate doctor, one who always greets you with the most genuine hug, followed by really *listening* to you. Due to my symptoms, she suggested a low dose of the pill. But considering even at 16 years of age I had refused to take the pill due to its many risks, I wasn't about to start. I had read about "natural bioidentical hormones." They were my preferred and <u>only</u> choice.

Between my doctor and my compound pharmacist, they designed a regimen consisting of testosterone, progesterone and estrogen, all bioidentical hormones. Finding the right dose for the testosterone was easy. The estrogen and progesterone proved to be a little more difficult. Considering my body type, i.e., tall, athletic, minimal body fat, and naturally small breasts, is the type that produces and sustains with very little estrogen, any change in estrogen is therefore felt immediately. I tried several forms, but each one came with side effects, side effects I was fortunate enough to tune into and tell my doctor about. She then quickly pulled me off of them.

What were the side effects?

I was first put on an estrogen pill. Within 10 days, I gained weight around my waistline, and my stomach was terribly bloated. I suddenly felt fat as a pig! (Eating too much soy can have the same effect, so beware.) And, as all women know, feeling F-A-T will no doubt lead to frustration and bitchiness! I also felt a bit hyper—not caffeine hyper, just a little wired. I knew the only thing I had changed was adding the hormones. I decided to check my blood pressure. Sure enough, it had skyrocketed from my average 115/60 to a shocking 165/75! (I realize the bottom number is more critical, but I still did not like the fact that my systolic pressure had shot up nearly 50 points.) Based on the research, I knew that about 8% of women have this reaction to oral estrogen. I stopped taking it without delay. Next, my doctor asked me to try an estrogen vaginal ring. Now that looked and felt like a child's play toy. I couldn't imagine being intimate with a man with that inside of me. Wow! *Talk about a distraction!* Besides being particularly awkward, it immediately made my stomach bloat, along with painful cramps. I pulled that, as well. I was then given an estrogen-based cream to use vaginally, with a varying dosage. Thus far, this option seems to work best for my body. As for the progesterone, it was actually triggering migraines. Each time I took a dose, the next day I had a migraine. Both my doctor and compound pharmacist agreed I would do fine with the minimal dose: 50mg once a day, for x-amount of days, cycled every six months. Although my migraines are not yet fully controlled, my joint pain is gone, no more hot flashes or night sweats, my strength in the gym is back to where it used to be, and my sexual passion is back in full glorious bloom.

Are these bioidentical hormones really worth the effort?
It does indeed take time and patience to find the combination that works best for your individual body, but if your hormones have declined, they're most certainly worth the effort. My goal is to help protect my female health, my heart, mind, body, and yes, my sexuality, via the bi-hormones. But there must be a proper balance. This requires tuning in to your body, *listening to your body*. Work closely with your doctor and compound pharmacist. And be sure they start you on them one at a time so you can monitor any possible side effects. But whatever you choose to do, please ladies, do NOT accept that awful-bloated-tummy-bitchy-dried-up-sleepless-always-tired-can't-remember-nothin'-lonely-lack-of-passion-sexual-desire as normal! It is not. Nor does it have to be part of the aging process! (An SES is the perfect complement to bi-hormones.)

Anything would be better than the way I feel now. My mood has certainly been horrendous—never mind the extra weight! I'll set up an appointment first thing. What about my husband? Can he benefit from bi-hormones?
Yes. After 40, men should be concerned with maintaining their hormones, primarily testosterone. A testosterone deficiency is exhibited by a diminished sexual drive and difficulty in getting and/or maintaining an erection. Lack of energy, loss of height, bone mass and muscle tissue, plus, being a bit more irritable are also common. But not all men lose testosterone. Some men don't get depressed; they maintain strength, energy, and muscle mass, and remain sexually active until the day they die. Either way, I would highly recommend that men over 40 get their blood work done to make sure their hormones are in order. Just as with women, bi-hormones are their best solution.

Migraines—*taking me to my knees!*

Didn't you say serotonin controls migraines? If so, why do you still have them?
Another excellent question. I have fewer migraines since I've been taking an SES, and even fewer since I started taking bi-hormones, but they're not yet gone completely. So I did some research. I found an extensive list of foods that may be triggering them. (Aspartame, alcohol, caffeine, sugar, and anything else that depletes serotonin can also trigger them. None of which I consume, though.) So, if your serotonin and hormones are indeed balanced, yet you still get a migraine, then I suggest you research the various foods. If, after that, and a migraine still comes pounding, do *not* take any pharmaceutical drugs to control them. *Why?* Because those drugs will cause other illness in your body—and they will also further deplete your serotonin, perpetuating even more migraines. It is a vicious cycle.

But the pain is absolutely excruciating! What can I do?
Trust me, I know this pain only too well. Mine feel like I have an ice pick being driven deep into the right side of my head. And, they tend to last no less than 12 hours. Through the course of trying to not only eliminate them, but also lessen the pain and duration, I've found that an ice wrap, one of those Velcro ice headbands that allowed me to secure it tightly around my head, works wonderfully to lessen the pain. And the colder, the better. Then I take an Alka-Seltzer extra strength cold medicine (minus the aspartame), two sublingual B-12/B-6, crawl into bed, slide my little black mask over my eyes to block out the light, make a conscious effort to slow my breathing down, and then—I simply lie still and *pray* for relief to come. Sometimes the pain is so unbearable I cry like a baby! As any woman knows, this, too, can somehow relieve the pressure. Moreover, believe it or not, ladies, *sexual stimulation*, whether flying solo or with the tender touch of your lover, has proven to help alleviate pain. Maybe it's simply the act of distraction, combined with the fact sexual arousal induces the release of our body's natural pain reliever, endorphins, but it works. I find this rather ironic, because so often you hear men complain that women avoid sex by saying they "have a headache." Truth be told, S-E-X can actually lessen their pain. But, again, only with the right partner, and most definitely, with the utmost compassion.

Observation: It's been over two months since I've cut out all poultry and cheese, which means I've added a lot more soy products to my diet. My migraines are now down to one every 60 days—and they strike with half the intensity. Better yet, I'm no longer feeling the need to take Alka-Seltzer! (Other than an occasional antibiotic, Alka-Seltzer is the only med/drug I ever take. I encourage you to first try plain baking soda.) I'm also down to bare minimum with the hormones, with no estrogen needed at all. I've also cut back on the soy. Due to the potential risk of getting uterine cancer from having too much estrogen, plus, the bloated/weight gain, this is a good thing. It's all about finding that balance.

Why would soy help?
Soy contains a group of plant estrogens (phytoestrogens) called isoflavones. And soy products, such as tofu, soy milk, soy cheese, veggie burgers, etc., contain these compounds. They're very similar in structure and function to estrogen. Thus, they have both anti-estrogenic and estrogenic effects. Studies show health benefits from eating soy can include cancer prevention, reduced risk of heart disease and osteoporosis—and a reduction in menopausal symptoms. (Update: It's now 7 months since I changed my diet. My migraines are all but gone!)

I have to be terribly honest and say it all sounds just too good to be true.
I'm sure it does. But, just remember, the research I'm sharing with you is based on "science" not diet or marketing hype. I encourage my clients to research on their own. Research the supplements I mentioned. Research the clinical studies on serotonin and its relation to high GI carb/sugar cravings, depression, ADD, binge eating, etc. I've also listed several books and Web sites at the back of my book where you can find further information.

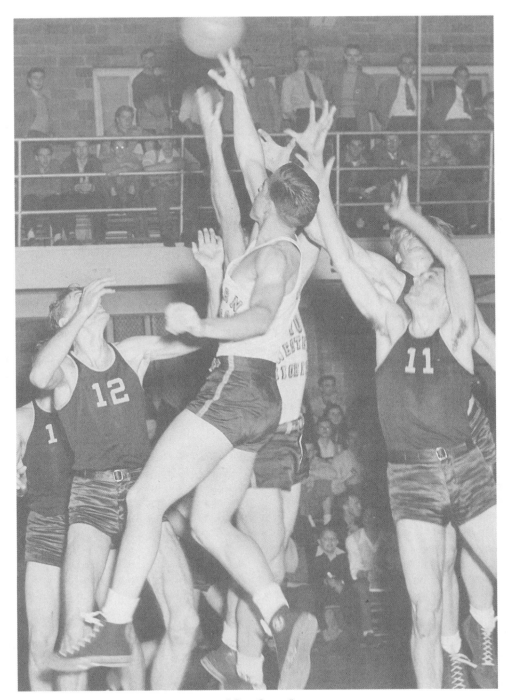

"Got Game"
Frank Gilman 1946

25

GENES…
Use 'em or abuse 'em!

You've shared so many amazing things with me, but I must ask, with regard to achieving this extraordinary health you speak of, isn't it really more about some people just having good genes?
No, and please don't allow yourself to fall for this myth. If you feel you were somehow shortchanged in this department, just push yourself harder. Clearly, some people have better genes than others—so what. I feel I am extraordinarily blessed when to comes to my genes, starting with my beloved grandmother. Harriet Vander Molen, born August 1,1897, was an amazingly strong (physically, mentally, emotionally, and spiritually), independent, courageous, and passionate Dutch woman. One of my earliest memories as a young child was waking up in the warm and loving embrace of my grandmother's arms. Rising with the sun—and before she even got out of bed—she'd do a couple of dozen leg lifts. Followed by a variety of arm exercises, then twisting on one of those old wooden squares to help keep her waist trim. Twenty minutes later, she'd go downstairs to have a Shaklee protein drink and read her Bible and daily affirmations. Little did I know how advanced she was. Little did I realize that my grandmother was fueling her body, mind, and spirit for the day.

What a great way to live life!

After her breakfast of hot tea, oatmeal with a side of prunes, home-baked bread with sweet real butter, she'd shower and then go to work. She was a personal caregiver and, among many things, she had to physically lift her patients several times on any given day. Being a widow for as long as I could remember, my grandmother worked happily into her seventies. After she retired, she traveled the world. She came to visit me several times in Florida, always eager to seek another adventure with me. (At only 22, I had plenty.) At 82, my grandma used to climb up on the roof of my building, boosting herself up two very tough ledges just so she could sunbathe topless with me. However, one of my favorite memories was when we were invited out on a 110-foot yacht for a sunset cruise to sip champagne and dine on fresh lobster. No big deal for most. But considering my grandmother didn't know how to swim, she was deathly afraid of the water. So what! She threw caution to the wind just so she could enjoy the moment with me. Oooh, how I miss her loving and adventurous spirit! She truly was amazing! Her motto was simple: *Try anything at least once!* What a great way to live life! She was also a very passionate woman. In her late eighties, she had men 20 years her junior, and some married, seeking her affections. Talk about genes! In fact, up until the day she died, men simply adored her. We should all be so fortunate to be desired at that age, or any age, for that matter.

My grandmother lived to be 93 years young and had nothing more than a touch of arthritis. All the while, she easily maintained her figure and her mental health. At 5'9", she was proud of being able to keep her weight at a slender 125 pounds. Plus, I never knew her to be sick. Moreover, she <u>never</u> took any pharmaceutical drugs. It was about a "healthy lifestyle" for her. If she were alive now, she would never give in to all these drugs! My grandmother knew, even way back then, that eating R-E-A-L food, and never skipping meals, was essential to good health. She took pride in growing her own garden. Vine-ripened tomatoes were always sitting on her windowsill. She rarely, if ever, drank alcohol, enjoying maybe a small glass of red wine on the holidays or at a Sunday dinner. She also knew the tremendous health benefits of a power nap. Her rewards for this lifestyle were living a long, happy, healthy, and fulfilled life. As I reflect, she really did live an amazing life. I'm forever grateful for that loving relationship.

My grandfather Cornelius Gilman, born September 2, 1891, was a strong, determined Dutchman. I never knew him, as he sadly died of colon cancer at age 69 when I was just a baby. Nevertheless, he and my grandmother passed their genes on to my father.

My father Frank at 6'2", 185 pounds, with black hair and hazel eyes, was a gorgeous, all-natural, all-American athlete (center, page 150) at Western Michigan University. In addition to his handsome good looks, he was a kind, soft-spoken, hard-to-anger, humble man, the type of man women adored. Similar to others of his generation, he smoked cigarettes early on, but eventually quit. He ate exceptionally healthy based on the AMA's recommendations back then, which of course, was "low-fat." Nevertheless, he never ate junk food. And just like his mother, I can't recall my dad ever being sick. If he was, it never slowed him down. He went to work every day, was never late coming home. He never stopped to hang with the boys, never disrespected his wife or ignored his responsibilities as a father. He'd religiously have two martinis with my stepmother before dinner so as to unwind. To bed by 11:30. Up by 7:15. This pattern never varied. My father was professionally driven, running his own successful lithography business. I'm grateful that he took tremendous pride in making sure his children were well provided for (*not pretentiously*), while quietly encouraging us to follow our own unique path. On the weekends, he used to love to do yard work, shoot hoops, swim, snowmobile, and water ski. Now, at 79, my concern is "where" my dad (and his wife) carry their extra weight, i.e., at their waistline. Unfortunately, they're still eating a low-fat diet—which equals too many carbs. Plus, other insulin stimulating factors. Prolonged high insulin levels lead to numerous health risks *far beyond* weight gain. And, just as I feared, though my dad's wise enough to avoid most pharmaceutical drugs, he's taking high blood pressure and cholesterol-lowering meds. Both of these issues are due to high insulin. Although he has a back that has caused him problems for 20 years, his high insulin levels (and the statin that his doctor has him on) worry me the most. Nonetheless, he still enjoys his yard work, grows his own little garden of fresh vegetables, travels, and plays a mean game of golf a couple of times a week—followed by an ice cold beer with his buddies. He's happy and enjoying his life. (Due to nerve damage, my dad conveyed my many concerns about statins to his doctor. Thankfully, he said he could stop taking it!)

With respect to my mother's parents, I only knew them for a brief time. But what I can remember was a lot of smoking and drinking. My grandfather died of a heart attack when he was in his sixties, with my grandmother dying in her early seventies.

My mother Barbara Holcombe suffered from mental illness and was institutionalized when I was barely two. I never knew her as I was growing up, but based on photos and family stories, she was an incredibly stunning, petite, creatively inspired, highly spirited, and very passionate woman of Belgian decent. She and my father had four children. Only now, at 46, have I been fortunate enough to actually spend time with her. I've discovered for myself what an amazing woman she really is. Her heart is so kind, reaching out to everyone with such compassion. Her emotions run even deeper. As for her diet, the meals she's fed are pretty old fashioned, i.e., meat, potatoes, veggie, dessert, skim milk, and coffee. For 73, she's done pretty well at keeping her little figure, but high insulin levels are never good. My other concern is that she smokes way too many damn cigarettes and drinks far too many sodas. *And why should this concern me?* Because the nicotine and the sugar-laden, highly caffeinated sodas play a huge role in further depleting her serotonin—and she eagerly consumes them all day long! This is distressing, because she's on powerful meds to help *stabilize* her depression, yet neither her doctor or psychiatrist inform her caregivers to keep her off these harmful, *serotonin-depleting* substances. (It may be impossible, but it's certainly worth the effort.) The saddest part of all of this, however, is how my mother cries to me, saying how sorry she is for not having been there for us—and how hard she's tried her entire life to "be normal." While I certainly understand she's on drugs to help balance her mentally/emotionally, I cry with her, and for her, knowing she's more normal than most people I meet on any given day. As for her not being there for us, it wasn't her fault. She's not alone, though, with her demons. My greatest torment is that I believed the many frightening stories my family told me. Thus, I waited far too long to go see her.

So, was I blessed with good genes? It depends on how you choose to look at it. For the most part, I'd have to say absolutely. And, I'm forever grateful. I also choose to focus on the positive. Regardless, I could have taken my so-called good genes and abused them. I could just as easily sit around and do nothing with them. It's the same with everyone else. Our genes are not a free ticket to good health, an attractive body, or a level of success. What truly matters is *what* you do with your genes. Once again, if you feel you were short-changed in some way, please do not give up, no matter your goals. Push yourself harder. Beat the supposed odds and make yourself proud!

I agree with you. It's just that I hear many of my friends use this as an excuse.
Yes, there are those who would rather find an excuse than face the challenge, a challenge that is well worth your efforts, a challenge that can be life-changing! Another common excuse is that it's "too late." Good news, people! It's <u>never</u> too late to start working out and living a healthier lifestyle! As a matter of fact, because we lose a quarter of a pound of muscle each year after age 30—which then changes our total body composition—you need now, *more than ever,* to start some sort of exercise program.

Is this why I'm suddenly gaining weight, even though my diet hasn't changed?
Generally speaking, yes. When you lose muscle mass, you naturally increase fat stores. Once this shift happens in your body composition, gaining weight is inevitable, and sometimes at an alarming rate.

Can't I just join a gym and do it on my own?
Of course. You can also opt to train at home. But keep in mind, the only thing worse than not working out is *wasting* your time when you do. And for those women who fear getting big and bulky, this is a myth. Women do not have enough testosterone for that to occur, nor will they be lifting the kind of extreme weight required to obtain that size. This is a far too common excuse some women use to avoid lifting weights. First of all, we each have different body types, so you'll train accordingly. Next, a healthy diet is critical to your success in the gym. The only way you'll bulk up is by training <u>without</u> also modifying your eating and drinking habits. (Properly balanced serotonin levels will help control your cravings and overall appetite, making your workouts much more effective.)

What do you focus on when you train?
When I train, my goal is never about how much weight I can lift; it is instead about proper form, technique, and consistency. That being said, I still like to feel a burn afterwards, so I have been known to lift heavy. I want to share the following story, only so women will better understand how lifting heavy does not equal big and bulky: I had just turned 40. I began dating a man who also weight-trained. He encouraged me to start doing squats. I wasn't quite sure why I hadn't done them before, especially since I had been training for over 20 years. Nonetheless, as a woman who never backs always from a challenge, I decided to try them. And, may I say, I absolutely fell in love, as it was such a powerful exercise! I started with the bar (45 pounds), needing to perfect my form. As the weeks went by, I worked my way up to 190 pounds. I then began to *warm up* with 225 pounds. Within nine months, I was able to free-squat 410 pounds for 6 reps. At 5'11" and 137 pounds, I was squatting over 3 times my body weight! (This was by no means a parallel squat.)

You're kidding? 410 pounds? That's amazing! Why did you push it so hard?
I wanted to see how far I could push my body and mind. You see, working out requires a lot of mental focus, as well. And I love the competition in my head. And you don't need to have a partner to compete. You can just as easily compete against yourself. (I also realize the risks involved when lifting heavy. I'm not about to risk injury, nor should you. Ever.) The other reason I pushed myself so hard was because my now ex-partner and I had just signed with Thane, one of the major infomercial companies. Although I was already in presentable shape, I wanted to see if I could push my body even further—and pushing the squats was part of that. Furthermore, and in all modesty, this was a huge accomplishment for me. It was also the best exercise I had ever done for my butt, legs, and total body conditioning. Free-squatting demands so many muscle groups to work that it is, without a doubt, one of the best exercises you can do.

More important than any amount of weight, I want you, the reader, to know that during this time frame my partner and I were dead broke. We were desperately borrowing from family and friends to keep our project moving forward, as well as to simply have enough to put food on the table. Then, once we were signed, we further struggled to raise the funding required to produce the infomercial. It got so bad we were actually living off my gas credit card. But, through it all, no matter how bad it was, no matter if there was enough money to eat or not, my priority was *always* to train. I would scrape together my last few dimes to pay the daily gym fee of $5.00. I'd only train two days a week, but I made my very limited time there work. It was enough to keep my mind and body strong. Those two little visits each week saved me in more ways than I can possibly tell you! Hence, for all those of you who may claim you can't afford to work out, I must respectfully disagree. You have no choice but to afford it! You have to take care of yourself, if you want to enjoy the other many wonderful aspects of your life, let alone, be around for those you love and care for.

So, fact or fiction? Does weight training make women big and bulky? Does it make women look any less feminine, less attractive, less desirable? You tell me. In case you didn't read the "Introduction," I'm the woman featured. Am I big? Bulky? Without feminine qualities? I sincerely hope not. (BTW: No "body-enhancing" Photoshop magic allowed. Moreover, if you did indeed skip the opening, please read it now.) Finally, please understand that my purpose in sharing this information with you, ladies, is to hopefully encourage you. I want to inspire you to want more, *to expect more from yourself!*

26

EXPECT MORE FROM YOURSELF!

Expect more from myself? What do you mean?

What I mean is that there are far too many women who sadly hide behind their designer outfits, yet never feel comfortable nor confident in a pair of shorts, a sleeveless dress, a bathing suit, and most assuredly, not naked! And to those women who think they don't need to work out because they already wear a size 2, well, I'm sorry to disappoint you, but this does not mean you're necessarily healthy, or sexually appealing. Being healthy means many things; at the very least, it includes a healthy metabolism and heart, strong bones, minimal body fat, low LDLs, high HDLs, normal blood pressure, hydrated skin/body, and having lean muscle mass that is firmly and beautifully sculpted. Now this, is what makes a healthy—and gorgeous physique—for women (and men).

Be proud of your naked body!

Ladies, wouldn't you like to be proud of your body both in and OUT of clothes? Wouldn't you like to stop camouflaging your problem areas with just the right outfit? Wouldn't you like to be proud of your body and all its little imperfections? *But why stop there?* Wouldn't you like to feel so gloriously sexy that you'd make love with the lights on, or maybe even with the added seduction that comes with making love in front of a mirror? And how about eagerly being on top, rather than shamefully hiding under the sheets or your lover's body? And, how wonderful would it be to take your lover to a secluded park and passionately play under the shade of a tree with a cool breeze blowing over your naked body? Better yet, how about feeling confident enough, ladies, to walk away from your lover, to leave the room <u>without</u> having to walk away backwards? Hmm? Wouldn't it feel absolutely empowering to be proud of your naked body, as you slowly and deliberately saunter across the room? Of course it would!

Okay, forget about all that talk of sex and mirrors. *Forget about everyone, but you!* My intentions here are pure and simple: I want every woman to be able to stand naked before a mirror and, using an additional mirror, look at themselves from all angles. I want each of you to be able to look at yourself from front to back, side to side, from every possible angle, and truly be happy with what you see! I don't care if you wear a size 4, 8, or 14, perfection is not, I repeat—*perfection is NOT your goal!* And, more importantly, please do not compare yourself to the airbrushed/Photoshop-inspired images you see in magazines. They are not reality! They are a marketing illusion! Instead, I want you to be *proud* of your naked female body, on <u>your</u> own terms! I want you to be *confident* in your body, in your appearance, in all that you are! You need to find what truly makes "you" happy! This will inspire and motivate you in many wonderful ways. And if you aren't happy with what you see before you, then push yourself harder! *Expect more from yourself!* Refuse to settle for less than what makes *you* happy!

From all angles? Ooh my! Are you serious?
Yes. We are all highly sexual beings. And our brains are our largest sexual organ, but as women, we sadly lose our sexual appetite and insatiable fiery passion when we feel overweight and out of shape. Well, not anymore. Time to change that! Don't let all the silly myths about weight training keep you from trying it. Weight training is about developing long, lean, yet strong muscles and bone mass. Those muscles you develop will help burn fat and calories long after you've left the gym. Weight training has also proven to help slow, if not reverse, the signs of aging. *What more could you ask for?* Combine this with a healthy life-style—and you can once again be that inspiring, sexually stimulating, *self-confident* woman!

But hold on, gentlemen! Not so fast! You are not off the hook here! Far too many of you have also allowed yourselves to get completely out of shape. Statistics verify the alarming pattern of obesity in men, starting as young as 20 and increasing steadily:

<u>2003 stats regarding obesity in men:</u>
24% age 20-34 • 25% age 35-44
30% age 44-54 • 32% age 55-64 • 33% age 65-74

These numbers are terribly concerning. And while we women certainly have our own issues, with all due respect, gentlemen, do you really think that big belly you're carrying around is attractive to us, let alone healthy? Do you think your 42-inch waist arouses us? What about your once beautifully sculpted chest and strong arms that are now weak and sagging? And we women most definitely like a nice firm ass as much as you men do, so *why* then did you let yours go soft? It wasn't so long ago, you were eager to get in the gym to make sure you stayed in shape. Suddenly, you no longer care. All those sports you played every weekend have also gone by the wayside. In its place, you find absolute bliss sitting on the couch all day with a beer in hand and a side of chips and salsa. Generally, this change in behavior happens after a man gets married. For some reason, there are men (and women) who fall into a certain comfort level once they're in a committed relationship. He begins to eat (and drink) more. He works out less. And less. He simply lets himself go.

Worst of all, he stops seducing the woman he fell in love with. No longer is he excited to see her at the end of his day. No longer does he give her the affection he once did when courting her. He doesn't understand that making love isn't just in the bedroom. Little does he know there are a *million other ways* to please the woman in his life.

For those gentlemen who may not be aware, it is not about flowers, candy, or expensive gifts. Though, such gestures are appreciated, it is, rather, about the *simplest* of things that should be part of any given day. It can be anything from picking up after yourself, putting down the toilet seat, taking out the trash without having to be asked, spending time with the kids away from the house, offering to go grocery shopping, helping with the laundry, asking with sincere intent how her day was, and then actually *listening* to her response, being willing to say you're sorry when you're wrong, a passionate hug for no reason (and with no further expectations), a tender kiss on her cheek as you leave the room, a hidden love note, a call in the middle of the day just to say how much she means to you, coming home early and making dinner, drawing her a hot bath with candles lit, to yes, wanting to give her a massage from time to time—minus penetration. While women, *without a doubt*, want to be sexually desired, we get tired of being sexually pawed at. We want to be acknowledged. Needed. Appreciated. Respected. Adored. We need to feel emotionally connected. We need to know you love and care about us for far more than what we bring to the proverbial bedroom.

Unfortunately, there are some men who don't realize that to seduce a woman's body, they must first seduce her mind. And that, dear gentlemen, is an all-day affair, not just moments before you hope to entice her out of her panties. Consequently, the woman feels unloved, unappreciated, worthless, and unattractive. She lashes out. She's hurt. Unhappy. Lonely. And angry. Rarely is the man able to understand her bitter reaction to his inability to express his affections. So, he, too, begins to feel unappreciated and unloved. This fuels an enormous, highly emotional chain reaction between them.

The heavier you get, the less desirable you feel.

This emotional stress that is so often found in relationships severely depletes serotonin. Your brain then endlessly tempts you with the foods that will elevate it. The emotional attachment to these foods is easy to understand, as the comfort you get from them is often the best part of your entire day. So you keep going back for more. The more you eat, the better you feel. You are also eating to fill the void. You eat to give yourself the happiness, the love you miss. The more you eat and drink to cover what your life is lacking, the heavier you get. The heavier you get, the less desirable you feel. The less desirable you feel, the less sexually inclined you are. Less sexual fulfilment leads to more unhappiness. More unhappiness leads to even more eating. More eating equals more weight gain. No wonder there are so many overweight people, with terribly unhappy and sexless relationships! No wonder both men and women are looking elsewhere to fulfill their emotional needs and satisfy their sexual appetites!

Gentlemen, let me ask you this: Don't you know that women are just as visually stimulated as you are? Don't you think that we want to be with a man who takes pride in his body, naked or otherwise? Don't you know that we want to be with a man who arouses us both in and out of the bedroom? Well, we do. We want to be with a man who loves himself (and us) enough to take the very best care of his body, mind, and soul.

Furthermore, guys, wouldn't you also like to once again look in the mirror and be proud of *your* naked body? Wouldn't you love to look great in and *out* of your clothes? Wouldn't it be wonderful to feel strong, confident, and desirable again? Wouldn't you love to feel virile again? Absolutely!

Christine, a beautiful friend of mine, admitted that unless she was willing to accept a bit of a belly on a man, she was never going to be able to date again. We laughed about this, but to be quite honest, it shouldn't be so rare to find a man in shape. Nevertheless, no one should have to settle for less than what they truly desire. Now *pleeease* don't go accusing us of being shallow, insensitive women. Women are fully and often painfully reminded that every red-blooded man wants a gorgeous, sexy, and intelligent woman on his arm. Women should want no less. Right? And I'm not saying what we want is right for you. Again, no one should have to settle for less than what makes them happy.

Oh, the truth can be tough sometimes! Question is, what can I do for my husband?
You know exactly what you can do for him—and yourself. Take everything that you learn here and put it to use. (Better yet, have him read this book.) Both of you need to make the commitment, once and for all, to take back your health. Stop procrastinating. There is no better time than right now! While healthy levels of serotonin will help you and your husband overcome your carb/sugar cravings, you will still need to make the *effort* to live a healthier lifestyle. This includes committing to a regular exercise program and seriously cutting back, if not eliminating, sugar, alcohol, caffeine, cigarettes, and drugs—pharmaceutical and over-the-counter. Eating healthy, getting plenty of sleep, and reducing your stress are all part of this lifestyle, as well. Losing the excess body fat will help you in many wonderful ways, but it's also about giving you your sexual life back. To *feel* passion for the one you love and then to be able to perform without anxiety, embarrassment, and/or risking your health can be so rewarding physically, mentally, and emotionally.

How do you feel about the sexual-enhancing drugs targeted toward men?
I believe ED (Erectile Dysfunction) is due to many factors, ranging from poor diet, being 20 pounds above your ideal weight, taking prescription/nonprescription drugs, excessive alcohol, smoking, lack of exercise, and so forth. But do you think your doctor would *ever* consider these factors first before suggesting you take Viagra, Cialis, or any one of the many sexual-enhancing drugs? Of course not. They don't make money that way. To reiterate, the pharmaceutical industry is a business. They are in it to make money! A lot of money, and always at your risk. ED, as with dozens of the other new so-called diseases,

diseases that are most often created by pharmaceutical drugs themselves, is making the pharmaceutical companies billions of dollars richer! Please keep in mind, though, serotonin controls many things in the human body. Libido is only one of them.

Are you saying serotonin controls our sexual desire?
Yes, serotonin controls sexual behavior/desire, but what I'm really trying to convey here is that far too many people allow themselves to get overweight. Among the other many serious health concerns that we've already discussed, one of the first things we lose is our self-respect. Losing our self-respect is *never* good, and once it happens, our sexual passion is not far behind. Eating yourself into oblivion is merely one side effect of this. When it comes to losing your sex drive, that can become a downward spiral. Reality is: Who wants to get all naked and naughty when they're carrying an extra 40, 50, or 100 pounds? How can you spend an entire rainy afternoon making love when you're grossly overweight, and thus, barely able to catch your breath? How can you think about sharing a romantic candlelit bubble bath with your lover if you're too heavy to even get into the tub? Who wants to think about making love in front of a mirror if they can't even stand the sight of their own naked body? I know I wouldn't.

Think back to not so long ago, when you were in shape, when you stood tall and proud of all that you were. Remember how confident you were as a single man (or woman) trying to seduce a lover? Think back to when you were proud of your body and how sexy you looked in your clothes—and out of them. Remember how great you felt with a lean, healthy body? Remember when you could wear any outfit you wanted without having to wear something to cover your ass or stomach? Remember how wonderful you felt and how much energy you had? Remember how physically and mentally strong you felt? Remember how proud you felt as you went about your day?

One of the first things we lose is our self-respect.

Reality is, we each have our own unique health goals. And you can achieve those goals, no matter your situation, no matter your age. But are you ready? I mean *really* ready? Are you ready to commit and do what it takes? How badly do you want it? Maybe you think it's too late or that you're too old to change. Maybe you're scared of failing again. Or maybe you simply don't care anymore. Some do not. And that's your choice. But if you want to live a long and happy life, one that is free of disease—especially if you want to be around for your loved ones—PLEASE make the effort to lose the excess weight! If you're reading this book, I'm going to assume that you sincerely desire a leaner, more attractive, and healthier body and mind. With these comes a healthy sexual appetite.

I'm ready to kick-start my love life! I know my husband would love me to, as well!
To reiterate, sexual energy is so much of who we are as human beings. I'm not saying that life is not complete without it, as I am sure there are many who maybe never liked it to

begin with, or who simply no longer want it. But if given the chance to be overweight and out of shape—or to have a body that you're not only proud of, but one that is also sexually arousing—well, which would you choose?

I choose the sexually arousing body!

I hope most would choose to live their life with love, with passion. If that should include sexual intimacy, all the better. For one moment, though, let's stop worrying about the visual aspect of being overweight and making love. I don't want you to think I'm so shallow that all I think about is what someone looks like on the outside. I'm creatively inspired in all aspects of my life, which makes me very visual, <u>not</u> just sexually speaking. That being said, I also need far more than just a gorgeous body. Nevertheless, no matter what your desires are, the human body can be one of the most beautiful things to look at. Please, take pride in yours and see what you can create.

Now I'm definitely ready to start working out, but I need a trainer. How do I know if a trainer is truly qualified?

I'm thrilled that you're willing to do what it takes. As for your question, please understand that just because someone is certified does *not* mean that they are qualified. I see way too many trainers who are sloppy, out of shape—some are downright fat. If I were looking for a trainer, I'd sure as heck want someone who shows me through their own physique how qualified they are. If they can't do it for themselves, how could they ever help me achieve my fitness goals?

Anything else I can do to make sure I get a good trainer?

I suggest you ask around the gym, starting with the manager. Tell them your needs. Don't be shy. You'll be paying good money for a trainer, and you want someone who can produce results, *without* injuries. After he or she makes their suggestions, I'd spend some time quietly observing those trainers as they interact with their clients. From there, make an appointment to talk with them to see how they think they can help you. After that, all I can say is you'll need to follow your instincts. Pick the one you feel most comfortable with. Try it for at least 12 sessions and see how you like it. Just remember, if you haven't ever lifted weights before, or if it has been some time since you were last in a gym, take it slowly. Don't let the trainer push you too hard, but at the same time, allow them to do their job. The fact of the matter is, you will be a little sore and you will feel some pain. But trust me, you'll get used to it. Your body will adjust. You'll even begin to look forward to going to the gym. In the meantime, your primary concerns at this point should be that you feel safe, secure, and confident in your trainer's abilities. With that in mind, I'd like to share the following quick story: A woman once screamed at me with such distaste, "Phoenix, you have the biggest ego I have even seen!" I was stunned by this comment. I was also hurt.

First of all, this woman barely knew me. Secondly, I'm rather reserved, not at all boastful. (If I should ever come across as boastful, *please* know it is <u>not</u> my intention, ever. My intentions are only to educate, motivate, and hopefully inspire others.) Nonetheless, I couldn't understand why she'd lash out with such a stinging comment. So, I asked her to please explain why she thought this. She replied, making a reference to the fact I so boldly used my own image on my products and business cards. *Excuse me?* This is what she based such a hurtful comment on? Obviously, I felt the urge to explain that it had absolutely nothing to do with my ego, but rather my "body" is my business. It was imperative that I was able to competently reflect my expertise not just through my spoken and/or written word, but also through my *physical* body. I expect others to equally reflect their expertise in their chosen profession. Does this make them egotistical? I should hope not.

Using my image on my products is also good business. Why would I pay a fitness model when I'm capable? As a photographer and one who knows a little something about product branding, it was equally important to start branding myself, at the same time trying to appeal to *both* sexes through my packaging. Which is why the images I choose to use always include both a man and a woman. But all of that is trivial; it means absolutely *nothing* compared to my most significant marketing strategy: **Inspire others!** I want to show the consumer that having a lean, healthy, attractive physique is NOT exclusive to those who are 20 and 30 years old. My intentions are to hopefully inspire others, no matter their age! And so, with a sincere, and, more importantly, *humble* desire to achieve that goal, I made Billy, a client and one of my dearest friends, pose with me. He's 53. He will, *undeniably*, inspire men of all ages! And, in all modesty, I hope that, at 46, I can equally inspire women. (Once again, if you did not read the "Introduction," please do so now. It will help insure your success.)

That man is 53? And that's you, at 46? Your bodies look unbelievable! I'm definitely inspired! You mentioned Billy's a client. I'm curious, was his diet always healthy?
Thank you for the compliments. And, yes, Billy ate remarkably healthy according to what he, and many others, had been told was healthy by the FDA and AMA.

Such as?
Billy ate plenty of healthy foods such as chicken, turkey, fish, etc., but he also had quite a taste for natural sugars and wannabe healthy fat-free carbs. He loved dried fruit, which is nothing more than crystallized fruit sugar. He ate a lot of fat-free yogurts, fat-free breakfast bars, Fig Newtons, coconut-dipped figs, bananas, grapes, honey, cereal, fruit juice, fat-free pretzels, assorted pasta dishes, and smoothies blended with lots of fresh fruit. He also enjoyed a daily Coke at midday to give him that much-needed boost, along with his weekend treat, Milano cookies. As you can see, Billy's carb choices were mostly from natural sugars, but they were *high GI carbs*. To make matters worse, drinking those carbs in a liquid form (smoothies, fruit juice, etc.) affected his insulin levels much quicker and more dramatically. (I hate to admit it, but while I easily avoided the dried fruit, fruit juice, and yogurts, as they gave me such a crazy sugar buzz, I did enjoy pretzels. *And why not?*

After all, they were "FAT-FREE!" Only now do I realize why I felt so bloated, thirsty, and fat after I ate them.)

Did Billy ever have any weight issues?
No, he never had any weight issues. But, as any man knows, no matter how hard you try, no matter how great the shape you're in, those love-handles can still be a problem. Billy was no different. It wasn't a big problem, but when he was eating all those sugar-laden carbs, they'd go right to his waist. Remember, guys, your waist is your insulin gauge. If you want to know how well your diet is working, just look at your waistline. Women generally carry their weight in several areas—from their hips, buttocks, and stomach—while men tend to carry all their excess weight in their stomach. Please understand, though, that you may not necessarily reflect this weight gain right away, if ever. But know this; damage is clearly being done to your body (and mind).

In all modesty, I'd like to say that since Billy has combined my nutritional program with his dedication, both in and out of the gym, he has lost all desire and cravings for those high GI carbs. This subsequently helped him gain far more lean muscle mass, while greatly *reducing* his body fat. He's also significantly improved his cholesterol panel.

Are you saying that SESs helped control his cravings for these carbs?
This is precisely what I'm saying. Once again, controlling the cravings equals less insulin spiking. Less insulin equals less fat stored, and more fat burned. All of this equals a much leaner, healthier body.

Does Billy have any other bad habits?
I have only two concerns with Billy. First of all, he eats way too many protein bars. While I know he genuinely believes his preferred bar is a healthy choice because the packaging claims a mere 2 net carbs, they are a perfect example of product deception. In addition to the excessive 240 calories per bar, the manufacturer hides their exorbitant amount of sugars in the glycerine and sugar alcohols, which, by the way, add up to 24g of carbs. A far cry from their professed 2g!

My second concern is Billy's love of caffeine. And while maintaining his serotonin levels, combined with my nutritional advice, has helped get him off all those numerous other insulin-producing carbs, which has subsequently led to much healthier blood panels, Billy is not quite ready to give up this habit. He, along with a lot of other men, love the jolt that comes from caffeine. And even though I've begged him to at least just *try* decaf, he refuses. Nonetheless, Billy has made so many other extraordinary changes in his diet that I leave him be. (That is, until tomorrow.)

As I said before, we can't be expected to do everything perfectly. After all, it is about moderation and making the best possible choices. It will require effort. Set small goals. Achieve them one by one. Then move on to the next. Remember, healthy levels of serotonin will help control the actual cravings. What's left is merely the "habit." Question is: *Are you ready to drop those unhealthy habits?* Some habits you may choose to hold on to. However, if you aren't happy with the way you look and feel, your unpredictable, stressed-out, depressed mood swings, or your inability to be intimate—well, then, this is where all those little things add up. Are the protein bars, flavored lattes, cocktails, fried chicken, cookies, crackers, sodas, or french fries really worth it? I hear so many people say they don't want to give up their pasta, chocolate cake, potato chips, etc., but they need to realize that their so-called emotional attachment to these foods is FALSE!

What do you mean it's false?
It's false because once you elevate your serotonin, your brain will no longer push you toward those foods. You will no longer desire them. And, best of all, you will NOT miss them! That love affair will no longer serve you. Now, if on occasion, you still want a treat, go ahead. But the actual *craving* will be long gone. Look, I encourage you to live as healthy a lifestyle as possible. How far you want to take it is entirely up to you. I suggest you at least pick your treats wisely.

Update, November 2004: After years of gently nagging poor Billy about the health risks associated with stimulants—and the fact it's nothing more than a "habit," since by boosting his serotonin his actual cravings were gone—Billy has *finally* given in! It's been two full weeks since he's had any coffee! Other than feeling a bit off for the first few days, he says he feels great, with a lot more energy! He also lost a quick few pounds. I told him that without all the water retention due to the insulin constantly being spiked, he would get even leaner than he already is. In addition, he's finally decided to listen to my concerns regarding protein bars. Wow! I am absolutely amazed! You have no idea how long I've bugged him about both. I am so proud of him!

A lesson to be learned here: Billy's probably the closest one to me and my research, but it shows you just how independent people can be. They have to find their own way, and do it in their own time. But, as long as they make the effort, this is what matters in the end. To reiterate, I don't expect Billy, or anyone else, to make all these changes overnight. As you can see, some habits can take years to break. But it can be done if you truly have the desire. (Another update, July 2005: It's now been 8 months since Billy cut out caffeine and protein bars. Not only is he leaner than ever before, but he doesn't miss them one bit. See, habits can be broken, if you're willing.)

And now, Billy kindly insisted on sharing his story, in his own words:

"Over the years, I've struggled, like most, with sugar cravings and finding a balance between diet and exercise. It's not that I was a junk food junky or hopelessly out of shape—I wasn't. I've worked out all of my adult life, but always seemed to carry an extra 5 pounds around my midsection. And for all the working out, and being as active as I am, I wasn't achieving that lean, muscle definition that I knew I could have. I also experienced

pretty extreme energy lows in the mid-morning and late afternoon. By 3pm I used to find myself actually having a Coke with a bag of pretzels just to keep my head from hitting the desk. Repeatedly Phoenix would tell me, "You're eating way too much sugar!" As a result, I decided to let her help me.

We started by tracking everything I'd consume in a week. I put it into a spreadsheet and broke it down into calories, carbs, protein, fat, and sugar. When we added up the natural sugar (plus the daily soda) that I was ingesting, combined with my carbohydrate intake, it was very illuminating. For example, orange juice, bananas, raisins, honey, and yogurt don't sound unhealthy, but they're terribly high in fructose, i.e., fruit sugar. And I was eating plenty of them. By eliminating them from my diet and replacing them with low GI carbs and adding more protein, I reduced my sugar intake from an amazing 173g per day to 29g! My carb intake went from 345g per day to 132g! My overall caloric intake went from 3,000 a day to about 2,050, which is right in line for my weight, height, age, and level of activity. My blood panels subsequently became much healthier, as well.

With Phoenix's expertise (and SES), not only was I able to drastically cut back my carb intake without any real effort, but my cravings for all those senseless high GI carbs also just seemed to vanish. No real effort, and I never missed them. This allowed me to get over the obstacles I just couldn't seem to conquer on my own. The end result was an almost immediate loss of about 7 pounds around my midsection and a substantial increase in muscle definition. My energy level is now consistent throughout the day, and I have far more energy for my workouts. Furthermore, I was an insomniac for nearly 10 years. I am, however, rediscovering what it feels like to sleep through the night. This is huge for me! I also found my ability to handle stress was greatly improved.

But even beyond those successes, having finally gotten off the caffeine and cut back on my protein bars, in two weeks' time—and with no other changes in my diet—I lost another 5 pounds. Better yet, I've now <u>finally</u> achieved the results I've worked so hard for. By the way, I'm 53 years old, 5'11", 185 pounds, with a 32" waist. My body fat is down to 9.4% and my LBM is 90.6%. I weight train no more than 3 to 4 days a week. My cardio exists of speed walking and riding my bike. And, I can honestly say, I've never felt better! Thank you, Phoenix, for all that you've done for me!"

It was my absolute pleasure, Billy! Thank you for making the effort to live a healthier life. And thank you for sharing your experience with my readers. You are an excellent testimonial—and a perfect example of what one can achieve—if they truly make the commitment. Your story, along with your phenomenal photos, will undoubtedly inspire men everywhere! That being said, I'd like to wrap this chapter up by saying:

The Lesson of the Day is...

Age is not
the determining factor
when it comes to achieving your health and fitness goals!

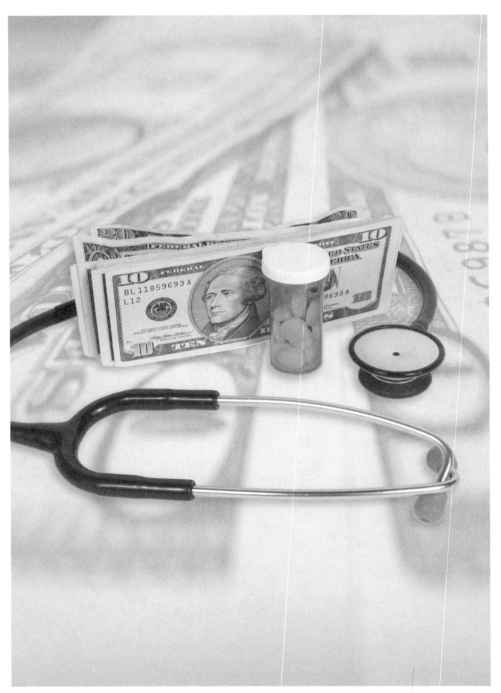

27

PHARMACEUTICAL DRUGS & THEIR SIDE EFFECTS:
weight gain, depression, loss of libido,
liver & heart failure, new disease, even death!

How do pharmaceutical drugs promote weight gain?
Pharmaceutical drugs, as well as nonprescription drugs (OTC meds, and that includes ordinary cold meds, pain relievers, etc.) are substances *foreign* to the body. They're NOT natural. They're chemicals and poisonous. As such, these drugs will, at bare minimum, trigger insulin. High insulin levels, as you recall, will lead to harmful cholesterol panels, increased water retention—and fat storage. These drugs will also deplete serotonin.

All pharmaceutical drugs deplete serotonin?
Yes, and although serotonin is a major neurotransmitter that controls many vital things within the body, side effects from these drugs can be far more serious.

I *encourage* weight gain (and depression) due to the fact these drugs deplete my serotonin, hence causing cravings for the foods that trigger insulin. Is this correct?
Absolutely. I'm so proud of you for making this connection. But remember, these drugs themselves, *trigger insulin*, causing all sorts of other health problems. They actually create new disease and perpetuate the very illnesses they are designed to so-call cure.

Our waistline is a gauge to judge how healthy our diet is, but it also reflects side effects from various drugs. Hence, one of the first things I ask a potential new client is, "What *type* of pharmaceutical drugs are you taking?" After all, this is one of the biggest factors contributing to why people either begin to gain weight, or why they can't lose weight, even though they're working out and eating well. Unfortunately, some clients refuse to acknowledge drugs may be a problem. They find it easier to blame me, or another health professional. These clients are also the ones who tend to believe their physicians are God. They absolutely refuse to question *why* their bodies are suddenly so bloated, why they're so damn depressed, with high blood pressure, and suffering from yet another illness every time they turn around. (Observation: Did you notice I didn't bother asking "if" they were on any such drugs? The reason being, is that there are very few people who aren't on at least one, two, or maybe even more pharmaceutical drugs. Worst of all, their doctors scare them into believing they need to be on a *lifelong* drug regimen!)

I thought these drugs helped cure disease?
Cure? Hardly! Appallingly, this is what the drug companies would love for us to believe. They mislead us into believing their drugs will cure us. This is not true. I repeat, *this is not*

true! Pharmaceutical drugs are NOT designed to heal or cure disease! And even if you can begin to afford these outrageously expensive drugs, they're designed for, and only capable of, targeting and <u>masking</u> the symptoms of disease. Herbs, on the other hand, have been used successfully for centuries in healing numerous ailments. Plus, no prescription is needed, and they're affordable.

Pharmaceutical drugs do <u>NOT</u> cure disease!

Are there other drug concerns?
Yes, too numerous to mention. All one has to do is listen to the disclaimers found at the end of drug commercials. Though they are stated way too fast for complete clarity, the drug companies and the FDA themselves are *fully aware* that their drugs are most often dangerous, if not DEADLY! (This was recently proven by the Vioxx scandal.) But don't believe me or trust these self-promoting advertisements. Do yourself a favor and buy a PDR and use it faithfully as your guide. Also, go to the FDA's own Web site and research the various and most often life-threatening side effects that come with any given pharmaceutical drug. Next, review the many lawsuits that are filed against the largest names in the pharmaceutical industry.

A perfect example is a very common drug called Lamisil. It's patented and produced by Novartis. Lamisil is a highly recommended drug to help get rid of simple nail fungus. But—*are you aware of the side effects from this drug?* Liver damage or complete liver failure! This is based on reports from the FDA themselves with regard to lawsuits brought against this drug. Yet these side effects are considered *acceptable* by the FDA! It is marketed freely to the public without any regard for those it will harm!

What I find equally disturbing is how Novartis advertises this particular drug. They use funny-looking cartoon characters with even funnier little voices, showing them attacking and crawling up under the nails. They make it seem so harmless, cute, and actually inviting to the consumer. Well, don't be fooled by this marketing strategy. The following is a list of the many side effects caused by Lamisil. These side effects are alarmingly very typical drug side effects—and all are *allowed* by the FDA:

"Early warning signs of liver damage induced by Lamisil are often minor, ranging from diarrhea, rashes, fever, stomach pain, and nausea. Initially these symptoms may seem minor, but can develop and become more severe, eventually resulting in liver damage. Darkened urine, loss of appetite, skin discoloration, and even fatigue all may be early signs of liver damage as well. Additionally, hair loss, yellowing of the eyes and skin, altered vision, and unusual bruising and bleeding are all possible side effects. Though Lamisil circulates briefly in the bloodstream, it remains in the fat cells of the skin and fingernails long after the patient has stopped using it, creating the possibility that liver damage may develop months after treatment has stopped."

Liver damage or complete liver failure just to get rid of some fungus?

Shockingly, these are very typical side effects that are associated with pharmaceutical drugs, both prescription and nonprescription. Another quick example is Nexium, *the Purple Pill.* This drug, which is touted every other minute via TV advertisements for treating Acid Reflux, has no less than 100 potential side effects! I had to laugh as I read the list of so-called rare, but nonetheless, potential side effects. The side effects listed actually utilized almost <u>every</u> <u>single</u> <u>letter</u> of the alphabet, and sometimes repeatedly.

Due to the fact 2.5 million children have been diagnosed with ADD/ADHD (a side effect of low serotonin), doctors are only too eager to prescribe drugs to treat them, primarily Strattera and Ritalin. I have to ask: *Are parents unaware that these drugs come with serious, life-threatening side effects for both kids and adults?* Side effects can include addiction, abnormal heartbeat, nausea, decreased appetite, insomnia, sexual side effects, liver and heart failure, to suicidal thoughts and behavior! One youth actually attempted suicide during the Strattera trials! These side effects are also clearly known by the FDA, but they are, once again, considered acceptable!

As of September 2005, the FDA finally issued a health advisory on Strattera after evaluating Eli Lilly's clinical trial data, data that showed it was, in fact, <u>increasing</u> suicidal thoughts and behavior in children (at 4 per 1,000). Considering the *millions* of kids on this drug, this is huge! Even one is too damn many! But, instead of pulling this deadly drug off the market, the FDA simply demanded that Lilly add a black-box warning. It will state: "This drug increases suicidal thoughts among youths." This is insane, if not intentional homicide! Parents, please STOP letting your doctor drug your kids! You need to remember that your child's diet plays a critical role in their ability to concentrate! Based on what you've learned here about serotonin and SESs, it is not necessary to risk their lives with these drugs! How pathetically ironic that parents lovingly teach their kids to "Just Say NO to Drugs"—all the while the medical industry is drugging them at an alarming rate!

Furthermore, let's all pause for a moment and quietly reflect: Have we all so quickly forgotten what it was like to be a child? Have we forgotten that, as a child, just by the pure nature of being a child, we all probably suffered from ADD/ADHD to some degree? And while diet indeed plays a major role in how children behave, they have a ton of energy that is not easily harnessed. So, instead of letting your kids watch TV or sit at the computer, they need to be encouraged or, if need be, *forced* out to play, and I mean P-L-A-Y for hours on end! In addition, do not waste another moment in getting them to eat healthier!

171

My god! Increases suicidal thoughts and behavior? The side effects are far worse than the so-called condition! Why would anyone take the chance?
Exactly. I am once again astounded by what the FDA considers safe to put into the marketplace. And then you wonder why those of us in the alternative healthcare industry get outraged when the FDA, FTC, and drug companies feverishly campaign to destroy us, or even shut us down completely. While they attempt to frighten the consumer away from buying dietary supplements, tens of *thousands* are dying each and every year from their "FDA-approved" drugs! Again, don't take my word on any of this. Buy yourself a PDR and review it. You'll be absolutely horrified to discover what the drug companies and FDA consider safe and acceptable. To help protect you and your family, you should use the PDR as your guide for any and all medications considered.

This is outrageous! Why is this allowed?
We should all be asking this *exact* question and equally demanding an answer from the FDA, FTC, AMA, drug companies, and our own doctors! Dare to question the incestuous relationship between these agencies! Dare to write your congressional representative and senator! Dare to hold these government and medical agencies liable!

Believe me, I'll start asking! I've also noticed there are suddenly so many new diseases. Why is that?
You're right. There's a new so-called disease discovered nearly every six months, ranging from ADD (Attention Deficit Disorder), AR (Acid Reflux), to ADHD (Attention Deficit Hyperactivity Disorder), to even Adult ADD (Adult Attention Deficit Disorder), to every type of anxiety/depression disorder. Two of the very latest diseases brought to the medical forefront are RLS (Restless Leg Syndrome. They can't be serious?!) and IRS (Insulin Resistance Syndrome). The headlines scream: *"The Newest Silent Killer!"* Hmm, no scare tactics involved here.

The real answer as to *why* we're suddenly being bombarded with so many new diseases is simple, yet terribly frightening: The pharmaceutical industry, selling over *$300 billion worth* of drugs each year, is BIG BUSINESS at its worst! And they're not about to stop searching for more ways to make even more money! One way to achieve this is by literally *creating* new diseases. Examples: Since when is having a little trouble focusing (ADD/ADHD) suddenly considered a disease? Better yet, since when is a flaccid penis (Erectile Dysfunction) considered a disease? These are, but a few. The list is endless! But these health concerns are not diseases; they are *conditions* that are most often due to an unhealthy lifestyle and—more often than not—actually caused by the prescription and nonprescription drugs you're currently taking. They are conditions that can most often be reversed by first getting off all such drugs and medications with the help of a qualified alternative healthcare practitioner, and by making serious changes in your diet and overall lifestyle. Good health will <u>not</u> be achieved by taking drugs! Once again, the prescription and nonprescription drugs that your doctor continually forces you to take to treat these conditions, will, in fact, create new conditions and diseases in your body! Furthermore, the more "conditions" the pharmaceutical industry can claim as a "disease," the more power and control they will have over that so-called disease. They get to develop and market even more drugs to *mask* the symptoms of that "newly designed" disease. Even more disturbing yet, is that, once the pharmaceutical industry makes those claims, once they turn that condition into a DISEASE, no one in the alternative healthcare industry can, in any way, diagnose, treat, cure, or simply try to help prevent that particular condition. *Why?* Big business at work, once again. The answer is simple: Greed! The FDA will do anything and everything to keep the power, control, and profits gained from treating any and all illness in the hands of the drug companies! (December 2005, I just learned firsthand how far the FDA will go to suppress us. They just classified the polylymaphatic delivery system as a "DRUG!" And, as such, no one in the supplement industry is allowed to further use this delivery system. *A drug?!* A "delivery system" is NOT a drug! My company spent nearly 2 years in R&D on this. What a waste of time and funds! Their endless abuse of power is astounding!)

Considering the FDA is financially supported in countless ways by the actual drug companies—which is unethical, *if not downright criminal*—they have so much to lose. Hence, the FDA works hand in hand with the pharmaceutical industry to annihilate any persons who attempt to threaten their monopoly and profit margins. And if I am fortunate enough to bring national awareness to this frighteningly sordid matter, as several others are trying to do, I will definitely be one they will want to silence. In the meantime, I will continue to do all that I can to educate, inform, and protect the consumer.

Once again, the pharmaceutical industry is NOT designed to cure or heal people. It is a proven fact their drugs are merely meant to target and mask symptoms. The drug companies themselves admit to this. They have, though, brainwashed patients, even doctors, into believing that their drugs are the ONLY effective treatment. Reality is: The pharmaceutical industry is an investment industry motivated *entirely* by the PROFITS of its shareholders. It is about the billions of dollars that are made by patenting their assorted drugs. It is not about curing disease!

What's even more disturbing is that, to expand their market, pharmaceutical companies continually search for new uses for their assortment of drugs. This is a new medical category called "pre-disease." They are scaring otherwise healthy people into believing they need to be on any number of their drugs to help avoid *potential* disease. A few examples of pre-disease drugs that are being heavily marketed are Fosamax and Actonel to prevent osteoporosis. And Plavix, a drug promoted to prevent stroke. Or so they'd love for us to believe. But *why* do they leave out the many serious side effects from taking these drugs? I'll tell you why. Because this, along with all their many drug claims, is nothing more than an insidious, self-serving marketing illusion!

Another example: Although aspirin is an OTC/nonprescription drug, Bayer has become the poster child for helping stop heart attacks. 50 million people have been convinced that simply by taking Bayer every day, they will either avoid a heart attack, or greatly reduce their risks for having one. *Really?* Where are the unbiased clinical studies to support this claim? And why do they conveniently forget to mention the side effects associated with taking an aspirin every day, i.e., stomach bleeding, kidney damage, even death? It also increases the odds of another often fatal condition; hemorrhagic stroke. Aspirin may offer some health benefits, but why aren't doctors promoting *living a healthy lifestyle* versus having to take aspirin to counter unhealthy lifestyle habits?

The aforementioned drugs are merely the tip of the proverbial iceberg. All one has to do is stay home and watch TV for a day to see that nearly every single commercial is a drug ad. These deadly drugs are cleverly promoted through million-dollar ad campaigns specifically designed to *frighten* you into going to see your doctor, who will then most definitely convince you that you must be on any number of their drugs. Considering that the majority of people blindly trust the medical industry, these endless fear-based ads are ferociously successful. As far as I'm concerned, based on what I know, and based on many other experts within the alternative healthcare industry, those involved in the drug industry are nothing more than legally acceptable drug dealers! All of them are in bed with the FTC and the FDA. While one hand despicably washes the other, profits for these organizations grow exponentially—and ALL at our expense!

Worst of all, most people will fall for their deception. Sadly, the elderly are the easiest victims when it comes to these drug peddlers. They, unfortunately, never question their doctor. They so willingly put their very lives in their doctors' hands, only to be abused in the worst possible way. And don't kid yourself, the medical industry is fully aware of how easy it is to manipulate the millions of seniors under their trusting care. That market alone is making them billions! Now, can you imagine the profits to be made off the baby boomers, as we creep into our later years?

Furthermore, one cannot possibly ignore the outrageous costs related to these drugs. The elderly are literally forced to go without food in order to take the drugs that their doctor insists they must take! Millions of seniors are going hungry, without heat or air conditioning, in an attempt to buy these drugs—drugs that, instead of healing them, are, in fact, killing them quicker! I have to ask: *Where will this end? How can this be allowed? Does no one care? Are we all so damn busy, so completely unaffected that we just turn our heads away and pray to God we never get sick?*

In the March 2005 edition of *Life Extension* magazine (a highly recommended publication) there is a very powerful article speaking out against the whole FDA/drug company scandal. They also included a chart outlining the most popular drugs and their costs, compared to supplements, markups, etc. Example: Xanax, is a tranquilizer used for treating and relieving anxiety, with a dosage of a mere 1mg. The cost of the generic active ingredient for 100 pills is only $0.02, while the drug companies sell it for $136.79! The drug companies *legally allowed* markup for this drug is a staggering 569,858%!

As previously mentioned, another successful strategy to broaden the pharmaceutical industry is to actually *create* new diseases with their current drugs. Because pharmaceutical drugs only mask symptoms, most, if not all, of the drugs that millions of people are currently taking for one health problem or another, will be the <u>cause</u> of many new diseases. This is a direct result from the drug's long-term side effects. A perfect example: One very common side effect from taking any pharmaceutical drug is the loss of sexual desire and/or function. But, rather than address the underlying reasons why their patients have suddenly lost all sexual desire or ability, it's far more beneficial financially to the drug companies to simply create a N-E-W disease. This particular new disease is, again, ED (Erectile Dysfunction). Another example: Cholesterol-lowering drugs. Numerous studies show that these drugs are known to actually *increase* the risk of developing cancer. The list is endless—and atrocious!

With regard to how many drugs some people are taking, as well as how drugs can create new disease, I felt it was important to share this news story: The makers of Botox, pharmaceutical company Allergan and Dr. Arnold Klein, a Beverly Hills dermatologist, were sued in August 2004 by Mike and Irena Medavoy. Their suit claims Irena was treated with Botox to help ease her migraines, but instead became "extremely ill," suffering from continued migraines, fever, respiratory problems, and hives. Some symptoms eventually subsided, but many allegedly did not. While this is a story well worth following on its own, my focus was drawn to the evidence brought forth by the defense team. They claimed that the dozen-plus pharmaceutical drugs Irena was taking, in addition to her Botox treatment, were the underlying cause of her symptoms, not the Botox. I was absolutely stunned when the lawyer read the number of drugs she was on. Literally, no less than a dozen! I don't recall the name/purpose of each drug, but they ranged from antidepressants, several for migraines, anxiety, others for insomnia, etc. More alarming was that the Medavoys were not even remotely aware of the side effects that were common to these assorted drugs.

Knowing what I know about the effects of taking just one pharmaceutical drug, I can't begin to imagine how the excessive amount of drugs are affecting her body and mind. At bare minimum, one of these drugs alone will deplete her serotonin, yet she's taking nearly a dozen. No wonder she's depressed, suffering from migraines, body aches and pain, unable to sleep, and highly stressed! Reality is, every single drug Mrs. Medavoy is taking comes with harmful side effects, creating a new condition or disease. When she complains of these new health problems, her doctor will simply prescribe another drug—which will create a whole new set of side effects, creating yet another new condition or disease, for which her doctor will, once again, prescribe yet another drug that will cause even more side effects. This is a frightening cycle, a cycle that is perpetual and terribly disturbing.

This is also a perfect example of people blindly trusting their doctor. *Why is it no one questions this?* How can two highly intelligent, educated people such as the Medavoys allow themselves to be so senselessly drugged *without* questioning it or being in the least bit concerned about the side effects of all these DRUGS? *How?*

I admit it's terribly frightening, but we've been brainwashed to believe that our doctor knows best. We accept what our doctor tells us—without questioning it. Apparently, this blind faith is not in our best interest.

Blind faith is never good! All I ask is that you learn to question your doctor's proposed treatment and do some research on your own. To reiterate, the pharmaceutical industry is a BUSINESS. Their business is disease. And it is one of the biggest scams on all of mankind! The endless promises of health touted by these pharmaceutical companies is not reality! Instead of renewed health, cures, or healing, most often their trusting patients are met with life-threatening side effects, new diseases, even death!

It's one thing if these drugs worked, even with such horrendous side effects, but they do not! To make this matter even more unsettling is the fact that the FDA, AMA, drug companies, and FTC will stop at *nothing* when it comes to trying to scare people away from alternative, all-natural methods of medicine! You see, the actual survival of the pharmaceutical industry depends on the elimination of any and all alternative health therapies, including dietary supplements.

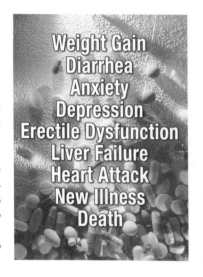

Weight Gain
Diarrhea
Anxiety
Depression
Erectile Dysfunction
Liver Failure
Heart Attack
New Illness
Death

Please understand I'm not saying doctors don't have a value. (Along with the few I've mentioned, Dr. Oz is a wonderful, but sadly rare example of what doctors should be like.) My sincere hope is that you learn to think for yourself, for your sake and for those you love. Do NOT take what these doctors say as gospel! Stop letting them put you and yours on all these senseless, ineffective, and harmful drugs! Research your options, starting with making sure you choose your physician with the greatest of care. You also need to realize that doctors have a stake in the drugs that are sold to you, their patient. Doctors get huge kickbacks from drug companies, ranging from lavish trips and dinners, free tickets to elite sporting events, golf vacations, etc. Drug companies spend on average $14,000 per year, per doctor, to seduce them into pushing their individual drugs. *And yet no one sees a problem with this?* Talk about a secure drug deal! This is exactly why you must be willing to respectfully QUESTION AUTHORITY! (Same for your vet, dentist, teacher, mechanic, lawyer, priest, accountant, etc.)

My doctor is always rushed, barely allowing me to speak. How do I approach him?
Politely demand that your doctor give you a moment to express your thoughts and concerns. Considering they're generally no less than 30 minutes late for our appointments, the least they can do is give us their undivided attention for a few moments, once they enter the room. Do not let their rudeness keep you from getting your much-needed answers. In addition, don't be afraid to question their diagnosis, treatment, medications, potential side

effects, etc. After you leave the appointment, go home and research so that you're better informed. Then either make an appointment with a new physician or call your doctor back. Tell him your concerns. Share your opinion. Be considerate, but demand answers. Dare to protect yourself—and your family. If you're not satisfied with his response, then insist on getting a second, third, even fourth medical opinion.

Some alarming medical statistics to ponder:

▶ 9,000 people die each year from aspirin, ibuprofen, and naproxen.

▶ 90,000 people die each year due to hospital errors.

▶ 106,000 people die each year from prescription drug side effects. Over the last decade, nearly 8 million have died from these drugs, with 191 million being injured!

▶ 250,000 people die each year when surgery goes wrong.

▶ 300,000 people die each year from alcohol.

▶ 450,000 people die each year from cigarettes.

▶ Tylenol (acetaminophen) can cause serious liver damage. Each year, more than 56,000 people visit the emergency room, and approximately 450 die.

▶ Celebrex has been linked to 10 deaths and 11 cases of gastrointestinal bleeding.

▶ As of October 2004, Vioxx, after 5 years and with over $10 billion in sales, has been pulled from the market due to an increased risk of heart attack and stroke.

▶ Rezulin was pulled off the market in March 2000, after 90 cases of liver failure were reported. 63 of these cases resulted in death, 10 required liver transplants.

▶ Bayer Pharmaceutical has voluntarily recalled its cholesterol-lowering drug Baycol, because it has been linked to nearly 40 deaths.

▶ Paxil, an antidepressant drug earning more than $3.1 billion, is addictive, causing severe withdrawal symptoms in consumers attempting to stop taking it.

▶ Eli Lilly has been charged with 300 lawsuits based on the side effects caused by Prozac. Charges allege Prozac can precipitate suicide in patients who are unable to break down Prozac's main ingredient, fluoxetine. In 1990, Lilly corporate executives convinced their scientists to alter records on doctors' experiences with Prozac. They changed any mention of suicidal thoughts to "depression" and suicide attempts to "overdose."

▶ Vioxx update: November 2004, the FDA and Merck are under extreme fire as evidence clearly indicates the FDA approved, promoted, and refused to recall Vioxx, even after they knew it was responsible for an untold number of fatalities. Thus far, 160,000 cases of heart attack and stroke have been reported! This is only the tip of the iceberg when it comes to the FDA working hand in hand with the drug companies only for profit! Just as with the Prozac scandal, those involved in this cover-up should equally be charged with intentional homicide!

▶ Vioxx continued: February 2005, the FDA has recommended that Merck *resume* sales of this proven deadly drug! Considering the evidence (the FDA and Merck were both *unequivocally* aware of the possibility that Vioxx would kill tens of thousands of people, not to mention cause thousands of heart attacks and strokes), how is it possible then, that the FDA would allow it back on the market? *How can this be?* I'll tell you how. It is solely because of corporate greed, because of the billions of dollars Merck (and the FDA) will make from selling this drug! The FDA's statement to support this deadly move claims they believe the number of people who can "benefit" from this drug far <u>outweighs</u> the possibility that others may suffer heart attacks, strokes, or even die! To further convince the public that this move is justified, the FDA is demanding Merck place a black box warning on the package. They're also asking physicians to properly warn their patients of the many risks associated with this drug. Oh, please!! They can't be serious! Most doctors don't even educate themselves to the deadly side effects of this, or any other drug, and yet they are suddenly going to care enough to warn their patients? I can't believe this rationalization! We've already seen just how many people have died from taking this drug. But the FDA willingly allows it to be sold? I'm sorry, but this can't possibly be considered acceptable medical treatment!

▶ Celebrex update: Pfizer announced in December 2004 that it has suspended use of its popular Celebrex medicine in a long-term cancer study, because patients who used it over an extended time showed an increased cardiovascular risk. However, the company said that it has no plans to pull the arthritis pain drug from the market.

▶ Naproxen update: In December 2004, Naproxen, sold over the counter by Bayer as Aleve, or in the prescription forms Naprosyn and Anaprox, have been found to increase risks of heart attacks and stroke by 50%! The FDA, though, as with so many other dangerous drugs, <u>refuses</u> to pull it from the market. Instead, they simply recommend the consumer should "consult their physicians and follow instructions on the labels."

This is unbelievable!
Yes, it's hard to believe, but the AMA, FDA, FTC, and drug companies see the previous statistics as nothing more than the "cost of doing business." They also have tremendous influence when it comes to keeping these alarming facts out of the headlines. As of December 2004, it was reported on CNN and stated by one of the FDA's very own, long-time employees that "The safety of the consumer is the FDA's *lowest* priority."

The list is incalculable of horrendous, but apparently *acceptable,* side effects of prescription and nonprescription drugs, and the other huge money-makers such as tobacco and alcohol! The FDA and FTC conveniently turn a blind eye, never ever considering a ban on these products! *Why?* Because far too many people would lose far too much money! Just the expenditures of the people who get sick from these products and/or drugs are far too big a business to throw away! Instead, these health risks are simply called acceptable and referred to as "The risks associated with treating diseases, with hopes to find cures." *Cures?* They know damn well these drugs will <u>not</u> cure disease! And when was the last time we heard of a cure? Polio, maybe! Nonetheless, it's all exceedingly disturbing, as the heartless, profit-motivated drug companies and the FDA clearly have no regard for human life! It is instead all about business and making BILLIONS of dollars from human suffering!

WARNING: As of May 2002, JAMA (*Journal of the American Medical Association*) reported that the potential dangers of newly FDA-approved drugs are *far higher* than initially believed prior to their going to market. An incredible 20% of new drugs will be labeled "dangerous" or will be pulled from the market! The report went on to say JAMA clearly admits that the safety of prescription drugs is inevitably "tested" on the public. The study concluded with this warning: "Serious Adverse Drug Reactions (ADR) commonly emerge after the FDA's approval. The 'safety' of new prescription drugs cannot be known with certainty until a drug has been on the market for many years."

Tested? *This is insane!* What are we, lab rats?

Yes, we are just that. My suggestion, as well as that of several other health experts, is that if you can't avoid drugs altogether, at the very least, avoid using any new drug. That includes drugs that have been on the market for fewer than 5 to 7 years.

How do dietary supplements rate?

Dietary supplements have had, on average, fewer than five confirmed deaths per year over the past 25 years in the U.S. Most of these were due to a single batch of genetically engineered tryptophan produced in the late 1980s. Some were due to ephedra.

I'm both infuriated and empowered by this information. I guess we're all simply too busy with our lives to take notice, that is unless it happens to us. What do you do when you get sick?

You'd better believe I do whatever it takes to stay healthy! Besides a few broken bones, I rarely get sick. On the rare occasion when I do, it's either a cold or flu, both of which I let run their course. I've taken antibiotics, but only as a <u>last</u> resort. (The over-prescribing of antibiotics is another serious issue.) I avoid all other meds, aspirin, cold or pain meds, OTC, pharmaceutical drugs, or otherwise. *Why?* Besides the fact that these medications most often make me feel worse, I also realize that every drug (and this includes OTC meds) I put in my body comes with harmful side effects, some deadly! At the very least, all such meds will deplete my serotonin. This is enough for me not to take them. Nonetheless, I make sure to be fully aware of any and all risks when taking these drugs. So should you. Research the many successful *alternative* options before you consider drugs or surgery. I also can't financially afford to get sick. Here's another example of how pathetic our healthcare system is: When I was finally able to afford health insurance, I was turned down because the carrier I had chosen, Blue Cross, considered me "high risk!" *Can you believe that?* Me, high risk? Now that—is funny! All because I got an abnormal reading on my pap smear. Even though this is pretty common for women, and even though I took an additional test and paid additional money to resolve this concern, they still <u>refused</u> me coverage. Instead of simply charging me a higher rate, I was flat out declined! My god, if I, with all that I do to stay healthy, in both body and mind, with no health issues whatso-ever, cannot get insured, how the hell do most Americans—who are most often borderline diabetic, overweight, pill-poppin', smokin', drinkin', depressed individuals—ever expect to get health coverage? And if you are fortunate enough to get coverage, the minute you make a claim, the carrier either cancels your policy, or jacks your premiums up so high that you can no longer afford it! Either way, they win. It is frightening to realize that health insurance is becoming a luxury that sadly only the very wealthy can afford.

I have absolutely no faith in the health insurance system. It is just another shameful scam on the American public. It cannot be counted on. All the more reason why you most defi-nitely need to do *whatever* it takes to stay healthy. Making sure I maintain my serotonin gives me the ability to do this, by making sure I eat a healthy diet. It keeps me away from sugar, alcohol, caffeine, etc. This is exactly why I encourage others to live a healthy lifestyle starting now, so as to hopefully avoid these medical risks. I also refuse to let myself worry, stress, talk, or think about such illnesses. Don't forget, what you focus your thoughts and spoken words on will manifest into your life. (*Science of Mind,* Ernest Holmes.)

Furthermore, with all the purported miracle drugs, why is everyone sicker than ever before? Hmm? *Where are all the healthy people?* Well, by now, you know the answer to that. Nevertheless, I'd also like to know why the medical industry doesn't promote "Preventative/Wellness" methods of healthcare instead of simply shoving their deadly drugs down on our throats? And why aren't those individuals who are <u>not</u> burdening the already floundering healthcare system, but instead going to great lengths to *prevent* ill-ness, compensated in some fashion? People should be able to write off any item and/or service that promotes Wellness of body and mind—be it gym memberships, exercise classes, supplements, etc. And to those who aren't so easily motivated to get healthy on their own, maybe a tax break might kick them into high gear. Either or, it's a win-win situ-ation, one that actually *rewards* Wellness!

As I write this chapter, I'm rather concerned about speaking such absolute truths against the almighty, ever-powerful FDA, drug companies, and FTC. It's a proven fact they will do *whatever* it takes to shut down and silence people like myself, people who dare to edu-cate and warn the public to their bureaucratic scams. There are also literally hundreds of examples of companies and individuals who have discovered all-natural cures for most, if not all, the major diseases. But the minute they start to share this extraordinary, lifesaving information with the public, the second they start to become successful, the FDA, FTC, and IRS rush in and heavily fine these businesses, shutting them down with lightening speed, confiscating their products, even putting some of these product developers in jail. And while these products are showing truly remarkable results with thousands of clients—with no side effects, no health risks of any kind—they are a dangerous threat to the survival of the drug companies. *Why?* Because these people and their all-natural products that are offering help and, yes, cures to the consumer, threaten all that the pharmaceutical companies thrive on! Without diseases, without the need for their thousands of expensive, ineffective, deadly drugs to treat these diseases (diseases that are most often created by the drugs themselves!) without the often senseless surgeries, the healthcare industry would suffer astronomical losses! It would, in essence, become obsolete. To reiterate, the healthcare system as it's designed today, is all about profits, NOT about curing diseases!

However, as of the Vioxx scandal (with a staggering 100,000 needless deaths!) and the many other drugs that are now subsequently being scrutinized, I sincerely hope that this will be the desperately overdue wake-up call that will bring down the FDA and the pharmaceutical industry as we know them. They need to be held accountable for all the lives they have destroyed, for the trust they have so easily and frighteningly abused, for the endless lies, deceit, and fraud they have perpetrated on the trusting consumer! As I see it, criminal prosecution is a must for all involved. I only wish there were more people like Dr. David Graham, the senior FDA scientist who had the conscience, and the *courage,* to blow the whistle on his own employer about Vioxx, a drug he knew would kill tens of thousands! Even after he was harassed, intimidated, and threatened by his supervisors, Dr. Graham never backed down and did what was right. Well done, Sir!

Because of all these concerns, and many more, you simply cannot sit in silence. You must be willing to educate yourself, to protect yourself and your loved ones. You must be ready to fight for what you believe, even if that means taking risks. As you know, change doesn't happen overnight. But we can sure as hell get a lot more accomplished when we present our grievances in numbers. Thus, please, take the time to educate yourself. Stop turning a deaf ear and praying it won't affect you. Dare to take a stand on this matter. It could very well save your life, or the life of someone you love.

I rarely meet one who feels as strongly as I do about the outrageous and illegal behavior of the FDA, drug and food companies. (As well as our federal government!) Bill Maher, HBO's host of *Real Time,* is my hero. I applaud him. I respect him for so boldly bringing awareness of these serious issues to his audience. He's a highly informed, passionate individual who has the guts to speak the ugly truths about these terrifyingly calculating agencies. Truth be told, our country would be a helluva lot better off with people like Bill, Oprah, and General Honore—with Senators Clinton and Obama leading us!

Fellow consumer activist Kevin Trudeau is equally someone who dares to speak up on behalf of the consumer and our constitutional rights; freedom of speech being his primary fight. Trust me, it's a fight well worth taking! As of February 2005, Kevin took his grievances one step further. He filed two separate lawsuits against the United States government and the FTC, charging them with "Breach of contract and publishing false and misleading information." He's basically giving them a taste of their own hypocritical medicine, demanding both parties be held to the same laws that they sue others for. I recommend you read his book, *Natural Cures "They" Don't Want You to Know About*. He also has a monthly newsletter. Both will open your eyes even further to the level of fraud within our government. I disagree with some of his opinions, as he surely will with mine, but what concerns me most is his latest diet book. He claims you can "Lose 30 pounds in 30 days—and all while eating virtually 'whatever' you want!" Well, you definitely know me well enough by now to know how I feel about that kind of claim. Moving on...

A hospital nightmare: December 2004, 1:30am, Billy called me, needing to be rushed to the emergency room. After waiting 3 stressful hours to simply get him admitted, it then took asking the nurses a dozen times to follow through on his pain meds. When they finally brought them, they stood around, calmly, casually, with no sense of urgency whatsoever, making small talk and jokes—all the while he was in *excruciating pain!* It wasn't just the pain meds, it was literally everything that needed to be done for him. Even more alarming, as the nurse was in the midst of injecting him with morphine, she suddenly stopped and asked, "Oh, by the way, you are indeed Mr. Ciampo, aren't you?" *Excuse me?* She couldn't possibly be serious? Talk about incompetency! She was halfway through giving Billy this drug before she bothered to make sure she even had the right patient! What if this drug had been something other than a pain medication? Hmm? *What then?*

This is awful! What do you suggest?
My suggestion here is to make damn sure you do everything possible to stay healthy and out of the hospital. If, by some misfortune, you do get sick and have to go, have someone with you watching your back! It could mean life or death. The fact is, 90,000 people die every year due to hospital errors!

Doctor claims: "McDonald's is a healthy choice!"
(Now I know you know better than to believe that!)

Another interesting observation: Nearly every nurse, doctor, and medical employee I saw was, at the very least, 25 pounds overweight. And, as I sat in the cafeteria, I found it further fascinating, and again all-telling, to see the types of foods not only the staff was eating, but also the visitors. It was another perfect example of watching what happens when serotonin is depleted. With stress being one of the major causes of depletion of serotonin, it's easy to understand why these people were consuming, and with great voracity, nothing but fries, sodas, bread, donuts, coffee, etc. Their brains were in a frenzy, forcing them to consume whatever foods/beverages it would take to elevate this calming brain chemical. And because the staff lives under this kind of stress daily, you can understand why so many of them continually eat this type of food and subsequently gain weight. I'd venture to guess they probably also suffer from, to some degree, in addition to the carbohydrate cravings, depression, insomnia, anxiety, and/or adult ADD—all symptoms of low serotonin.

Speaking of hospital food, if you believe the medical industry has your best interests at heart, then explain how McDonald's was ever allowed to set up shop in hospitals across the country? *How is that possible?* A doctor interviewed eagerly defended this by saying it was "good for their patients, as McDonald's is a well-known comfort food. It seems to help in the recovery process." WHAT?! I couldn't believe he actually said this, moreover, he expected the public to believe it! This business decision, a poor one at that, was based entirely on financial greed—and ignorance.

As I was closing this chapter, I recalled a medical condition I had years ago. It wasn't anything serious, just some swelling in my fingers that just happened to occur after a minor surgery. Coincidence? I doubt it. Nonetheless, I went to my primary caregiver who proceeded to run a few simple blood tests. His medical diagnosis: Raynaud's disease, a lifelong condition. He advised me my only treatment was one of two drugs, both also lifelong. Considering I wasn't about to take his word without first doing some research, I went home and immediately looked it up online, especially the drugs he was suggesting I take for "life." Not only did my symptoms barely fall under the guidelines of Raynaud's, but I was further shocked at the side effects that were common to those drugs. Liver failure was only one of the many potential risks! I wasted no time in calling him to discuss other options and to have him explain how he came to his conclusion. He admitted there was nothing that actually "confirmed" his medical diagnosis; it was, rather, because the other few tests had come back negative. Wow! Now that's a helluva way to diagnose a patient! He was not even sure of what I had, but yet he insisted I risk my health (and life) by using dangerous drugs for the rest of my life! All the more reason why I am immensely grateful that I have learned to think for myself. I listen to my body, and I dare to question others, no matter their profession. And thank goodness, because it's been 10 years and all symptoms are long gone. I hate to think what might have happened had I listened to him and taken those deadly lifelong drugs.

I feel the need to summarize this chapter by restating the following facts:
• The drug companies are *publicly traded* corporations. Their motive is, first and foremost, to make a profit. • The FDA and FTC both work hand in hand with the drug companies. Their priority is not the welfare of the consumer, but rather it is about their profits. • Drug companies, without hesitation, dangerously manipulate, and thus, falsify their clinical studies to suit their selfish needs. • Both prescription and nonprescription drugs are designed to be capable only of targeting and masking symptoms. These drugs do not cure illness or disease. • Both prescription and nonprescription drugs will, indisputably, create new disease and illness in the body. They will also deplete serotonin, leading to depression, anxiety, cravings, obesity, insomnia, ADD, ED, heart disease, etc. • If you want to get well and/or stay healthy, you need to get off all drugs.

ATTENTION: *If you suffer from an illness or have symptoms of an illness, consult your physician. If you're currently taking prescription drugs or OTC medication, don't stop taking them or replace them based on any information or recommendations appearing in this book without first consulting your medical doctor.*

PART II

CARBOHYDRATES
&
THE GLYCEMIC INDEX

All carbohydrates are sugar.
But they're ranked quite differently,
based on how quickly they affect blood sugar levels.
This ranking of carbohydrates is called
The Glycemic Index.

28

WHAT IS A CARB?

All this fear of carbohydrates, but I'm not even sure what a carb is.
Carbohydrates supply our bodies with the energy they need to function properly. They are the primary source of blood glucose. Blood glucose is a major fuel for our cells. Blood glucose is the only source of energy for red blood cells and our brain.

Where do carbs come from?
Carbohydrates are either plant-based or fruit-based. They are found in starchy and non-starchy vegetables, breads, bagels, cereals, grains, sweets, pasta, fruits, milk, yogurt, and many other dairy products. Carbs can be real or man-made. Avoid man-made carbs.

Aren't there two specific types of carbs?
Yes. Carbohydrates are divided into simple or complex carbohydrates. Simple carbs include table sugar (sucrose), milk sugar (lactose), and fruit sugar (fructose). Simple carbs, those found in such foods as cookies, candy, sodas, white bread, most breakfast cereals, fruits, fruit juices, milk (more so skim and fat-free milk), etc., quickly affect the body, causing blood sugar levels to rise too high. This response causes insulin levels to spike, perpetuating carbohydrate cravings, fat storage, depression, and so forth.

Complex carbs, those found in whole grains and vegetables, though still made up of sugar molecules, are made up of longer, more complex chains. They're slower burning, slower to metabolize into energy, which means they do not affect blood sugar levels in such a dramatic manner. Either way, when you eat simple or complex carbohydrates, they are converted into glucose. This glucose is then either used immediately to supply energy to the body, or it's stored in the form of glycogen.

How does the body use carbs?
Carbs are fuel for the body and mind. The body requires a continuous intake of carbs to feed the brain properly. The brain uses glucose, a form of sugar, as its primary source of energy. The brain actually uses over 2/3 of the carbohydrates circulating in the bloodstream while you're resting. To maintain this high demand, the body continually takes carbohydrates and converts them into glucose. To reiterate, any carbohydrates that are not used right away by the body will be stored in the form of glycogen for later use. But if all of the glycogen stores are full, guess what? The extra glucose is converted into fat. Bottom line: If you eat more carbs than your body can use, the excess will be stored as body fat. Another reason you must limit your carbohydrate intake, choose your carbs wisely, and increase your level of exercise. The more physically active you are, the more (good) carbs you can afford to eat.

29

GOOD CARB? BAD CARB?
Which is it?

First and foremost, all carbs are *not* bad. The carbs you need to avoid are the highly refined, processed carbs such as breakfast cereals, pasta, candy, white bread, white rice, snack foods, etc. In other words, *high glycemic carbs*. Unfortunately, one of the most popular, but equally unhealthy, carbohydrate foods is shown in the previous chapter. And, yes, that would be bagels.

Bagels? I thought bagels were a healthy choice?
Sorry, bagels are one of the worst choices when it comes to carbs, for the mere fact that to get them to taste so moist and delicious, they're highly refined. Which means that as soon as you eat them, they turn into blood sugar, spiking insulin dramatically. If you insist on having a bagel, you're far better off eating a whole grain bagel along with some sort of healthy fat and lean protein. Eggs, butter, avocado, or tomatoes, turkey, cheese, etc., are all great choices, as these foods will help lower the blood sugar response compared to eating just a plain bagel. And make sure you "combine" these foods, never eating your carbs first, or alone, as you want to avoid spiking your insulin. I also recommend you eat your protein first, as it will signal your brain that food is coming and will, as a result, help control your appetite naturally.

Diets like Atkins make it seem like all carbs are evil. Are they?
Once again, all carbs are not evil. With regard to Atkins, he did not condemn all carbs. People often misinterpret his recommendations. It is primarily during the induction stage of his program that he asks you to seriously limits carbs. And that meant eating only 20g of nonstarchy carbs per day. His goal is to put the body into ketosis. The theory of ketosis is that, by depleting the body's glycogen stores (which are from carbs), you force your body to use its stored body fat for fuel. Personally, and among other concerns, I think that's far too few carbs for the body and mind to function on.

What is the glycemic index?
The glycemic index (GI) was created in the early 1980s by a team of researchers. It is a guide for helping control diabetes. The GI is widely accepted in Canada, England, and Australia to help control not only diabetes, but also as an overall diet strategy. Just recently, the U.S. has come to realize the importance of this nutritional breakthrough.

How does it work?
The GI ranks, on a scale from 1–100, the speed at which carbohydrate foods are converted

into blood sugar. Pure glucose is the benchmark, with a rating of 100. Carbohydrates that break down quickly during digestion have the highest GI value. This conversion triggers the rapid release of insulin. Insulin's primary role at this time is to protect the brain from this dangerous overload of sugar.

Can you please explain it again?
All carbohydrates are recognized as sugar by the body, but they're ranked quite differently based on how quickly they affect blood sugar levels. On this scale of 1–100, 1–54 is considered low GI. 55–70 is considered medium GI. 71–100 is considered high GI. Please note, this only measures quantity, *not quality*. For example: While white bread has a higher GI than a chocolate bar, the candy would send your insulin levels soaring for hours. High levels of insulin, especially over long periods of time, are extremely harmful to your health. They can lead to insulin resistance, type 2 diabetes, and heart disease. Insulin is a hormone, and when it's elevated, it will upset every other hormone. Insulin also encourages the storage of body fat. Remember, insulin is the trigger that opens fat cells.

Insulin actually opens fat cells?
Yes. To reiterate, insulin stimulates the body's 30 billion fat cell receptors and deposits carbohydrate energy directly into their interiors. This is how the body stores fat. With every meal, blood sugar levels rise. The key to maintaining a lean, healthy body is to keep your insulin levels stabilized. Therefore, please consume complex/low GI carbs, as they cause the least amount of insulin production. That being said, though the GI rating of foods is what you need to concern yourself with most, it's not perfect either, as eating too many low GI carbs can equally trigger insulin. And on the other hand, you can actually help *lower* the GI rating of a high GI food by eating a good quality fat and protein along with it.

Is this what all those "net carb/impact carb" products are referring to?
Yes. These products are claiming you only need to count a certain number of carbs. But please do not fall for this deceptive marketing ploy. While I agree there are carbs that are better than others, as well as carbs that affect blood sugar levels at different intensity (simple versus complex), all carbs break down into sugar once consumed. At the end of the day, I want to know how many total carbs I've eaten.

My bigger concern is that since the food/nutritional industry has finally shifted from the all-consuming "fat-free" movement, it has done a 180-degree turnaround to literally everything claiming to be LOW-CARB. From low-carb milk, low-carb yogurt, to carb-friendly cookies! Not to mention every restaurant advertisement is touting their low-carb menus. Everyone has jumped on this bandwagon. This could all prove to be highly beneficial in the war against obesity, but only if the consumer really understands what low-carb means. Unfortunately, this is rarely the case. I find it a fascinating study to watch people as they grocery shop. It's all-telling and rather frightening. It also confirms my fears about what this whole low-carb/net carb movement is going to do to our obesity rate. Please allow me...

Sugar-free cookies?
Ah, a dream come true!

I was out shopping with Cookie, a beautiful 10-year-old girl that I mentor. As we stood in the checkout line, I quietly observed the woman ahead of us. Her basket was filled with junk food. Oh, she had quite an assortment of goodies, ranging from several bags of sugar-free candy, Keebler's Carb Sensible Chocolate-Chip Cookies, SnackWells CarbWell Fudge Brownie Cookies, sugar-free cookies, low-carb crackers, low-carb chips, to a dozen low-carb Hershey chocolate bars. Which, by the way, were claiming a mere 2 net carbs. But hold on a minute! Do not be overly critical when judging this woman's choices. After all, I knew that, based on what she was buying, i.e., all LOW-CARB and/or SUGAR-FREE, she *believed* she was doing the right thing!

You see, this woman clearly believed, based on her items of choice, that she was buying foods that would keep her thin, or at least keep her from gaining any more weight. How terribly wrong, though! She's going to be in for a big—and not so pleasant surprise as she starts to pack on the pounds. This disturbing scenario is a perfect example of most Americans' buying habits. Sorry to say, but most people tend to believe whatever food manufacturers claim on their labels. They assume they're being honest in their claims. This woman, and millions more just like her, will focus on buying all these bogus low-carb, net/impact carb, sugar-free foods and then wonder why the hell they're getting fatter and moodier than ever!

Are you starting to see *why* all this deceptive marketing is going to further fuel obesity, type 2 diabetes, heart disease, and cancer? Beware! This has quickly become the next multi-billion-dollar opportunity for food manufacturers! And with the FDA and FTC setting few, if any regulations, a manufacturer can, in fact claim "low-carb/sugar-free" without any such proof. And without standards or regulations, how can one determine what is truly low-carb or sugar-free? This is just one of many reasons why I wrote this book: To help educate the consumer so they can hopefully make wiser and healthier choices.

Aren't the net carb claims found mostly on diet food and protein bars?
These claims are now found on all health bars, as well as everything from chips, crackers, cookies, milk, bagels, yogurt, cereal, to even ice cream. And this is exactly why you need to seriously question the legitimacy of these claims. Compare "real carbohydrate" claims to these invented, processed foods. Do you see them claiming on a tomato: "Only 3 Net Carbs!" Or on a bag of mixed greens: "Only 2 Impact Carbs!" No, of course not.

What about protein bars?
To reiterate, I'd like to believe the protein bar market was originally created to provide a healthy way for athletes to get extra protein. But due to the phenomenal success of this market, these so-called health, nutritional, and meal replacement bars have become nothing more than over-hyped, overpriced candy bars. Reading the various labels is

proof enough. They're loaded with all kinds of additives, a ton of hidden sugars, HFCS, chocolate, fillers, etc. They are not a healthy choice, and they're definitely NOT a free food! Meaning: You cannot eat them all day long and think they won't show up on your hips or thighs! Among many things, they will most certainly perpetuate cravings.

I see so many overweight people, people who clearly have never seen the inside of a gym, yet they're filling their grocery carts with these bars. I know darn well, though, based on the clever, million-dollar marketing strategy put forth by the manufacturers, the consumer is seduced into believing they're doing the right thing. Once again: Please, eat *real* food instead of these highly processed bars! (I must admit I eat a protein bar on a *very rare* occasion. But I also realize they are nothing more than an expensive candy bar with added protein.)

Even personal trainers can be fooled!

As I close this chapter, I'd like to share the following, as it's a perfect example of just how easy it is to be fooled with product labels, their various claims, be it with regard to low-carb, sugar-free, or otherwise: Sylvester Stallone's company, *Stallone*, recently came out with an alternative to the standard, highly processed protein bar. It's a ready-to-eat, deliciously creamy, high protein pudding that comes in either milk chocolate or vanilla cream. Each individual 6.4 ounce can contains 20g of quality protein, a mere 1g of carbs, 2g of total fat, 0 trans fat, 330mg of potassium, only 100 calories, 5mg of cholesterol, free of lactose, but, a whopping 420mg of sodium! Now I realize endurance athletes need to replenish their sodium, but 420mg in one little serving is awfully high, even for athletes—and especially for the average consumer. An 8 ounce serving of Gatorade has only 110mg of sodium, and it's the highest of all the sports drinks.

My primary point here, though, is that they also claim the pudding is SUGAR-FREE. Now, as you have learned, nothing that sweet can be truly sugar-free. So, if it's not naturally occurring sugar or they didn't physically add sugar on the front end, then how can they claim sugar-free? Easy. They used sucralose, an <u>artificial</u> sweetener.

While I absolutely love Mr. Stallone's unique concept behind the very convenient packaging of a protein snack, my concern is with the high sodium, and the sucralose they're using to sweeten the product. As mentioned earlier, sucralose is chemically altered and the subsequent health risks are numerous! This would have made for an excellent protein alternative to bars had they used far less sodium—and stevia, Lou Han Guo, or some other all-natural extract—in lieu of sucralose.

The ironic part of this story is that only days after reviewing this pudding, I saw a trainer in the gym eagerly devouring two of Stallone's protein puddings. (Which = 840mg of sodium and god knows how much sucralose in one sitting.) All the while, he was raving to his client about how terrific it was, because "not only was it high in protein, but better yet, it was also *sugar-free!"* The client was, of course, just as eager to go buy some. And as much as I wanted to say something, it wasn't my place. Unfortunately, as you can see, even most fitness experts aren't aware of the rules (and yes, trickery) behind the manufacturers claims of their products being so-called "sugar-free."

My suggestion would be that, first and foremost, manufacturers be held to the strictest of guidelines as to declaring what is truly in their foods. Then, instead of the endless deceptive "sugar-free, fat-free, low-carb, net-carb" product claims, they should honestly, and accurately, state the "GI Rating" on all their products, as the GI is the critical factor in whether or not insulin is triggered. I believe this will, in fact, be the next big wave in product labeling. Will they be honest, though, is the real concern.

30

GLYCOGEN'S ROLE

What is glycogen?

Glycogen is created when the body converts glucose into storage. It plays a major role in controlling blood sugar levels. Glycogen is the form in which carbohydrates are stored. And, as I mentioned earlier, carbs are the body's preferred choice for fuel. They're readily available and quickest to burn. However, it takes about 20 minutes of moderate to intense aerobic exercise (with oxygen) versus anaerobic exercise (without oxygen) before your body will shift from burning glycogen to a slower burning, more efficient fuel. That fuel being stored body fat.

Is weight training considered anaerobic?

Yes, and because weight training is an anaerobic exercise and, therefore, won't actually "burn fat" as you train, it will, though, help build the lean muscle tissue needed for your body to burn fat/calories long after you leave the gym. This is also why I prefer that my clients do their cardio after I train them, as their bodies will be primed and ready to burn body fat. For those who don't have time to do both on the same day, I highly recommend they do their cardio first thing in the morning—and on an empty stomach. Training on an empty stomach, no matter the exercise, will help insure that your body utilizes body fat as fuel instead of carbs/glycogen. On the other hand, all the training in the world won't matter if you're not eating a balanced diet, especially eating enough quality protein so that your muscles can grow.

Where is glycogen stored?

Glycogen is stored in the liver and the muscles. The liver's capacity to store carbohydrates in the form of glycogen is limited to only a 12-hour supply, approximately 100g of glycogen. The muscles have the capacity to store between 250–400g of glycogen, depending on our own unique muscle mass and physical condition. Liver glycogen is able to supply energy for the entire body, while muscle glycogen only supplies energy to muscles. Consequently, the liver's glycogen reserves must be maintained on a continual basis. This is why we need to eat healthy carbohydrates on a continual basis.

If the body has an excess of glucose and all of the glycogen stores are full, the extra glucose is converted into fat by the liver and stored as adipose tissue, i.e., body fat, throughout the body. Unfortunately, the glycogen stored in the muscles is inaccessible to the brain. Only the glycogen stored in the liver can be broken down and sent back to the bloodstream so as to maintain adequate blood sugar levels for proper brain function.

Is this why we crave high GI foods?
Yes, and no. The previous chapters explained in great detail the relationship between crav-ings and high GI carbs. However, it's also about the brain believing it's being starved. The brain will do whatever it takes to survive, and this includes consuming its own vital organs, as occurs in low-cal dieting. Thus, it will create noise, i.e., a *craving*, pushing you toward high GI carbs, because they are the foods that break down *quickest* into blood sugar. And blood sugar is the preferred food of choice for the brain.

But I thought cravings were caused by low serotonin?
Yes, they are. To reiterate, when serotonin levels are low, we *subconsciously* crave the types of foods that break down quickly into blood sugar, i.e., high GI carbohydrates. These foods can range from bagels, chips, candy, pastries, cereal, fries, pizza, to ice cream, fruit juice, smoothies, etc. All these foods are high GI carbs and they all break down into sugar. They not only elevate insulin and, subsequently serotonin levels, but they also provide the quickest blood sugar for the brain.

If I spike my insulin, I'd be forcing my body to store fat instead of burn it, right?
Exactly. Now you're getting it!

I realize now that serotonin really is the key to eliminating high GI carbs!
Maintaining healthy levels of serotonin will, unquestionably, control your cravings for high GI carbs. This will lead to <u>controlling</u> your insulin levels. Controlled insulin levels means less fat stored, *more fat burned*.

Is this the serotonin-insulin connection you spoke of earlier?
Yes. It is the proven science, the *solution* we've all been waiting for. When you are able to support healthy levels of serotonin, you'll be able to help control these cravings effort-lessly. You'll easily begin to eat healthier, which means less insulin spiking. Without the high insulin levels, your body will have *less* ability to store fat and instead begin to <u>burn</u> its fat stores.

What are some other benefits from eating low GI carbs?
Most low GI/complex carbs have these special advantages for those trying to lose fat: They keep your insulin levels stable, they fill you up quicker, keep you satisfied longer, and they help burn *more* body fat and <u>less</u> body muscle.

What do you consider to be the healthiest carbs?
I suggest grains, legumes, starchy and nonstarchy vegetables. And because nonstarchy vegetables are highly fibrous, they'll lower the GI of your entire meal.

How many carbohydrate grams should I eat daily?
The daily number of carbs that is required will vary greatly, depending on each person's level of physical exercise, body composition, overall health condition, metabolism, age,

as well as eating and lifestyle habits. On days when you're more physically active, you'll need more. On days when you're more sedentary, you'll need less. You'll need to find your own number that your body (and mind) can thrive on, without gaining body fat or losing vital energy. Remember, your brain needs blood sugar to survive. But because carbs are the food group you need to closely monitor so as to avoid gaining body fat, allow me to suggest: I'm going to respectfully assume that most people reading my book will be those who want (and need) to lose body fat. Most will have excess weight at their mid-section. They also won't be physically active. So, I suggest starting with 15 to 20g of low GI carbs per meal, with approximately 7–9g per snack. Once you start exercising (which will be right away, right?), you'll need to slowly add more carbs. The aforementioned is at least an excellent place to start.

Should I count how many carbs I eat daily?

Yes, you need to count all carbs for the first few months. *Why?* A single piece of white bread (which, by the way, is not a low GI carb) can easily have 25g of carbs. Or how about a bowl of white rice at 37g of carbs? Better yet, how about a multi-bran chex cereal at a whopping 41g of carbs? This doesn't include the milk and fruit most will add to the cereal. Nor does it include the glass of orange juice at 25g that usually accompanies this cereal. So you see, counting carbs is a fantastic way for you to realize just how many carbs you consume on any given day. When you're forced to actually *count* the amount of carbs you eat, you can't help but see why you've gained weight. BTW: Don't worry about craving or even missing any of those high GI carbs, the carbs you *think* you can't live without. Maintaining healthy levels of serotonin with an SES will help you control these cravings, cravings that are simply a side effect of low serotonin. You will be astonished at how you no longer desire or need those trigger/comfort foods.

Do you count carbs?

To be honest, no, I don't. Maintaining healthy serotonin levels control my desire and any and all cravings for carbs. It also controls my overall appetite. It allows me to eat healthy, and to eat less. Please note, when I speak of eating less, it's not so much about eating *less* food, as in counting calories, but it is, instead, about eating just enough food for my body and mind to remain healthy—and all without effort or ever feeling deprived. Therefore, I do not count carbs (or calories). That being said, and for all the reasons listed above, I still want you to count your daily carb intake for at least 60 days. This process will help you tremendously in better understanding where all your carbs are coming from. All of this combined will further help you reach and maintain your weight loss goals.

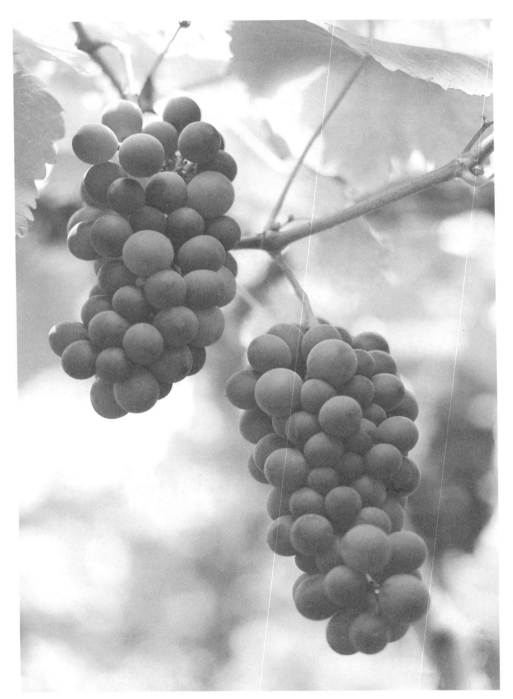

198

31

CRUCIAL CARBOHYDRATE FACTS

▶ Simple carbs (fruit and candy) and complex carbs (vegetables and grains) are both broken down in the digestive system into one-sugar molecules.

▶ Simple carbohydrates consist of 1 to 2 linked sugar molecules. Complex carbohydrates consist of 3 or more linked sugar molecules.

▶ All carbohydrates are recognized as sugar by the body.

▶ Fruit, though natural, is still a carbohydrate and high in fructose. Avoid eating fruit alone, or first. Instead, combine it with a healthy fat and quality protein. (I mix my fruit with salads, turkey, crab, eggs, etc.)

▶ When trying to lose excess body fat, eat only one serving of a low GI fruit per day.

▶ Carbohydrates are the only nutrient group that quickly converts into blood sugar.

▶ Unlike carbohydrates, your body will let you know when you've eaten enough fat and protein.

▶ Liquid carbohydrates, i.e., milk, fruit juice, smoothies, etc., are absorbed by the body much quicker than solids, which gives them a higher GI response.

▶ Carbohydrates are the only food group you need to count closely.

▶ Excess carbohydrates will be converted into and stored as body fat.

▶ Never eat carbohydrates alone. Instead, combine them with a healthy (non-damaged) fat and quality protein to help lower the GI.

▶ Include at least one complex/low GI carb with every meal.

▶ The rougher the grain or flour, the lower the GI.

▶ Avoid foods made with white flour.

▶ Though pasta, cereal, and bread are considered to be complex carbs, they are *highly refined man-made* carbs. Avoid man-made carbs as they require no digestion time, which means they quickly break down into blood sugar, thereby affecting insulin levels dramatically.

▶ Avoid eating over-ripe fruit, as it's highest in sugar.

▶ Adding vinegar or lemon juice to carbs will help lower the GI.

▶ When snacking, avoid eating carbs alone, especially high GI carbs.

▶ Even though some food may be considered to be a low GI carb, it may, nevertheless, still be high in useless carbs, sugar, etc., and thus, provide empty calories. Example: Some candy has a low GI. It is not, though, a healthy food choice.

▶ You can eat more of low GI foods—or less of high GI foods—and still achieve the same blood sugar levels.

▶ With regard to fruit, berries have the lowest GI.

▶ When considering insulin levels, it's not only the GI you should be concerned with, but also the amount and type of overall carbohydrates consumed.

▶ The brain requires a continuous supply of blood sugar, i.e., glucose, to survive. This fuel can only come from carbohydrates. For that reason, you need to eat a healthy diet consisting of complex carbs with every meal.

A quick summary:
Complex/low GI carbs:
▶ Are more satisfying
▶ Keep you fuller, longer
▶ Help curb your appetite
▶ Are the best fuel for your body and mind
▶ Can help lower the GI of an entire meal
▶ Can reduce the amount of insulin needed, thereby lowering risks for type 2 diabetes
▶ Equal a smaller rise in blood glucose levels after meals, which equals less fat stored
▶ Make fat harder to store—and easier to burn
▶ Can prolong physical endurance
▶ Combined with regular exercise and maintaining serotonin, can produce tremendous weight loss results and much better overall health

NOTES

32

EXCELLENT LOW GLYCEMIC CARBS

The following is a list of low (to medium) GI carbs. They're some of the healthiest choices when it comes to carbs. Once again, whether low, medium, or high GI carbs, don't ever eat them alone. Always combine them with a healthy fat and quality protein.

Fruits:

Blueberries	Strawberries	Mulberries
Blackberries	Raspberries	Cherries
Oranges	Kiwi	Grapefruit
Pears	Peaches	Apricots
Plums	Apples	Melon

Grains:

Barley	Brown rice	Bulgur	Couscous
Oats	Polenta	Rye	Semolina
Whole grain products	Wheat germ	Wild rice	

Beverages:
Tomato or other vegetable juice (Fresh only and beware of sodium. They're also a "liquid carb" which means they'll affect blood sugar levels more dramatically.)

Vegetables/Legumes/Beans:

Artichokes	Arugula	Asparagus	Bean sprouts
Black beans	Black-eyed peas	Broccoli	Brussels sprouts
Butter beans	Cannellini beans	Cabbage	Carrots (raw)
Collard greens	Celery	Cucumber	Eggplant
Garbanzo beans	Garlic	Green beans	Jicama
Leeks	Lentils	Lima beans	Lettuces
Mushrooms	Mustard greens	Navy beans	Okra
Onions	Parsnips	Peppers	Pinto beans
Radishes	Red peppers	Kale	Shallots
Spaghetti squash	Spinach	Split peas	Tomatoes
White beans	Sweet potatoes	Yams	Watercress
Acorn squash	Red kidney beans	Butternut squash	

Nuts/Seeds:

Almond	Walnut	Cashew	Macadamia
Brazil	Pumpkin	Sunflower	Flaxseed

Dairy:

Cream cheese	Feta	Goat	Ricotta
Mozzarella	Swiss (limit)	Soy milk	Whipping cream
Organic soy yogurt (no added sugar)		Cottage cheese (watch sodium)	

All-Natural Sweeteners:

Stevia	Xylitol	Ki-Sweet	Lou Han Gou

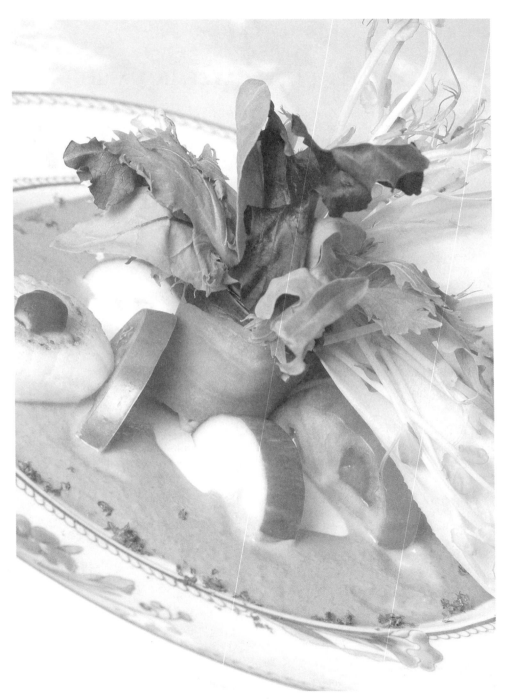

33

SUGGESTED FOODS...
My personal choices

In all modesty, people often ask me what I eat to stay so lean and healthy. This is even more flattering, considering my age. Therefore, I felt it might be helpful to dedicate a chapter to the foods I have in my own home, to show you which foods best fuel both my body and mind. Please understand, however, that it was while writing this book, particularly chapter 23, that I had no choice but to rethink my diet. It was easy enough to stop eating poultry, butter, and cheese, but I've yet to give up eggs and shellfish for precise dietary needs, i.e., healthy dietary fat and cholesterol. In the meantime, though the foods that are listed are wonderfully healthy choices, the meat and cheese products are those foods I "used" to eat on any given day prior to this very personal commitment.

That being said, my first rule is to buy *real* food, food that is fresh and organically grown. But with the latest health buzz on organic foods, be aware that the FDA does not have any set guidelines when it comes to food manufacturers who make these claims. This also pertains to range-free, cruelty-free, etc. This leaves the market wide open to certain manufacturers who will surely abuse this loophole. This is another reason why I'm so strongly committed to changing my diet. Even if I want to buy organically grown, range-free dairy products, I really have no idea if the manufacturers' claims are true. My concern is that I may still be contributing to the torment of these farm animals, as well as eating food that is harmful to my health. (To those who claim they can't afford to buy organic, my groceries run about $60 per week. *That's less than $10 per day, and eating 5 meals per day!* Can't get any cheaper or healthier than that.)

Next, I make sure I do NOT buy the things I know I shouldn't eat. *Why tempt myself?* I encourage you to do the same. On the other hand, there is absolutely no effort for me eat this way, as long as I maintain my serotonin. I <u>never</u> feel deprived or hungry. Ever. The following foods are what I have found to work best for me, be it physically, mentally, or emotionally. They are exceptionally healthy choices, but they are also "my personal" choices. They may not be your favorite foods, but they will definitely give you a better idea of what you should be eating.

My groceries include the following:
- Vanilla or banana whey protein powder (aspartame/sucralose-free, low-carb/sugar)
- Blueberries, raspberries, strawberries, blackberries, apples, grapefruit, mango, melon
- Fresh salmon, sardines, catfish, mahi-mahi, crab, shrimp, lobster, scallops
- Organic chicken, ground turkey, tofu, free-range, antibiotic/hormone-free eggs

- Organic, all-natural almond, peanut, and sunflower seed butters (no sugar added, no hydrogenated fats/oils)
- Feta, goat, mozzarella, cottage cheese, ricotta, Muenster, cream cheese, and limited Parmesan and Swiss (white, fresh cheeses are best versus aged or yellow)
- Herb salad greens, collard greens, spinach, eggplant, celery, kidney and black beans
- Brussels sprouts, spinach, broccoli, asparagus, red/yellow peppers, bean sprouts
- Yams, acorn/spaghetti squash, portobello and shiitake mushrooms, hearts of palm
- Green olives, capers, avocados, tomatoes, seedless cucumbers, alfalfa sprouts
- Whole grain oatmeal (unsweetened), whole grain bread, whole grain crackers
- Unsweetened fresh whipping cream (lowest in carbs), organic soy yogurt (low-sugar)
- Coconut water, lite coconut milk (low in carbs/sugar, healthy fat)
- Decaf green tea, decaf hazelnut/vanilla tea
- Macadamias, almonds, walnuts, pecans, sunflower and pumpkin seeds (unsalted, raw or dry roasted only)

Many of my clients say they don't know what to eat for a snack (or a meal), so I've included some of my favorites. Again, rather than eat a lot at one sitting, I choose to eat light, but more often. Some of these are snacks, some are meals. The key is to be creative and always combine a healthy fat and protein along with a complex/low GI carb.

- Mini spinach wraps w/ chopped grilled shrimp (or lobster), feta, cilantro
- 2 eggs, medium portobello mushroom, alfalfa sprouts, olive/grapeseed oil, pepper
- 1/2 cup oatmeal w/ 1 scoop protein powder, 5 walnuts crushed, heat, add nutmeg
- Turkey patty, 1/4 cup cottage cheese over spinach, olive/grapeseed oil, parsley, lime
- Chopped shrimp, crab, avocado, 1/4 cup mango, crushed macadamias, cilantro, lime, tossed, serve cold.
- 2 scrambled eggs w/ shaved broccoli, side of tomatoes, buttered whole grain toast
- Broiled salmon, buttered acorn squash, herb salad w/ olive/grapeseed oil
- Sardines on 4 whole grain crackers w/ crumbled feta
- 1/2 small baked yam, 1 egg, goat cheese, rosemary, pepper (before 3pm)
- Broiled catfish, collard greens and tofu sautéed in olive oil, sprinkle of Parmesan
- Shaved cucumber, mozzarella, sprouts, diced shrimp, olive oil, capers, lime
- 1/2 avocado, diced tomatoes, crab, blended w/ pepper, olive/grapeseed oil
- Walnuts, mozzarella, shiitake mushrooms, green apple slices over spinach, heated
- Shaved asparagus w/ tips, grapeseed oil, pepper, lime, topped w/ crab (or mahi-mahi)
- Goat cheese, turkey, strawberries, hearts of palm over herb salad greens, olive oil
- Whole grain toast w/ sliced tomato, melted mozzarella, green olives, pepper
- Sliced tomatoes, 1/4 cup cottage cheese, topped w/ 2 tbsp yogurt
- Muenster cheese, 1/4 cup blueberries w/ unsweetened fresh whipping cream
- Vanilla protein drink w/ 1 tsp sunflower seed butter, 1/4 cup blueberries on the side
- 1 tbsp peanut butter on half an apple (or 2 celery sticks), 1 hard-boiled egg
- 1/4 cup of assorted raw nuts and seeds (a daily snack)
- 1 serving of walnuts (about 12) sprinkled w/ Parmesan, slightly heated

Favorite flavor enhancers:
- Extra virgin olive oil, grapeseed oil, flaxseed oil, real butter (organic/unsalted)
- All-natural organic mayo, balsamic vinegar
- Fresh cilantro, rosemary, basil, parsley, dill
- Lemon, lime, pepper, sesame seeds, cinnamon, nutmeg, stevia, xylitol

* Though I don't care for garlic, it has many extraordinary health benefits.

Note: It has long been my personal choice not to eat most meat. To reiterate, however, it was while I was in the midst of writing this book, that I knew I had to make better choices. I'd love it if you, too, would at least *consider* eating a kinder, much healthier, and more compassionate diet. But if you should choose to continue to eat meat, red or white, please limit it (especially red meat) and select only those products that are lean, free-range, organic and free of nitrates, fertilizers, pesticides, antibiotics, and hormones to help insure healthier meats, whether beef, lamb, turkey, duck, chicken, pork, etc.

Below are the newest items to be added to my grocery list. They are my vegetarian choices in lieu of eating any more chicken, turkey, and cheese. (Due to certain dietary needs, I may still eat goat cheese.) They're extremely healthy, excellent in taste, low in carbs and sodium, sugar-free, high in protein, and, best of all, *animal-friendly.* Although I was never fond of the taste of meat, I've long enjoyed veggie burgers. But only recently did I try veggie sausage patties and veggie spinach burgers. And I must say, they were both really very good. They tasted so good, in fact, I challenge the female readers to prepare these vegetarian foods for their families and see if they notice. I guarantee, most will not. So you see, for all those of you who say you can't live without meat, there are many other choices. Also available is everything from meatless ribs and meat balls, to vegetarian hotdogs, turkey, even corn dogs. The corndogs and wings are obviously higher in carbs, but they're still healthier choices than the meat-based products. Therefore, won't you please at least consider the many kinder, healthier options? And again, if your grocery store does not carry vegetarian foods, ask them to please start.

- Extra firm organic tofu, baked organic lemon tofu w/ spinach and lemon
- Baked organic Thai tofu (watch the sodium content)
- Veggie burgers, veggie spinach burgers, veggie sausage patties and links
- Soy yogurt, soy cheese (There are many assorted cheese flavors, but I must be perfectly honest and admit that this cheese can't possibly compare to a nice feta, goat, blue or provolone. Nevertheless, I prefer the shredded 3 cheese blend called *Soy-Sation*. It's healthy and animal-friendly.

* Whether you become a vegetarian or simply cut back your meat and dairy, you need to make sure you get enough quality protein throughout the day. I recommend a perfect protein powder, but make sure it's sweetened with stevia <u>not</u> sucralose/Splenda, HFCS, or aspartame. However, among other health concerns, too much soy may make your stomach bloat. Therefore, I choose to use a high-end whey protein powder.

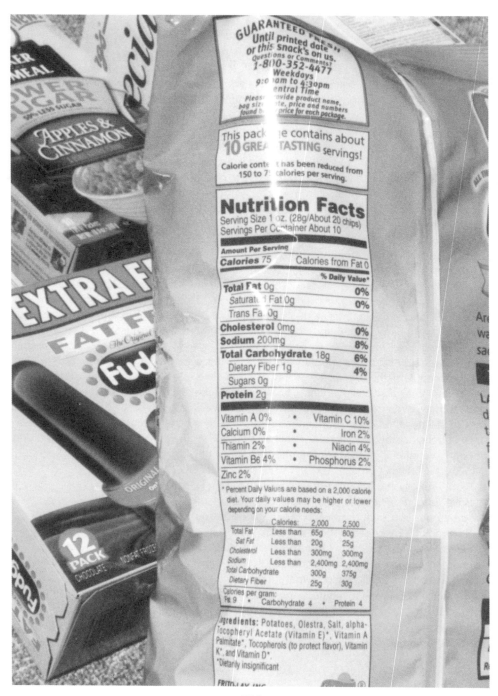

GUARANTEED FRESH
Until printed date
or this snack's on us.
Questions or Comments?
1-800-352-4477
Weekdays
9:00 am to 4:30pm
Central Time
Please provide product name,
bag size, date, price and numbers
found by the price for each package.

This package contains about
10 GREAT TASTING servings!
Calorie content has been reduced from
150 to 75 calories per serving.

Nutrition Facts

Serving Size 1 oz. (28g/About 20 chips)
Servings Per Container About 10

Amount Per Serving

Calories 75   Calories from Fat 0

	% Daily Value*
Total Fat 0g	0%
Saturated Fat 0g	0%
Trans Fat 0g	
Cholesterol 0mg	0%
Sodium 200mg	8%
Total Carbohydrate 18g	6%
Dietary Fiber 1g	4%
Sugars 0g	
Protein 2g	

Vitamin A 0%	•	Vitamin C 10%
Calcium 0%	•	Iron 2%
Thiamin 2%	•	Niacin 4%
Vitamin B6 4%	•	Phosphorus 2%
Zinc 2%		

* Percent Daily Values are based on a 2,000 calorie
diet. Your daily values may be higher or lower
depending on your calorie needs:

	Calories:	2,000	2,500
Total Fat	Less than	65g	80g
Sat Fat	Less than	20g	25g
Cholesterol	Less than	300mg	300mg
Sodium	Less than	2,400mg	2,400mg
Total Carbohydrate		300g	375g
Dietary Fiber		25g	30g

Calories per gram:
Fat 9 • Carbohydrate 4 • Protein 4

Ingredients: Potatoes, Olestra, Salt, alpha-
Tocopheryl Acetate (Vitamin E)*, Vitamin A
Palmitate*, Tocopherols (to protect flavor), Vitamin
K*, and Vitamin D*.
*Dietarily insignificant

FRITO-LAY INC.

34

HOW TO READ A NUTRITIONAL PANEL
Don't be fooled!
Know what you're eating!

With so much deception, how will I ever really know what I'm eating?
As we discussed earlier, food and beverage manufacturers are required to provide certain nutritional facts on their products. While this information has, unfortunately, proven to be far less than truthful, you still need to read the label to get an idea of what you're eating. Then learn to *listen* to your body. If something is sweet, ask *why*. If you feel a sugar/adrenaline rush after eating something, ask *why*. If you suddenly feel thirsty, read the label again and look for the amount of sodium. If you feel bloated, ask *why*. If you unexpectedly feel agitated, ask *why*. Read and reread food labels until you really begin to understand how and why foods and beverages play such a critical role in your physical, emotional, and mental health.

As hard as I try, why is it so difficult to get through a grocery store without buying junk food? I can't seem to resist!
You're not alone, as it is a well-known fact grocery stores spend a great deal of time and money displaying their assorted foods and beverages in a very precise and manipulative manner. They strategically place processed/high GI carbs at the front of the store and center aisles, while R-E-A-L food, i.e., seafood, meat, vegetables, etc., are on the outside aisles and in the rear of the store. Assorted chips, cookies, alcohol, flavored drinks, candy, bagels, etc., take front and center, placed at the beginning of each aisle. Don't forget, every checkout line is loaded with candy and other junk food. Well, understand this: It is not a coincidence. THIS IS ALL FOR A REASON! Those in charge know these foods are *impulse* items, trigger foods. They also know these foods are *addictive!* Their motive: Sell this junk with no regard for our health. It is, once again, all about PROFITS! These foods perpetuate cravings, contributing to excessive fat gain, type 2 diabetes, depression, heart disease, cancer, etc. Beware of these marketing tactics!

Excuse me? You say candy doesn't tempt you? That's great to know. But how about this: The latest marketing ploy by grocery stores is having warm, wonderfully fresh baked bread placed on huge racks right at the entrance of every checkout line. This bread is so fresh, the steam is literally rising from it. So, as you patiently wait in line, trying to avoid the many other temptations placed before you, the smell of this bread is an even bigger tease! I ask you: *How many people can ignore this temptation?* And how many people, who had no desire for bread, end up grabbing a loaf, based solely on this clever manipulation? And if the bread isn't tempting enough, the stores are also now placing racks of Krispy Kreme donuts at the beginning of the aisles! I am simply amazed at the lengths the grocery stores go to control their unsuspecting customers. Again, buyer beware!

But hold on a second! That's not all. The most recent marketing ploy by the grocery stores is to have food on the actual turn aisle, at the end of where your groceries are bagged. It's not just any food, either. Oh, no, definitely not. It's only those foods that the store knows are addictive. Foods such as cereal, candy, soda, chips, etc. The first time I saw this, I had to laugh. I mean, come on, *where does it end?* You've done your best to get through their manipulative aisles, you've succeeded in ignoring their attempts to seduce you with the endless rows of candy, fresh baked bread, and sinfully sweet smelling donuts, only to have them, at the checkout line, once again, so brazenly tempt and tease you with another bunch of sugar-laden, high GI carbs while you're trying to pay for your groceries! Worse yet, it doesn't stop there. If you're able to ignore whatever the chosen item is on display, an item that is literally shoved in your face, the cashier actually *asks* you if you'd like to purchase it! Once again, how many people will be able to refrain from this shrewd manipulation and endless temptation? Not many, I'm afraid.

Now that you are hopefully better informed as to these tactics, you will next need to know how to read, to interpret a food label. The following is the order in which I, personally, read a label. This will determine what I buy and subsequently put into my body. Nevertheless, before I even begin to read the label, and depending on the food source, I will check to see if the food is organically grown, range-free, hormone/antibiotic-free. You must also keep in mind that the FDA does not enforce the law that says all the ingredients in pack-aged/processed foods must be listed. These are, of course, the hidden ingredients that food manufacturers <u>don't</u> what us to know about. These are the very ingredients that these companies sneak into our food, ingredients that further insure we get addicted, coming back for more, and all the while make us fat, depressed, and sicker than ever! With all that in mind, the following is how (and why) I read a nutritional label:

1) Ingredients:
I first look to see what the product is made of. This is where you'll find exactly what ingre-dients are in the product. This will let me know if I even want to buy this particular item. This section will list everything from the primary ingredient source (ranging from chicken, pork, beef, cheese, to flour, grains, starch, caffeine, hydrogenated fats, etc.) You'll also find additives, colorings, and the many <u>hidden</u> sugars, alternative sweeteners, and artificial sweeteners, such as aspartame, sucralose, HFCS, sugar alcohols, molasses, glycerine, etc., in this section. To reiterate, there is an exact science behind how these ingredients are listed. The ones listed first are the ones in *heaviest* concentrations, and so forth down the line. Please read this list with great consideration.

2) Total Carbohydrate:

Next, I look at how many total carbs are in a product. The number shown is based on a single serving. I look to see how many milligrams or grams are in each serving. Although complex and simple carbs affect the blood sugar levels at different rates, all carbs break down into sugar once consumed. Consequently, I focus on the <u>total</u> number of carbs versus just the amount of sugar. It's also important to note that I'm choosing healthy complex/low GI carbs, NOT processed/refined carbs. It's effortless for me to eat this way, because I maintain my serotonin, which subsequently controls cravings and overall appetite. Thus, I don't *ever* count carbs. If I did, I'd prefer a range of 5–15g of carbs per serving, with 20–30g total per meal, and about 10g per snack. This works for me, based on my body type, level of exercise, metabolic rate, and age. (Studies suggest the body requires approximately 60g of carbs for it to merely function properly.)

3) Serving Size:

Keep in mind that nutritional facts are based on a single serving size. This data is then broken down into precise categories. The total numbers shown reflect only that one serving size. Example: A small bag of chips may easily have 2 servings per bag. As a result, if you were to eat the entire bag, you'd have to double all the numbers shown to get the TOTAL number of carbs, sugar, sodium, fat, etc. Another example is a particular brand of protein powder. On their front label, they claim in huge letters: *"46g of PROTEIN!"* Not quite. But you'd have to read the nutritional panel to see that it would take 3 large scoops to actually get those 46g. *Deceptive marketing?* Not really. Misleading is more like it. Manufacturers realize that most consumers only read the front of the label, believing whatever the label claims. Compared to many of the other protein powders, 46g is huge! Hence, you buy it, naturally thinking you're getting more for your money. However, unless you read the serving size, you won't realize it takes twice, maybe three times, the amount of product to get that amount.

4) Net Carbs/Impact Carbs:

I completely ignore this number. I advise you to do the same. Once again, while carbs certainly affect blood sugar levels differently, some burning slower and longer than others, there is no accurate way to measure this claim. Without any FDA regulations, as to what truly determines low-carb or net/impact carbs, *consumer beware*. Focus on eating healthy complex/low GI carbs, combining them with healthy fats and proteins, and then account for the <u>total</u> number of carbs—not just their erratic claims of only net carbs/impact carbs. As I stated earlier, this is merely another deceitful marketing practice being imposed on the far too trusting consumer. My concern is how many (total) carbs they're claiming. Even that is often inaccurate. And, because of all the deception, I rely on what they claim for the amount of carbs and sugar, along with their ingredient list. I also pay very close attention to the order in which the ingredients are listed. All of this information combined, will give me a much better idea of what is in a particular product. (Food/beverage manufacturers should be required to declare the "GI Rating" of all their products. This would help consumers make far healthier choices.)

5) Sugars:

To reiterate, I concern myself mostly with total carbs, as all carbs "turn into sugar" once consumed, but I still look at the amount of sugar the product is claiming to have. You also need to realize that the number of grams of sugar a product claims does not distinguish between sugars that are naturally occurring and those that are refined (or artificial). Though I'd like to avoid all types of sugar and sweeteners, it's nearly impossible. I do my best to limit my intake to 0–3g of sugar per serving.

WARNING:

"No Sugar Added" or "Sugar-Free" only means that the manufacturer didn't actually add sugar on the front end when making this product! Please, please, please, do NOT fall for this marketing ploy! It does NOT account for the carbs that will turn into sugar once they are consumed. It does NOT account for the sugars found naturally in the product. Nor does it account for alternative/artificial sweeteners, i.e., aspartame, sucralose, maltodextrin, neotame, maltitol, etc., that they may use to sweeten this so-called "SUGAR-FREE" product. This is just another example of clever and misleading marketing tactics.

Example: Smucker's Sugar-Free Jam. How can jam, which is made from fruit, possibly be sugar-free? Easy. It's not. It's made from fruit, which contains fructose, i.e., fruit sugar! But, because Smucker's did not physically add sugar to this product, nor do they have to account for the naturally occurring sugar, they can legally make this "sugar-free" claim. Even more disturbing, is that when I was out buying a bunch of this junk food to take a photo for this chapter, I made sure to grab this popular sugar-free jam. When I read the ingredient section, I was absolutely stunned to see they use ASPARTAME in their alleged wholesome food!

Another example: How can a package of cookies claim to be sugar-free? Again, the manufacturer either did not physically add sugar on the front end or they used artificial sweeteners. Either way, once consumed, the body will recognize the exorbitant amount of high GI carbs in these cookies as S-U-G-A-R.

6) Other Carbohydrate/Sugar Alcohols:

Beware! These items are listed below the area where you would normally look for carbs, sugar, protein, etc. Go to the bottom. Read the fine print. This category is relatively new and found only on professed carb-friendly foods. To be honest, I have no idea what "Other Carbohydrate" are. It seems to be merely another marketing attempt to hide additional sugars, at the same time, hoping we get addicted to their foods. After all, it's the sugar that makes things taste so good and keeps us coming back for more.

Sugar Alcohols: Food manufacturers claim they don't affect blood sugar levels. Many believe otherwise, as it's still a form of sugar. Nonetheless, sugar alcohols perpetuate cravings. To reiterate, they also play havoc on the digestive system, causing flatulence (gas) and diarrhea. Make sure you read the fine print. Avoid sugar alcohols.

7) Dietary Fiber:
Dietary fibers are indigestible (complex) carbs that pass through the intestinal tract without being absorbed. This is because the bacteria present in the digestive system lacks the enzymes required to break down this fiber. The fiber content means these particular carbs are slower burning and much slower to affect blood sugar levels. Fiber also helps curb food cravings and makes you feel full. Due to its many health benefits, the <u>higher</u> the fiber, the better. Many health experts claim you can subtract the amount of fiber from the total amount of carbs to get the "true" number of carbs. However, I still say a carb, is a carb, is a carb. No matter their source, simple or complex, all carbohydrates are recognized as sugar by the body. Thus, I believe all carbs need to be accounted for. *Why?* Because, at the end of the day, if my body hasn't used the carbs for fuel, they'll be stored as fat. Moreover, with all the marketing deception, I don't believe most of what I read. This is why it's crucial to learn to listen to your body.

8) Protein:
I like to see at least 7, 10, maybe even 14g of protein per serving. This will depend on the food source. Your protein needs will vary, depending on whether you want to build muscle, have more endurance, or lose weight, as well as how many times a day you eat. Women generally need about 20g of protein per meal, with men around 28g. (To be more exact, go to muscletech.com/CALCULATORS/PROTEIN/Protein_Calculator).

9) Total Fat:
Again, because of the types of foods I buy, I rarely, if ever, look at the fat. I don't stress over the amount fat, as long as it comes from a good dietary source. Saturated, polyunsaturated, and monounsaturated fats are all needed for a healthy body and mind. Perfect examples of saturated fat; butter, cheese, eggs, sour cream, mayo, chicken and turkey fat. Excellent sources of monounsaturated fat are found in the following oils; olive, almond, canola, hazelnut, peanut, oat, and grapeseed. The following oils are wonderful sources of polyunsaturated fat; flaxseed, primrose, herring, salmon, sardine, wheat germ, and sesame oil. I get most of my fats from butter, nuts, seeds, extra virgin olive oil, organic mayonnaise, eggs, cheese, avocados, and sardines.

I realize far too many of you are still scared of eating fat, especially saturated fat. But you need to know there's a huge difference between eating the above fats versus the (damaged) fats you find in french fries, fried onion rings, donuts, pastries, etc. The body *needs* fat to rebuild bones, hair, hormones, cells, enzymes, muscles, and neurotransmitters. To reiterate, eating *healthy, non-damaged* fat does NOT make you fat, because it does not trigger insulin. So please, eat fat, but choose your fats wisely.

WARNING: Fat-Free/Low-Fat:
Avoid all foods that make this claim, as they are loaded with sugar, HFCS, corn syrup, etc. And if these foods aren't loaded with sugar, the fat-free snack foods often contain olestra, an indigestible fat substitute that causes serious side effects. BEWARE!

10) Sodium:
Though sodium is needed to help control body fluids, maintain normal blood pressure, nerve, and muscle activity, I stay relatively low, from 0–250mg per serving. I also <u>never</u> add salt to my food, as I get plenty through the foods I eat. Too much sodium can lead to high blood pressure, osteoporosis, stomach cancer, and other serious health risks. At bare minimum, too much sodium will make you extra thirsty and retain water, i.e., bloated. Unfortunately, we women too often equate this feeling to being F-A-T! Therefore, when you're trying to get lean, these sodium side effects will most assuredly discourage your dieting efforts. Just realize, though, that this is occurring from too much salt. Drink more water, flush your system, and move on. Then be sure to avoid salty foods—and throw away your salt shaker.

11) Calories:
Based on the healthy foods I choose, I never ever count calories. Low-calorie dieting is one of the worst ways to try to lose excess body fat. That being said, carbs are the only calories you will need to count, as an excess will be stored as fat. However, if your serotonin levels are properly maintained and you combine healthy fats and proteins with complex/low GI carbs, your body will tell you when to stop eating. The key is to *listen to your body*. But, you must remember that no matter what method you choose to attempt to lose weight—low-fat, low-carb, even stomach stapling—they will inevitably fail if you consume more calories than your body needs. Thus, maintaining your serotonin levels is absolutely crucial to successful "long-term" weight loss. (Don't forget, determining your BMR will provide you with a base to work from.)

12) Calories from Fat:
I equally do not count calories from fat. I eat plenty of healthy fats. This is, once again, because of the foods I choose, along with keeping my serotonin maintained.

13) Cholesterol:
As for cholesterol, and because of the healthy foods I eat, I never look at it. Medical experts and their subsequent findings, clearly show that we must "eat" cholesterol to shut down the body's internal clock from producing its own. If you don't, your body will make cholesterol from carbs and this will <u>not</u> be a good form of cholesterol. Therefore, you need to eat a good dietary cholesterol with every meal, which can be found in foods such as eggs, shellfish, red meat, cheese, poultry, fish, and butter. I believe this to be true, as I mentioned earlier, I eat a ton of cheese, love shellfish, butter, enjoy a dozen eggs a week—and yet my cholesterol panels are fine. My focus with respect to a healthy cholesterol panel is to AVOID any insulin-producing foods, beverages, or substances. Maintaining your serotonin will help you do this effortlessly. Beyond that, having a healthy heart comes from living a healthy *lifestyle*.

14) Vitamins, Minerals, and Other Information:
This lists the various vitamins, minerals, and nutrients in the food and their daily percent

values. It's best to try to average daily 100% DV for vitamins A, C, calcium, fiber, and iron. (To be honest, based on the healthy foods choices I make, I never read this.)

Additional Label Verbiage:
The FDA claims they regulate the phrases/terms used on product packaging. But, based on what I know, I seriously doubt this so-called regulation. All one has to do is look at the hundreds of net/impact carbs and sugar-free labels to realize this. Below are several of the more common marketing attempts to explain what a product contains, as well as how the food manufacturers attempt to seduce you into buying it. This is all based on a single serving. You'll need to know what that serving size is.

▶ *Sugar-Free*: The product has to contain less than 1/2g of sugar per serving. However, and I cannot say this enough: Sugar-free only means that the manufacturers did not physically add sugar on the front end. It does NOT account for the carbs that will *turn into* sugar once consumed, nor does it account for the sugars found naturally in the product. And it definitely does not account for the harmful artificial sweeteners they use!

▶ *Reduced-Sugar:* 25% or less sugar per serving than the principle food

▶ *Calorie-Free/No Calories:* Contains less than 5 calories per serving

▶ *Low-Calorie:* Contains 1/3 the calories of the original version or a similar product

▶ *Lite:* Contains 1/3 the calories or 1/2 the fat per serving of the original version

▶ *Fat-Free/No-Fat:* Must contain less than 1/2g of fat per serving

▶ *Reduced-Fat/Lower-Fat:* 25% or less fat per serving than the principle food

▶ *Low-Fat:* Contains less than 3g of fat per serving

▶ *No Preservatives Added:* May contain *natural* preservatives, but none "added"

▶ *No Preservatives:* Contains no preservatives, chemical or natural

▶ *Low-Sodium:* Contains less than 140mg of sodium per serving

▶ *No Salt/Salt-Free:* Contains less than 5mg of sodium per serving

▶ *Good Source of Fiber*: 2.5g to 5g per serving

▶ *More/Added Fiber:* Contains 2.5g or more fiber per serving than the principle food

▶ *High-Fiber:* 5g or more fiber per serving

Definitions:
10g = 10 grams
10mg = 10 milligrams
10mcg = 10 micrograms
2 tsp = 2 teaspoons
2 tbsp = tablespoons
1 serving size = the amount of food that can, in theory, fit in the palm of your hand

35

A SUMMARY OF HEALTH TIPS
THAT WILL HELP KEEP YOU
LEAN & HEALTHY

I hope you realize I've tried to share this information with you in an easy-to-understand type of dialogue. (It's also based on actual conversations with various clients.) Nothing is worse, though, than when you finally get motivated to improve your health and you go out and buy the latest diet/health/fitness books, only to discover that far too often these books are filled with over-the-top medical jargon that even those individuals in the health industry can't comprehend. I promise that if you read this book and then read it again—until you really get it—your life will *forever* be changed. Guaranteed!

Keeping that in mind, I wanted to summarize some of the health facts we just talked about. Hopefully, this list will help you understand it all even more than you already do.

- 98% of all attempts to lose weight will inevitably fail, unless you're able to properly maintain serotonin, a major neurotransmitter.

- Serotonin is depleted by everything from stress, alcohol, sugar, high GI carbs, lack of deep restorative sleep, processed/refined foods, artificial sweeteners, prescription, nonprescription, and street drugs, OTC meds, nicotine, caffeine, ephedrine, dieting (especially low-fat dieting), lack of exercise, etc.

- People often feel as if they are addicted to certain carbs, because these foods increase the production of serotonin, a wonderful, mood-altering brain chemical.

- When serotonin is depleted, our brain will force us on a *subconscious* level toward high GI carbs. Its primary goal is to both boost serotonin, a major neurotransmitter, and provide the quickest fuel to the brain. Both of which are achieved by consuming high GI carbs.

- To boost serotonin in this manner, however, insulin must first be triggered.

- Insulin is the hormone that opens fat cells. Hence, causing the body to store fat.

- A diet high in processed/high GI carbs = high insulin levels/low serotonin levels.

- A diet high in sugar = high insulin levels/low serotonin levels.

- A diet high in caffeine/stimulants = high insulin levels/low serotonin levels.

- High insulin levels = high fat storage ratio, water retention, abnormal thyroid and hormone function, harmful cholesterol profile, plaqueing of the arteries, high blood pressure, increased risks of cancer, heart disease, stroke, type 2 diabetes, etc.

- Low serotonin = high GI carb/sugar cravings, bulimia, obesity, rage, sudden outbursts, mood swings, ADD, ADHD, extreme agitation, anxiety, panic attacks, PMS, insomnia, alcoholism, headaches, migraines, chronic body pain, lethargy, decreased libido, OCD, irritable bowel syndrome, memory loss, schizophrenia, suicidal behavior, etc.

- Controlling cravings = less insulin.

- Less insulin = less fat stored, more fat utilized as fuel.

- Less insulin = lowering risks for obesity, high blood pressure, heart attacks, stroke, cancer, type 2 diabetes, etc.

- Less insulin = healthier cholesterol and thyroid panels.

- More body fat = less lean muscle mass (plus, higher triglycerides and increased risks for type 2 diabetes, heart disease, cancer, stroke, high blood pressure, etc.)

- Less lean muscle mass = slower metabolism/lower BMR, less calories/ fat burned.

- More lean muscle mass = faster, more effective metabolism/higher BMR. *Why?* Muscle is a metabolically active tissue. (8 times more active than fat cells.) It requires a precise number of calories daily to maintain itself. Therefore, the more muscle you have, the higher your BMR. This equals far more calories/fat burned (24/7), even while your body is at rest.

- Proteins and fats build muscle tissue.

- Carbohydrates do not build muscle tissue.

- Carbohydrates are the preferred fuel choice for the muscles (and brain). They're readily available and quickest to burn.

- It takes about 20 minutes of moderate to intense aerobic (not anaerobic) exercise before your body will shift from burning glycogen to a slower burning, more efficient fuel. That fuel being stored body fat, i.e., free fatty acids.

- Do cardio first thing in the morning—and on an empty stomach, as your body will burn more fat versus carbs. Second best option: do cardio right after you weight train.

▶ Eat sugar, crave sugar. Eat sugar, wear it as fat. Eat sugar, be moody, anxious, depressed, and with low, sporadic energy levels. Eat sugar, increase your risks for perpetual health conditions!

▶ Calories in excess of our energy needs will be stored as fat, especially an excess of carbs, as carbs need to be used immediately as energy or they'll be stored as fat. Whereas with protein and fats, the body can utilize these foods for rebuilding the body's cells, hormones, enzymes, muscles, neurotransmitters, etc.

▶ 1 pound of body fat = 3,500 calories. To lose 1 pound of fat, you must burn or reduce your calories by 3,500. The most effective method to lose body fat—and keep it off long-term—is by building LBM and eating healthy.

▶ Maintaining healthy levels of serotonin = controlling high GI carb/sugar cravings and binge eating, reducing body fat, water retention, anxiety, panic attacks, alleviating mood swings, aggression, depression, SAD, ADD, ADHD, OCD, PMS, suicidal behavior, migraines, chronic pain disorders, while improving sleep patterns, sexual behavior/ desire, etc.

▶ For those individuals who smoke, take drugs (pharmaceutical and/or recreational), eat sugar, processed/refined foods, drink alcohol, caffeine, sodas, consume HFCS, corn syrup, aspartame, neotame, sucralose, and other artificial sweeteners, eat a low-fat/fat-free diet, along with living a sedentary lifestyle—and yet don't have a weight or health problem, BEWARE! Don't let this fool you! The serious health risks associated with living such an unhealthy lifestyle can literally take years to surface. Damage is indeed being done at the cellular level and you will, sooner or later, reap what you sow.

▶ If you want to live a long, happy, and healthy life, you must live a *healthy lifestyle*. This healthy lifestyle is, though, completely dependent upon you being able to properly maintain your serotonin.

▶ To help insure you achieve and maintain healthy levels of this major neurotransmitter, find a quality SES and take it faithfully each and every day.

▶ Maintaining your serotonin will, undoubtedly, help you live this much-needed healthier lifestyle. But you must also be <u>willing</u> to make the effort, to break old unhealthy habits, and you must exercise! Please do not wait until you're sick, suffering with heart disease, diabetes, or on your death bed before you decide to live this healthier lifestyle! Please make the effort starting today—for you, and all those you love!

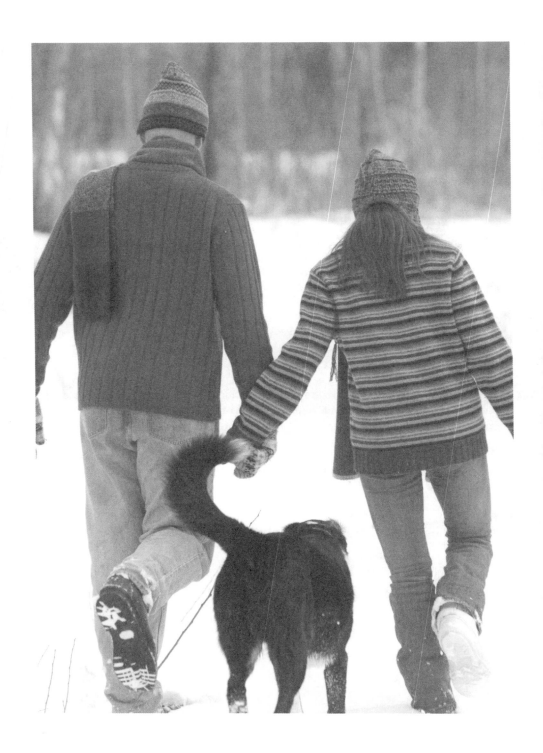

PART III

300+ PERSONAL HEALTH TIPS

for body, mind & spirit

36

PHYSICAL HEALTH TIPS

▶ Food is fuel for your body and mind. How well you nourish them will determine how well they run. Question is: How healthy do you want to be? How good do you want to feel? How long do you want to live?

▶ Help save your *own* life by living a healthy lifestyle! Watching the horror of Katrina's victims should be all the evidence you need to make damn sure you're healthy enough to save yourself, your loved ones—and your beloved pets!

▶ Sugar is your diet downfall. Eat it, wear it as fat. Eating sugar makes you *crave* more sugar. Sugar is highly addictive. Sugar has absolutely no nutritional value. Avoid sugar at all cost. It's that simple.

▶ Fat-free and low-fat foods are loaded with sugar, usually in the form of HFCS (high-fructose corn syrup). This is the worst form of sugar.

▶ Do not buy any foods or beverages that claim they are low calorie, low-fat, fat-free, sugar-free, carb-free, low-carb, or net/impact carb.

▶ Cravings are not about being addicted or weak-willed. They are, however, a side effect of low serotonin. Binge eating is also not about being weak-willed, but again, due to low serotonin.

▶ Whether simple or complex, <u>all</u> carbohydrates are recognized as sugar by the body.

▶ Please do not ever buy larger-sized clothes to accommodate your weight gain. This only perpetuates further weight gain, as you will, unfortunately, find new comfort in the larger sizes.

▶ Eat fruit in its *natural* state, as it will keep the fiber intact and lower the GI. Breaking fruit down, turns it into nothing more than a pure fruit sugar liquid, spiking insulin levels dramatically.

▶ Healthiest fruit? The berry family: blueberries, strawberries, blackberries, raspberries, etc. They're highest in antioxidants and lowest on the GI scale.

▶ Beware and limit fructose (fruit sugar), lactose (milk sugar), and sucrose (table sugar).

▶ Make sure to eat plenty of dark, leafy green vegetables, as well as yellow and red vegetables. Each and every colored vegetable brings its own unique health benefits.

▶ If a food or beverage is sweet, ask *why!* Read the label. Educate yourself.

▶ Buyer beware: Don't fall for the snack food companies' marketing tricks. If they claim sugar-free, this only means that no sugar was added. They don't have to account for the excessive carbohydrates that turn into sugar once consumed, the food's naturally occurring sugars, or artificial sweeteners.

▶ Eating healthy fat does not make you fat. *Why?* Because it doesn't trigger insulin.

▶ Clean out your cupboards. Either donate all your fat-free/low-fat foods to your local homeless shelter or throw them away.

▶ 98% of all diets will inevitably fail unless you're able to maintain healthy levels of serotonin. Be sure to take an SES faithfully.

▶ Set realistic weight loss goals. Don't set yourself up for failure.

▶ It's not just about losing excess body fat, it's about achieving lifelong quality health.

▶ You really *are* what you eat.

▶ Avoid foods made with white or bleached flour.

▶ Do not add salt to your food. You get plenty of sodium naturally through your diet.

▶ Find a well-trained naturopathic doctor, one who is highly educated—and practices both Eastern and Western medicine.

▶ Take your selected dietary supplements faithfully. They can't help you if you don't take them on a regular and consistent basis. In case you aren't aware, herbs are cumulative in affect. The longer you're on them, the greater the health benefits.

▶ Learn to read and understand nutritional panels found on all foods and beverages.

▶ Avoid all rice, potatoes, pasta, bread, and anything made with white flour when you're trying to lose excess body fat. Once you're close to your desired weight, eat only long grain, or wild rice; whole grain bread; and sweet potato or yam; but limit them. Also, always combine them with a healthy fat and quality protein—and eat them early in the day. (I choose not to eat any rice, potatoes, pasta, and definitely not any white bread, as it keeps me much leaner. I do, however, eat yams.)

▶ When eating sushi, please enjoy the fish <u>without</u> the rice (sashimi). Not only is this white rice, but most often the chefs add sugar to it to enhance the flavor.

▶ Too much sodium is directly related to high blood pressure. Reducing sodium intake is good for all overall health, as well as helping to limit excess water weight.

▶ It's one thing to "want" to lose weight, it's entirely another matter to actually <u>do</u> what it takes. So, be serious. Be committed. Please stop cheating yourself.

▶ The best thing to do when you feel bloated is to drink more water.

▶ Just because something is "all-natural" doesn't mean it's necessarily safe. And just because you buy something at a "health food" store doesn't mean it's healthy.

▶ Drinking water helps your mind and body in so many ways, but it also helps transport fat out of the body as waste.

▶ Nearly 70% of all doctors tell their patients <u>nothing</u> about adverse side effects when they are prescribing a drug.

▶ Read the warning labels on all medications! It's horrifying to realize what the FDA, FTC, AMA, and drug companies consider safe!

▶ <u>Latest statistics</u>:
  • 450,000 people die each year from cigarettes
  • 300,000 people die each year from alcohol
  • 250,000 people die each year when surgery goes wrong
  • 106,000 people die each year from prescription drug side effects
  • 100,000 people die each year from auto accidents
  • 90,000 people die each year due to hospital errors
  • 20,000 people die each year from risky sexual behavior
  • 17,000 people die each year from illicit use of drugs
  • 0 people die each year from marijuana

▶ According to the American Cancer Society, 30% of all cancer deaths are attributed to dietary factors.

▶ Carbs that trigger insulin have proven to cause cancer cells to multiply, especially cancer cells related directly to breast cancer.

▶ Shockingly, the fastest-growing market for antidepressants is preschoolers. Please make sure your children are eating a *healthy diet* before you put them on these dangerous, if not, deadly drugs!

- A Harvard University study revealed the rate of increase of depression in children is an astounding 23%! Remember, diet is directly linked to depression.

- Obesity rose 33% in the last decade, with 65% of Americans now overweight.

- Obesity-related deaths are slowly, but surely, becoming the #1 preventable death.

- Dare to question your medical doctor. I have many elderly friends who, unfortunately, believe their doctors are God. Sadly, they take whatever medication they're prescribed, never stopping to question the side effects or interactions with the many other drugs they're already taking. Please, *learn to think for yourself!*

- Make sure you're getting enough protein, specially when you're training. Your muscles need sufficient protein to grow.

- Avoid processed foods. Eat "real" food. And eat organic foods whenever possible.

- Take the stairs. And walk to do your errands as often as possible.

- The only thing worse than not working out is *wasting* your time when you do.

- Our emotional state of mind is directly related to what we eat.

- Regular exercise is one of the best ways to slow, even reverse, the signs of aging.

- The body is made up of two components: LBM (Lean Body Mass) which includes muscles, bone, blood, and organs and FM (Fat Mass) which consists of the body's fat stores. FACT: The more you exercise, the more you will increase your LMB, while *decreasing* your FM. The more LBM you have, the higher your metabolism, more efficient your body will be at burning fat and calories. When you diet and don't exercise, you will lose minimal FM—and LBM. When you lose LBM, you slow down your metabolism, making it even harder to lose FM.

- Be patient in reaching your fat loss goals. It's genetically impossible to lose more than 1 or 2 pounds per week. You can lose more, but you're losing mostly water and LBM.

- Need more fiber? Eat more nonstarchy carbs, legumes, lentils, prunes, nuts, etc.

- Do not allow others to distract or hinder you in reaching your weight loss goals. Be around people who inspire, encourage, and motivate you. Unfortunately, misery loves company. Choose your companions wisely.

- A quality protein drink can be the perfect midday snack.

- I know the clothing style for the younger kids is the baggy look, but please, do not follow this trend. Learn to create your own unique style. This grunge look only allows you to gain weight without guilt, as you can so easily hide the extra pounds under those excessively baggy clothes. Never forget how attractive the human body can be if properly taken care of. Stop hiding it. Be proud of your body.

- There is no more efficient, more effective way to develop a lean, toned, sexy body than with weight training. Do yourself a favor and try it for 6 months before you judge otherwise. If you've never tried it before, please hire a qualified trainer to assist you.

- Far too many women avoid weight training for fear of getting big and bulky. This will not happen. First of all, women do not have enough testosterone for this to occur, nor will they be eating the enormous amount of calories required to achieve such muscle mass. Furthermore, weight training is about developing long, lean, yet strong muscles and bone mass. Added bonus: Your metabolism will stay high for hours, long after you've stopped exercising.

- Exercise is a natural way to stimulate growth hormone, help alleviate depression, suppress appetite, lower your risks for heart disease, osteoarthritis, osteoporosis, type 2 diabetes, and other serious health conditions.

- Do not drink tap water. Buy quality filtered water or double-filter your home water. Plus, drink *before* you get thirsty, on a regular basis, and at least 2 quarts daily.

- Muscles have memory, so when training, vary your routine. This will also help you from getting bored.

- If you don't like to go to the gym, speed walk, swim, golf, work in the garden, or play ball with your children. Just get outside in the fresh air and get your body moving.

- Maybe it's the tomboy in me, but I love to do yard work. I love the feel of dirt in my hands as I pull weeds and repot plants. And I so enjoy the stress release of a chain saw as I trim shrubs. When the day is done, I've gotten some exercise, a little sun, and I feel like I've done something productive.

- The body needs 8 hours of *quality* sleep each night to rebuild. If less than, at the very least, it will deplete serotonin. Cravings, weight gain, depression, anxiety, and aging more rapidly are just a few of the many side effects. Research also shows that the hours from 10pm to 6am rejuvenate the body/mind best.

- For those who claim they don't have time to work out, with all due respect, you'd better find the time now or pay the price later. You'll have no choice, but to find the time for all those doctor visits.

▶ Ladies: For those round, firm buttocks, combine squats, single dumbbell (plié) squats, deadlifts, leg presses, lunges, cable kickbacks, pelvic thrusts with weight, and seated abductors. Slow. Focused. Intense. Anywhere from 7–20 reps per set, 3 sets each. This will vary depending upon your goals. (In theory, though both will sculpt, heavier weight/lower reps build larger muscle mass. Lighter weight/higher reps for leaner, less mass.) To be rather bold, if you really want an ass that you're proud of, and one that turns heads, devote one training session a week to this. The gluteus maximus (buttocks) is a very responsive muscle group, but you must be consistent with your workouts and eat healthy. BTW: There's a huge difference between having a big butt versus one that is firm, cellulite-free, and beautifully sculpted. And no, "butt implants" are not an option.

▶ Do not judge your fat loss success by weighing yourself, especially if you're training with weights, as muscle weighs more than fat.

▶ With regard to the healthy lifestyle I've suggested, you will lose inches long before you lose pounds. Losing the excess body fat should be your primary focus.

▶ Free squats are one of the best exercises for the overall body.

▶ Find a friend to work out with. Competition motivates and inspires!

▶ When training, it's intensity, technique, and consistency that you should focus on.

▶ Developing a fit, healthy body is not just about losing fat. It's about building and maintaining lean muscle mass, strong bones, and a healthy cardiovascular system.

▶ Are you one of those people who enjoys a Coke? Do you have any idea just how harmful this soda is for you? Here are a few examples: 1) Most highway patrol officers carry two gallons of Coke in their trunks to remove blood from the highway after a car accident. 2) The active ingredient in Coke is phosphoric acid, which has a pH of 2.8. Phosphoric acid will dissolve a nail in about four days. 3) To carry Coca-Cola syrup (the concentrate), a commercial trucker must use the HAZARDOUS MATERIAL cards reserved for highly corrosive materials. So, still feel like Coke is the *real thing*?

▶ Walking 10 minutes prior to a meal will help curb your appetite.

▶ You don't need to join a gym to achieve a great look. Combine a floor routine, i.e., push-ups, donkey-kicks, lunges, squats, sit-ups, etc. Walk with your dog. Use ankle weights, dumbbells, jump rope, do yoga, surf, hike, etc. The key is to be creative.

▶ Write down all the reasons for which you want and need to lose weight. Include both the many wonderful benefits of achieving your weight loss goals, as well as the countless health risks, diseases, emotional and mental trauma that will afflict you if you don't.

Use this list to empower you through this amazing journey. Just remember: *All things are possible!* But you must first believe in yourself! Use the power of your mind to envision your weight loss goals. See yourself, as you want to be. See yourself doing all the things you desire. This is where visualization can become life-changing. You must be able to truly "see yourself" in this movie in your mind. Now, passionately stay focused on those images and never lose sight of them.

▶ Stop eating (especially carbs) 3 hours before bedtime. If you absolutely have to eat something, I finish my day with a small protein drink or a handful of raw nuts.

▶ Beware of condiments, as they're most often high in sugar, sodium, and chemicals.

▶ Eat eggs, eat the whole egg, and eat them often. They're a perfect protein, a healthy source of both dietary fat and cholesterol, and they're low in calories and carbs.

▶ Be sure to eat good dietary cholesterol to keep your body from making its own from carbohydrates. That is not a healthy form of cholesterol.

▶ Eat breakfast. Don't skip lunch. In fact, eat every 3 hours. People often think that the less they eat, the thinner they will be. Wrong! You must eat for good health. Furthermore, low-calorie eating puts your body into a starvation mode.

▶ Turn off the TV. If not, do some leg extensions, standing dumbbell curls, lateral raises, ab crunches, pelvic thrusts, squats, and push-ups as you watch your favorite show.

▶ The 8th leading cause of death is infections, infections that are due to the lack of cleanliness in *hospitals!* Do whatever it takes to stay healthy!

▶ Buy a PDR (Prescription Drug Reference) and refer to it faithfully.

▶ The best time to have surgery is early in the morning, and early in the week.

▶ 7,000 people die each year due to medication errors. Be sure to double-check your prescriptions!

▶ The safest, most effective way to boost serotonin is by taking dietary supplements, not pharmaceutical drugs.

▶ There are many serious health concerns regarding the ingredients in toothpaste (and mouthwash). All one has to do is read the warning labels to know there is good cause: "If swallowed, please call the Poison Control Center immediately!" The warnings are even more frightening if you have young children. Please consider changing to an all-natural toothpaste and mouthwash.

▶ Our skin is our largest organ. Therefore, beware of cleaning solutions, facial peels, nail polishes/removers, acrylic liquids, soaps, deodorants, sunscreens, bug repellents, hair sprays, gels, and hundreds of other products that contain cancer causing agents. What we put in and "on" our bodies is absorbed into the bloodstream and subsequently processed by the liver. Read all labels, not just food labels! You'll be amazed at what's in these various products. Buy all-natural products. I also recommend that you wear rubber gloves when cleaning, as household cleaning products are even more harmful. Breathing their toxic fumes is equally unhealthy, so please consider wearing a mask to reduce inhalation.

▶ With regard to the above concerns, it will be nearly impossible to avoid all such poisons. Therefore, cleanse your body on a regular basis with all-natural products.

▶ To help minimize the spread of germs and bacteria, wash your hands (and that means with soap!) after using the bathroom, no matter your business. And when using a public restroom, *touch nothing,* and use a paper towel to open the door upon leaving.

▶ Some old but wise advice: Eat your food much slower. Put your fork down in between bites. Converse with those you're dining with. Enjoy your food. Don't inhale it. This gives your body a chance to tell your brain that food is coming. Most people eat way too fast, not allowing their body to even realize that they're full.

▶ Though a great protein source, there are many studies that show cow's milk is not meant for human consumption. Those concerns are now much more serious due to all the hormones the cows are given, not to mention the disgusting so-called food they're fed. Never to forget, if you drink cow's milk, *you support the veal industry.*

▶ Eat when you're hungry, not out of emotion. This is why serotonin must be balanced.

▶ Get off the fat-free/low-fat, low-cal, and wannabe low-carb diets without further delay.

▶ Both high and low levels of estrogen can effect brain chemistry, thus depleting serotonin and increasing carbohydrate cravings, depression, rage, heart disease, etc. Women should be aware of this, particularly as they near perimenopause and menopause.

▶ Learn how to read and truly understand a "Supplement Facts" panel found on all dietary supplements. First, look for actual ingredients used. Watch for stimulants, fillers, aspartame, etc. Make sure the extracts are standardized, and with a GMP (Good Marketing Practices) or better rating. Compare serving size to the amount of product actually required to meet the serving size. Some are as high as 8 pills/2x per day! In addition, to keep competitive in the market place, companies are starting to offer only a two-week supply. This may give their products a lower retail price, but the unsuspecting consumer needs to realize they're actually paying more *for less.*

▶ Taper off stimulants, as all stimulants become depressants. *Why?* Because they deplete serotonin, which causes depression. They also perpetuate the vicious cycle of cravings, fat gain, and the production of the worst form of cholesterol.

▶ Eat less, but more often, preferably 5 to 6 times per day (3 meals with 2 to 3 snacks), and 3 hours apart. It will keep your metabolism going strong.

▶ Please beware of all the hip new, highly caffeinated, sugar-laden beverages. They're loaded with either sugar and/or caffeine. (*And then our government wonders why we are a nation that is overly stressed, overweight, depressed, and unable to sleep!*)

▶ Avoid caffeine, ephedrine, nicotine, alcohol, sodas, diet drinks, lemonade, flavored drinks, fruit juices (even those that claim "no sugar added"), iced tea, etc.

▶ Parents need to diligently watch out for the hidden sugars in so-called healthy fruit-based drinks that are marketed to their children. They're loaded with sugar, naturally occurring or otherwise.

▶ "Trail Mix," so often thought of as health food, usually contains too much sugar. The sugar is found in the raisins, carob/chocolate chips, dried fruit, yogurt-covered almonds, etc. Please beware of the carb/sugar count on these products. I make my own trail mix to avoid the sugar.

▶ The first way to *not* eat unhealthy foods is not buy them. Keep them out of your house. *Why tempt yourself or your family?*

▶ Use *real* butter. Organic, unsalted butter is even better. Avoid using any and all butter substitutes, i.e., shortening, margarine, etc.

▶ Beware of ALL prescription drugs, more so the latest "lifelong" drugs that doctors claim we need—thyroid, cholesterol-lowering, acid reflux, etc. Their self-serving claims are based solely on GREED! This is nothing but big business at work!

▶ Why is it that NO one ever questions the fact that the <u>Food</u> and <u>Drug</u> Administration resides—and makes laws—under one highly questionable business partnership? A serious conflict of interest, and another frightening link to this bureaucratic monopoly!

▶ A quote by Philip Morris, the tobacco king: "There are no safe cigarettes." So, please, stop smoking and avoid second-hand smoke! An SES will help control these cravings.

▶ An SES will help control many cravings. But you must be willing to break old, unhealthy habits if you want to achieve lifelong health. You must make a conscious effort to change your lifestyle.

▶ Your body needs good, healthy fat to burn fat. It's also a fantastic fuel source.

▶ Menopause is not a disease. It's a natural stage of the aging process. Ladies, please find a doctor and compound pharmacist who are especially trained in all-natural/real hormones, i.e., bioidentical hormones.

▶ One tablespoon of flaxseed oil daily is recommended, as it's high in essential fatty acids. It's the richest source available of omega-3 fatty acids, which are proven to provide protection against heart disease, cancer, and arthritis.

▶ Recent studies suggest magnesium deficiency may be a leading cause of heart disease. Foods highest in magnesium? Tofu, peanuts, spinach, and broccoli.

▶ Adding vinegar or lemon juice to carbs will slow down the rate at which they turn into blood sugar. Adding hot sauce/peppers will help lower the GI by approximately 25%.

▶ There are good fats and bad fats. Eat plenty of good fats, which are found in nature, i.e., eggs, chicken, turkey, nuts, seeds, fish, olives, avocados, butter, lean meat, etc. Bad fats are those that are man-made.

▶ Lose weight gradually. Don't rush it. The faster you lose the weight, the more lean muscle you will lose.

▶ Use stevia or xylitol instead of sugar, corn syrup, HFCS, or any artificial sweeteners.

▶ I know we're all rushed these days, but please sit down when you eat. Standing up or eating on the run encourages you to eat too fast and eat more than you really need.

▶ Learn to *listen* to your body.

▶ Margarine was originally manufactured to fatten up turkeys. The only problem was, it was killing the birds. Researchers behind the project were desperate not to lose their money, so they decided to add some color to it and sell it as a substitute for butter. While there are numerous health risks, the most disturbing fact is that margarine is only one molecule away from being *plastic!*

▶ Do not grocery shop when you're hungry.

▶ Eat plenty of "whole" grains versus refined/processed grains.

▶ Oils are hydrogenated in order to harden them. Examples: Coconut, palm kernel oil, margarine, etc. Their chemical structure is altered to form trans-fatty acids. Avoid hydrogenated oils, hydrogenated fats, and trans-fatty acids. Avoid eating deep-fried foods such as fries, and baked goods such as doughnuts, cookies, crackers, etc.

▶ Want some help naturally curbing your family's appetite? Serve smaller portions, and use smaller plates, bowls, utensils, cups, etc.

▶ Buy organic, free-range foods whenever possible. You will pay a little more, but it's definitely worth the few extra dollars spent.

▶ Learn to read and understand all food labels. Avoid HFCS, sucrose, aspartame, saccharin, sucralose, maltodextrin, fructose, corn syrup, sorbital, maltitol, molasses, etc. These sugars are hidden in over 90% of all processed foods. (Considering many food companies are being less than honest when it comes to actual ingredients, *dare to question* everything that you read. Listen to your body and mind.)

▶ Beware of total grams of carbs per serving. Remember, once consumed, all carbs break down into sugar.

▶ Make it a habit that every time you look at a food item, the first thing you do is read the nutritional panel. Learn to really understand what you're eating. It will empower you—and help keep you healthy!

▶ Read carefully the actual ingredients used, i.e., pork, beef, white flour, aspartame, HFCS, sugar alcohols, hydrogenated fats, chemicals, preservatives, dyes, etc.

▶ Beware of flavored bottled water that claims it's sugar-free, as these are often sweetened with aspartame!

▶ Beware of the grocery store's numerous marketing tactics to seduce you into buying sugar-laden, addictive junk food.

▶ Once you get rid of all the toxins from eating processed food, you will be amazed at just how good you can really feel when you eat healthy.

▶ Find (your) ideal body weight. Don't obsess with the scale. In fact, stay off the scale!

▶ Not so many years ago, the average size for a woman was an 8. It's now a 14. To further exasperate this growth, there are clothing manufacturers who manipulate their sizes to make their female shoppers "feel better" about themselves. While I am all about making people feel better, this is not the way. Beware of this deception.

▶ Speaking of sizes, you do not need to lose a lot of weight to make phenomenal changes in your physical appearance and overall health. There was a time in my life when I partied too much, ate the recommended low-fat diet, and didn't train nearly as much with weights. It's easy to understand why I was not as lean. Although I only weighed about 15 pounds more than I do now, it was a HUGE difference in sizes. At 5'11", I went from a size 11/12 at 152/155 pounds to a size 3/4 while weighing 137/140. So you see, the scale is not an accurate way to measure your success.

▶ Whether you wear a size 8, 12, or 16, dress for your body shape. While I still encourage you to lose the excess body fat, at least wear clothes that complement your body, whatever the size.

▶ Think of your metabolism as a slow but steady fire. Do not let the flame go out. *Why?* Because it makes your body store fat.

▶ Success in your fat loss goals should be measured by the following: Lower heart rate and blood pressure, decrease in LDL (bad cholesterol) and triglycerides, higher HDL (good cholesterol), and, of course, changes in total body composition. (Using extra virgin olive oil is a great way to help raise HDL, the *good* cholesterol.)

▶ Keep healthy snacks in your purse, briefcase, car, etc. (Unsalted, raw or dry roasted almonds, macadamias, walnuts, pecans, sunflower and pumpkin seeds are ideal.)

▶ Studies suggest that broccoli and tomatoes are two of the best cancer-fighting foods.

▶ BMI (Body Mass Index) used to be considered the best way to measure body fat. Unfortunately, it doesn't account for those who train with weights and would thus, weigh more due to larger muscle mass.

▶ Do not skip meals, as it shuts down your metabolism. I cannot stress this enough: You need to force yourself to start the day with a healthy breakfast and then fuel your body every 3 hours with a healthy snack or smaller meal. This, is what kicks your metabolism into high gear, not stimulants!

▶ When dining out, don't feel obligated to order a main dish. Appetizers can be far more entertaining and a lot less filling.

▶ No matter your desire or goal, it's never too late to start.

▶ Warning: Protein bars are loaded with various forms of sugar/artificial sweeteners, often disguised in the form of glycerine, aspartame, HFCS, sucralose, and sugar alcohols.

▶ Chew your food slowly and stop eating before you actually feel full.

▶ If you don't have anyone to work out with, no problem. Use your own creative imagination to motivate yourself. Trust me, it works.

- There are various advanced machines to measure body fat, but I believe one the most efficient methods is by using a tape measure and keeping track of your waistline.

- Another exceptional test for fat loss success: Get naked and look in the mirror from all angles! Now, *do you like what you see?*

- By the time you're thirsty, you're already dehydrated. When you think you're hungry, more times than not you're actually dehydrated.

- Eat a diet high in fiber (about 25g per day) and drink plenty of water to help cleanse the body of waste. When the intestines are free of waste, body fat and water retention are reduced much quicker. Your bowels should move once per day.

- Colon health is extremely important. At any given time, your colon can hold 3–15 pounds of fecal matter. This is toxic material. It also slows down your metabolism and makes it harder for your body to properly absorb nutrients from the food you eat. There are many herbal supplements that can help cleanse your colon. In addition, I suggest you find a certified colon therapist for regular colonics.

- Don't eat when you're upset. It will only add to your misery. Instead, go for a walk, call a friend, take a hot shower, soak in a bubble bath, meditate, walk your dog, embrace your lover.

- Do not judge your beauty or self-worth by what advertisers flaunt. What you see in magazines is NOT reality!

- *Want to look younger?* Put down the junk food! Processed foods, and those that are high in sugar, are major contributors to wrinkles and speeding the aging process!

- Avoid roasted/ready to go chickens, as they're basted with brown sugar, honey, etc. And do not eat processed or deli-style/pre-packaged meats.

- Bananas have many health benefits, but they're also high in sugar (14g). Eat them as green as possible—and then limit them, especially when you're trying to lose weight.

- When diabetics need to quickly raise blood sugar levels, the recommendation is to drink either skim milk or fruit juice. *Still doubting the high sugar effect of these drinks?*

- Please do NOT have cosmetic surgery to please anyone but yourself—and only after you've dedicated a year to living a healthy lifestyle, which would include, at the very least, weight training and a diet void of sugar, high GI carbs, etc. Personally, I would

235

never consider going under the knife if it was something that I could improve with weight training. The following two procedures were definitely out of my control. Regardless, when you're ready to move ahead, choose your doctor with the greatest of care. Confirm that they're board-certified plastic surgeons. Check with the Medical Board for any complaints/legal actions filed against them. Interview no fewer than five doctors. In their legal docs, agree to "mediation" not arbitration. Listen to your inner voice. If it doesn't feel right for whatever the reason, get up and walk out! Don't go through with it, even if you're already on the operating table! Trust me, I went against my instincts and paid the price dearly. August 2002: When things went wrong with my breast augmentation, rather than the plastic surgeon admitting he misjudged his work, he suddenly claimed I had a "SUNKEN CHEST CAVITY!" A pathetic lie to cover his incompetence. January 2003: Although it was a very personal procedure, I was assured it was common and, more importantly, with few risks. But when things went horrifically wrong, rather than the ob/gyn admitting to his mistake, he insisted I had a "FLESH-EATING DISEASE!" This was another blatant and viciously cruel lie, a lie told solely to protect his incompetence. Look, I know mistakes can happen, but it's *how* these doctors chose to handle their mistakes that I find terribly disturbing. Plastic surgery is a booming industry that is frighteningly filled with doctors who lack the surgical skills required to keep you safe, let alone come close to delivering the cosmetic results you were promised. Far too many of these doctors (and general surgeons) have no sense of conscience, nor does the Medical Board hold them liable in any way. That board, a board that was specifically designed to oversee doctors and to help protect patients, is a joke! No wonder people sue. So, please, go under the knife only if it's absolutely necessary. And then it's vital that you hold whatever doctor you choose, plastic surgeon or otherwise, accountable for their numerous promises so freely proposed to seduce you into becoming their trusting patient. (Although I was in the midst of this business venture, I felt a desperate need to try and help save others from what I went through. My idea was to publish a magazine that would educate the consumer about the latest cosmetic procedures, various options and risks, best doctors, etc. With Billy's help, I designed a full magazine concept. I then met with publishing mogul Larry Flynt to discuss partnering with me. While I was certainly flattered that Mr. Flynt even took the time to meet with me, I was further pleased that he was actually impressed with my concept. Unfortunately, he was not taking on any more magazines.) Nevertheless, do your homework and listen to your inner voice!

▶ The best way to reduce cellulite? Avoid processed/refined/high GI foods, drink plenty of water, do regular cardio (even if it's only a brisk walk), and build lean muscle mass via weight training. Please stop wasting your money on useless creams!

▶ Definitely do not waste your money (or hopes) on the ridiculous $139 jeans that claim they can get rid of cellulite. I'm absolutely stunned the consumer is desperate enough to put their faith in this, and spend their hard-earned money to fall for this marketing scam. Obviously they are, as the stores can't keep them in stock. *Pleeease* stop looking for the magic pill, oops, I mean magic jeans! If you simply accept the fact that getting a lean, healthy, and sexy body requires change, effort, and consistency, you could be on your way to a life free of excess weight and dieting. Not to mention feeling exceedingly proud of yourself for having accomplished all such goals!

▶ Avoid eating dried fruit, as it's nothing more than crystallized fruit sugar. It's best to eat fruit in its natural state.

▶ Great sources of protein: Organic eggs, chicken, turkey, fresh white cheese, cottage cheese, fermented soy products, nuts, lean meat, fresh salmon, tuna, mahi-mahi.

▶ Due to various health concerns, avoid eating red meat. Better yet, become a vegetarian and live healthier, while helping stop the killing of millions of innocent farm animals! At the very least, *please eat with a conscience!* This goes for fashion, as well. Please do not wear fur! There are wonderful synthetic alternatives. (furisdead.com)

▶ When dining out, rather than filling up on bread, which will spike your insulin and encourage your meal to be stored as fat, order a small selection of fresh cheeses in lieu of the bread. It will help curb your appetite without the insulin spiking. Or, if you insist on eating bread, ask for whole grain bread. Pour olive oil on to a plate, grate fresh mozzarella cheese, add pepper to season. Use that to dip your bread in. It's delicious, healthy, and it will help lower the GI of the bread.

▶ Best sources of omega-3 fatty acids: Fresh salmon, rainbow trout, mackerel, flaxseed oil, tuna, herring, and sardines. Eat them often.

▶ Ladies: You do not have to be a size 4 to be beautiful, sexy, or desirable. But obesity can increase serious health risks by over 50%! Please, challenge yourself! Do it for yourself! Make yourself proud by losing the excess body fat!

▶ It's not the "fat" in ice cream that you need to be concerned with, but rather the amount of SUGAR. If it's not damaged fat, you're actually better off with it left in, as it will help lower the blood sugar response. Either way, this is not a good food choice.

▶ Portion size is an easy method to help control your diet. Stick with portions that can, in theory, fit in the palm of your hand.

▶ NEWS FLASH: *We are far more than our wrinkles!* Do not give in to society's pressure that growing old is somehow unacceptable or unattractive. Wrinkles are part of who we are. Each one tells a story. I'm sure we would all very much like to discover the proverbial fountain of youth, but until that fountain is found, try to grow old gracefully and with pride, instead of fighting it with endless, often risky surgical procedures and monthly injections of Botox! Besides making people look rather freakish, I guarantee that not so long down the road, the long-term side effects from those many poisonous injections will arise! If you want to fight the aging process, *live a healthy lifestyle!* Put down the damn fries, sodas, coffee, cocktails, cigarettes, and exercise regularly!

▶ Do not have liposuction unless you have dedicated at least one full year to eating healthy, along with a regular exercise program. If, after that time, you're still unable to lose those last few pounds, consider a minor touch-up. But do <u>not</u> use this procedure as a quick and easy way to diet! It is a gruesome procedure that can be extremely dangerous. And unless you change your lifestyle, it will only be a *temporary* fix. If you really want a leaner and sexier body, eat right, and start working out. Once again, I believe weight training is the most effective long-term way to reshape your body.

▶ If you truly have the desire to eat one of your forbidden foods, first ask yourself *why* you want it? Did you have a stressful week, a restless night's sleep, drink the night before? As all these things deplete serotonin, it would, therefore, be considered a craving. You can either give in to the craving, or take another dose of your SES. Either way, move on. Don't give up on yourself. It's about moderation/determination.

▶ One in 50 American adults are 100 pounds overweight! Equally shocking, three out of five children are considered obese! Children need to be taught at an early age exactly how food affects their physical and mental well-being. Parents need to help break the cycle of obesity and depression for their children—and themselves.

▶ Most cereals are excessively high in carbs and sugar. And the recent marketing of breakfast cereal bars is equally as bad. READ THE LABELS. If you have time to pour a bowl of cereal, you have time to eat some cottage cheese with tomato and slice of chicken, or veggie sausage patty with eggs over spinach. Or how about crab meat and avocado, served on whole grain toast? Mix it up and be creative!

▶ How is it we ever came to believe that sunlight was bad for us? Sunlight causes our body to produce melanin. Melanin is the pigment responsible for turning our skin brown. It's a *natural protector* from cancer. Recent studies indicate that sunlight can actually help protect you from cancer of the breast, colon, ovary, bladder, womb, stomach, and prostate. Sunlight is also a powerful and natural mood enhancer. SAD (Seasonal Affective Disorder) is caused by the lack of sunlight. It directly affects our serotonin, thus causing mood swings, even depression. So, why then, has skin cancer incidence *gone up* since the introduction of sunscreen products? Please allow me: For starters, sunlight provides us with our main source of vitamin D. It is a powerful cancer fighter. Scientists have long known that this nutrient strengthens our muscles and bones, and boosts our immune system. Ten minutes of daily exposure to sunlight will supply us with all the vitamin D that we need. However, sunscreens <u>block</u> the body's ability to produce vitamin D. Even more alarming is that these products themselves contain strikingly harmful chemicals that have shown to stimulate tumor growth and fuel cancer cells.

Personally, I love the sun. I lived in Florida for 15 years and laid out as often as possible. While I rarely lay out anymore, I still enjoy the sun, reaping its many wonderful benefits through boating, yard work, walking my dogs, or reading/picnicking at the harbor. And no, I never use sunscreens for all the reasons listed above. Plus, my particular skin type allows me to tan easily, without burning. I also use common sense—making sure I don't over do it. My best advice: Enjoy the sun in moderation. Avoid getting burned. Get at least 10 minutes of sunlight daily. See a dermatologist for regular check-ups.

▶ Researchers found total obesity-related healthcare costs varied greatly from state to state, ranging from Wyoming with a low of $87 million, to an extraordinary $7.7 billion in California! (I'm sure California's huge population has a lot to do with this statistic.)

▶ Being thin does not necessarily mean you're healthy, nor does being overweight necessarily mean you're unhealthy. It is about living a "healthy lifestyle."

▶ AVOID fast food! If you can't, choose your food wisely. Eat veggie burgers, salads minus croutons, broiled instead of fried, eat the meat with no bun, avoid sauces, juice, coffee, fries, and desserts. Drink water instead of soda.

▶ Question authority! Do not take the advice of your vet, doctor, AMA, FTC, FDA, etc., as gospel. *Research on your own!* Get a second, even third opinion before making any decisions. It could save your life or the life of someone you love.

▶ Do NOT reply on our government to protect you! Have 2 weeks worth of food and water set aside for an emergency. I'm absolutely horrified, ashamed, and deeply distraught by the unconscionable suffering endured by those caught in Katrina's path! The individuals who failed those thousands of helpless people need to be held accountable!

▶ For those who say they don't have time for breakfast, MAKE TIME! Easy options: Whole grain toast with all-natural peanut butter, 1/4 cup blueberries. Or heat up a Teflon-free pan for veggie sausage patties, with side of cottage cheese, tomato, and olive oil. Or 2 eggs with collard greens or spinach, scramble, top with Swiss cheese. Done. Delicious. All in less than 4 minutes—and healthy! The key is to be creative. (I used to use microwave ovens, but I no longer can ignore the potential health risks. Nor should you.)

▶ When I desire something sinfully sweet, I mix water with 1 scoop of banana protein powder. Add lots of ice and blend. Top with nutmeg or cinnamon. It's sweet, creamy, delicious—and guilt-free! (1 tbsp of all-natural peanut butter is also an added option.)

▶ Overweight or otherwise, don't allow yourself to live in baggy sweats and oversized shirts, as it can encourage overeating. Dress with pride. It will do wonders for your emotional and mental state of mind.

▶ Too many parents stress about giving their children "breakfast food." Breakfast food does not have to consist of the typical cereal, Pop-tart, or cinnabun. My rule is to eat whatever I like, as long as it's a healthy choice. I often have a turkey patty over spinach with cottage cheese and avocado. Or maybe half a yam, one egg, tomato slices, topped with goat cheese. Once again, learn to think outside the box. Breakfast should be far more than just sugar-laden cereals, bagels, breakfast bars, or hazelnut lattes with Krispy Kreme donuts.

▶ Herbs have been successfully used for centuries. They have few, if any, side effects. They can actually *heal* rather than mask symptoms. Research. Then use them selectively for good health. (I'm thrilled to report that dietary supplements account for an estimated $17 billion in sales a year. It's wonderful to see Americans are seeking *alternative* healing methods.)

▶ Simple things to improve overall appearance: Dress and walk with pride. As it's needed for good health of body and mind, get some sun on your body, even if it's just 15 minutes a day. Also, hygiene, hygiene, hygiene. Be meticulous in grooming. Smiles are terribly important to our self image, as well as to how others perceive us. Have your teeth professionally cleaned and whitened. Brush and floss regularly. And, if needed, braces or veneers can work wonders.

▶ MEN: Take pride in your appearance. Dress with style. Eat healthy. Go to the gym. Get regular manicures/pedicures. Shave, trim, tweeze, or laser excess body hair—that means back, shoulders, nose and ear hairs. And, with all due respect, whoever said all that underarm or *other* body hair was necessary? Besides being rather unsightly, it's a breeding ground for bacteria. Above all, live with a conscience.

▶ LADIES: Step outside your comfort zone. Dare to change your hair color and style. Buy a new wardrobe. Be edgier. Sexier. Freer. Stop worrying about what others think. Dare to be yourself. Take time for yourself away from the husband and kids. It will refuel you in many wonderful ways. And please, devote as much attention to your physical, mental, and emotional health, as you do to your loved ones and your career.

▶ One of the easiest ways to appear thinner is through your posture. Stand tall, head high, shoulders back, stomach in. A strong, confident posture alone can make you far more attractive. You'll exude a newfound confidence, which can be quite intoxicating to the opposite sex, and you'll easily look 10 pounds thinner. Then make sure you wear clothes that flatter your body, no matter your size. Just because you may be a bit heavy, just because you may have a problem area or two, doesn't mean you can't dress with sensational style!

▶ There are few things more beautiful than the human body. Take pride in yours. Challenge yourself to see what you can create.

- It's nearly impossible to feel sexy, let alone capable of performing sexually, if you're obese. In addition to having better health, far more energy, and feeling absolutely wonderful emotionally, wouldn't you also like an active and fulfilling love life? *Wouldn't you?* Maybe this will motivate you to lose that excess body fat. I hope so. (Now I'm sure there are those few who will claim they can indeed feel sexy and enjoy sexual intimacy to its fullest with an extra 100 pounds. If this is the case, I'm sincerely happy for you. But I would still encourage you to please lose the excess weight.)

- Guys, before you go on any SED (Sex-Enhancing Drug) be it Viagra, Levitra, or Cialis, remember that each of these drugs comes with serious side effects. Speaking of Cialis, *"The Weekender,"* how is it, the drug companies, can develop a drug that makes a man sexually capable for up to 36 hours—but they can't cure PMS or the common cold? While I certainly appreciate a man wanting to please his lover, drugs aren't the answer. Furthermore, wouldn't you agree that the millions of dollars spent by drug companies to develop SEDs, could be far better invested in finding cures for cancer and AIDS? Regardless, the frightening reality is, there has long been a cure for cancer (and most other deadly diseases), but the medical community will <u>never</u> disclose it, as treating the millions who get cancer is a huge *business,* worth billions!

- The latest research for sexual enhancement drug therapy is focusing on triggering the "desire" aspects in the mind rather than just increasing the physical attributes of the penis. I find this truly enlightening, as this is exactly what SESs can do, <u>minus</u> the many risks associated with pharmaceutical drugs. After all, serotonin is the brain chemical that governs sexual behavior.

- There are numerous studies on the extraordinary healing benefits of hydrogen peroxide. So extraordinary, in fact, that it has shown to actually kill the herpes virus, plus, successfully treat many other diseases. When used in conjunction with DMSO (Dimethyl Sulfoxide), it has been shown to have even greater benefits. Of course, the medical industry would never tell us this, as it would cut into the billions of dollars they make on treating such "lifelong" illnesses. Also, are you aware that chicken pox, a form of herpes, will show up on herpes testing 30 to 40 years later? And, who, of my age group, hasn't had chicken pox? I believe this contributes to why so many people test positive with the herpes, yet never show any symptoms. Whether someone has herpes or not, everyone should read "Never an Outbreak" by William Fharel.

- Want to live a long, happy, and healthy life? <u>Practice safe sex</u>! STDs do not care what kind of car you drive or how much money you have! Ladies, there are far too many men who will say and do just about *anything* to convince you to have sex without a condom. Beware of this—and please do not fall for their shameless pleas!

- A healthy, active, creative, and monogamous sex life with someone you love can be tremendously rewarding physically, mentally, and emotionally.

241

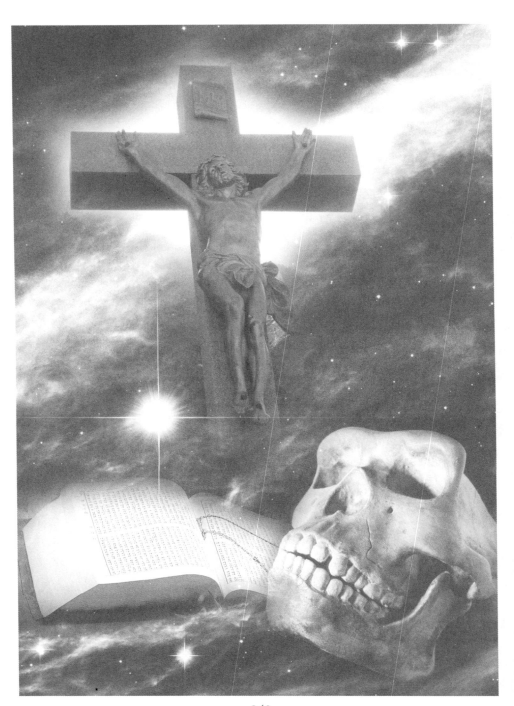

242

37

MENTAL, EMOTIONAL & SPIRITUAL
HEALTH TIPS

▶ Challenge yourself. Believe in yourself. Make yourself proud.

▶ Live a life that is true to yourself.

▶ Make a difference.

▶ Live honorably.

▶ Give of yourself. It does wonders for your mental, emotional, and spiritual health.

▶ Say what you mean, and mean what you say.

▶ Try to perform at least one act of kindness each and every day.

▶ Take a few moments for yourself each day.

▶ Work out for your mind; your body will follow.

▶ If you are overweight, or simply unhappy with your appearance, do not call yourself names. Do not put yourself down, not even in jest.

▶ Your thoughts (and words) have tremendous effect on your health. Be extremely conscious of them.

▶ Try to eliminate stress from your life as much as possible.

▶ Love is best expressed through actions, not words.

▶ Be around people who make you happy, who encourage and inspire you to be your best.

▶ No matter what you have, no matter what you feel you lack, *be grateful*. Gratitude can produce miracles.

- Choose your friends with the greatest of care—*then treasure them daily.*

- Never settle for less than what you need/want/desire.

- Learn to forgive. And, though, forgetting is often not possible, do your best to learn from it—and then move on.

- Find your purpose in life. It's there, right in front of you, waiting for you to grab hold.

- Be aware of how you awaken. Meaning: Don't wake up with a traditional alarm clock. That sudden jolt puts your body immediately into a high-stress mode. It's a terribly unhealthy way to start your day.

- Remember, *these* are the good ole days.

- If there is no one to spoil you, *spoil yourself.*

- Learn to think outside the box.

- Respect yourself. And while you need to respect others, defend your honor when others disrespect you or those you love.

- Being late is not fashionable. Be considerate of others.

- One of the greatest statements of truth is from Florence Scovel Shinn: "Life is a game that cannot be played successfully without the knowledge of Spiritual Law." We all use this law everyday. It's either working for us, or against us. Her book, *The Wisdom of Florence Scovel Shinn*, should be a <u>mandatory</u> read in school. It is life-changing!

- Turn off the music. Turn off the TV. Calm your mind. Be quiet. Learn to listen to your inner voice. This voice, what women know as intuition, is a Higher Power gently guiding you. (To open your mind—and empower your body at the same time—try yoga.)

- That feeling of doubt we all get means STOP! <u>Every</u> <u>single</u> <u>time</u> I ignore this gut feeling, every single time I ignore that soft, barely there little voice, I regret it. Once again, I believe that voice within us is our Spirit Guide, a Higher Power trying to guide us, to protect us. We all have this instinct. Learn to tune into it. Do not ignore it.

- Affirmations are extraordinarily powerful. They can literally change your life. Say them daily. Better yet, consider recording them in your own voice onto a tape or CD. You can then listen to them as you fall asleep and upon waking. The mind is most receptive at these times.

▶ Visualize what you want in your life. You must see, feel, and believe in it before it can manifest into the physical plane.

▶ Pray—and give humble thanks. Then sincerely expect your prayers to be answered. The so-called secret to successful praying is *believing* your prayers are already answered.

▶ We attract what we feel/vibrate. The Law of Attraction is always at work.

▶ Pay very close attention to what you "think and say," even more when you're angry. Your thoughts and spoken words are powerful forms of creative energy waiting to manifest in your life. So, please, be overly aware of the words you use each and every day. They literally form your life. (*"As a Man Thinketh, So Shall He Be."*)

▶ Circumstances don't make a man, they *reveal* a man.

▶ Change your words; change your life. There is <u>nothing</u> that can affect your life as dramatically, as coming to understand the power behind your spoken words. Use your words with care, caution, direct intention, and then watch your world change.

▶ Change your perspective. Stop complaining. Both can change your life.

▶ Discover the amazing power behind these few words: "I'm sorry. Please forgive me. I made a mistake. I love you."

▶ Remember the incredible power of a hug.

▶ Learn to be a good listener.

▶ I've learned that so often people want what they aren't willing and/or capable of giving of themselves. Remember, you only get what you give.

▶ Empathy is, unfortunately, not a trait that most people know how and/or are willing to express. Yet it is absolutely crucial to healthy, fulfilling relationships.

▶ Discover who "you" really are. And then learn to love all that you are.

▶ Look <u>beneath</u> the color of one's skin. Look <u>beyond</u> one's age. We are far more than the color of our skin. We are far more than a number.

▶ I'm not a religious person, more spiritually driven. Either way, I try to live a life that is true and just. One of the greatest quotes I've found to live by is a classic, yet still very much relevant: "Do unto others, as you would have others do unto you."

- Stand up for what you believe in.

- This above all, to thine own self be true. — Shakespeare

- Stimulate your mind daily, be it through reading, art, music, etc.

- Unfortunately, our society far too often views women as being over the hill and no longer worthy even at a mere 30 years of age. We need to remind ourselves that we are all more than just a number. With this in mind, here is an empowering quote by Antonio: "Ladies, age is not a handicap. It is a *privilege*, not a condition."

- Gentlemen, please understand that women want and need to be heard. We want to know that you're at least making an effort to understand us. This compassion will go a very long way with the lady in your life.

- Give more. Expect less.

- Stop idolizing TV/movie stars/professional athletes. Create your own brilliant life!

- When it comes to your career, do what you love to do. Discover what truly inspires you, and then find a way to make a living from it. There are few greater rewards than doing what you love, and getting paid for it.

- Learn to be alone, *without* feeling lonesome.

- NEVER GIVE UP!

- Dare to dream. But, more importantly, dare to do. — Scotty Christensen

- Be a leader. Don't follow the crowd.

- Without trying to sound morbid, please allow me: I want you to look into your future. See yourself on your deathbed. Now—do you honestly think you'll be saying, *"Oh, how I wish I had watched more TV!"* I seriously doubt it.

- I strongly suggest you limit the amount of news you take in, be it in the form of print, radio, and/or TV. It is nothing but "Doom and Gloom!" The media likes to keep us in a perpetual state of panic. How can we expect to be happy, upbeat, and enthusiastic about life if we are bombarded with nothing but death, disease, murder, terror alerts, deadly flu viruses, insects, asteroids, and so forth?

- Trust and respect are earned, <u>not</u> freely given.

▶ Find a hobby. Be creative. Discover your passion.

▶ Dare to be different.

▶ Learn to think for yourself.

▶ Each day is a new opportunity to make new choices, to change your life.

▶ Stop being a victim. You have the power to live your life as you choose.

▶ If you're not getting the affection, love, respect, or consideration you think you deserve from others—give it to yourself. *You are deserving*, even if others have yet to notice, or are simply incapable of giving you what you need.

▶ Time goes by far too quickly to waste a single second. Try to live in the moment each and every day, as happiness is most often found in the littlest of moments.

▶ The most important part of any relationship is not what you get, but what you give.
— Eleanor Roosevelt

▶ Expect miracles.

▶ Tell those you admire/respect/love how much they mean to you. Tell them often. Do not wait until it's too late.

▶ Do not judge or criticize others. What you put out, comes right back to you.

▶ Have issues that concern you? Write your senator or congress representative and let them be known. Do not sit in silence! Dare to make a difference!

▶ VOTE! Let your voice be heard. Now more than ever you need to stand up for your rights or those rights will slowly, but surely be taken away! It's already happening.

▶ Pick your fights wisely.

▶ With respect to dating, while it may seem like there are far too few good men or women available, there is also no time to waste on those who do not fulfill all that you need/want/desire. Nonetheless, before you feel incomplete, please look *within* for love, contentment, and self-worth. And don't be afraid to be alone. Learn to enjoy your own company. Hopefully, you will then be much more selective when choosing a lover.

▶ Find a charity that is personal to you, and then give to it regularly—be it donations of your personal time and/or money.

▸ Mentoring children through my life has given me tremendous personal satisfaction. It also makes me seriously question our government and its various regulations. On one hand, the law demands a license for everything from driving a car, motorcycle, hunting, fishing, to owning a gun, etc. And yet, when it concerns one of *the most important responsibilities* a person will ever take on, i.e., bringing a new life into this world, a life that will either gracefully benefit our society or be a burden, there is no such testing, evaluation, requirement, no proof of competency—be it financially, mentally, or emotionally. I find this amazing. Please, consider all factors before taking on parenthood. It is not meant for everyone, nor does it make you less of a woman (or a man) if you should choose not to take this path. Personally, I think it should be a prerequisite to mentor a child for a minimum of one full year before you have a child of your own. First of all, it would immensely help millions of children in need, while at the same time giving you a much better idea of what parenting would actually be like. I think far too many people get caught up in the "baby" stage and how adorable kids can be at ages 3 and 4. But, they seem to forget to look at the much bigger picture and all that it will really require to raise a healthy, emotionally sound, loving, confident, educated, and productive young adult. So, please, won't you consider mentoring a child *before* you sign on to that life-long commitment? Then, if and when you are ready to become a parent, will you please consider adopting instead of spending tens of thousands on fertility treatments?

▸ Don't wait for Christmas to give to those you love, or those in need. Instead, spread this holiday spirit *throughout* the year. And when Christmas does come 'round, focus on giving to children, especially those children (and families) who have less than you do. Personally, as of 2004, I have boycotted buying gifts for adults, as this holiday is so much against who I am. Not that I don't love to give—I do. But I choose to give throughout the year, not on this far too commercialized, over-hyped holiday. Christmas is shoved in our face before Halloween. We are manipulated into believing we must spend our every cent, or feel guilty. Again, this holiday cheer, sense of joy, love, and giving should be spread throughout the year, not just reserved for Christmas.

▸ When asked how you're doing, reply, "I'm doing absolutely fantastic!" Even if this may not be true, said often enough, you soon will be, as your words shape your world.

▸ Have something or someone to care for, to love, to nurture. It could be as simple as a plant, a fish, adopting a homeless dog or cat, or mentoring a child in need. It will do wonders for your heart and soul!

▸ Studies have proven that owning a pet can actually help both alleviate depression and lower blood pressure.

▸ If you have a dog, walk her/him daily. It's a fantastic way to get you out walking, and they'll love you for it. However, please avoid the heat of the day and don't drag them alongside your bicycle.

▶ If you don't have a dog, please, consider adopting one from your local animal shelter. Never will you find such a loyal and loving friend! More importantly, *you will save a life!*

▶ Weight loss supplements and diet food are now available for our pets, primarily dogs. PLEASE! Just as with humans, first make sure you're giving your dog enough exercise and feed them a healthy diet before you put them on a diet. Rather than just one large meal, feed them two smaller meals (one in the morning and one late in the day). This will help boost their metabolism. Make sure your pet's food does not contain road-kill, animal parts, euthanized or diseased animals, which are disgustingly (yet legally) allowed to be put in pet food. *And we wonder why our pets are all getting cancer and other life-threatening diseases!* This is not just a concern with the cheaper brands of pet food. These ingredients are found in the biggest names in the industry. Feed your beloved pets *real* food. If this isn't possible, use either Nutro Natural Choice or Flint River Ranch food as a base, topped with a variety of cottage cheese, tofu, *cooked* eggs, shaved broccoli, avocado, etc.

▶ If humans had the ability to express *even half* the compassion, forgiveness, loyalty, and unconditional love that most animals give us each and every day of their life, this world would be a much kinder, gentler place in which to live.

▶ We won't drink tap water, so why give it to our pets? Please filter their water. If you can't do this, at least run the water for 30 seconds before you fill their bowl.

▶ Visit your local nursing or retirement home and make a new friend. <u>Visit them often</u>. While you will give them such joy, it will make you greatly appreciate what you have. It will also remind you how very important exercise and balanced nutrition is today.

▶ Life is short. Live it well! But most of all, live it with compassion, integrity, and gratitude. (In memory of the thousands who perished on 9/11 and in Katrina's wake.)

▶ Be a true and loyal friend, lover, spouse...

▶ Be careful who you do, because Karmic Law is just and true—and <u>always</u> at work.

▶ Lonell, ex-professional baseball player, once said to me, "The reason most marriages fail is because a man will marry a woman he can live with—instead of marrying a woman he can't live without!" How profound! How very true! To my complete dismay, though, Lonell went on to say, "Then again, men are only as faithful as their options." Ooooh, what terribly unsettling commentary that was, as options can be endless in this very sexual world. I believe, however, that the ability and/or *willingness* to be faithful is based on one's level of character and integrity. Men (and women) either have such strength of character or they do not. It is a choice, <u>not</u> an option. It is also about being a M-A-N, not a boy. Nor is it about using the far too often lame excuse that they are "men" with so-called needs, and are, therefore, entitled to infidelities.

With all due respect, gentlemen,
the next 3 health tips are dedicated to the ladies.
I completely understand, however, that these concerns may affect you, as well:

▶ Ladies, considering online dating has become so prevalent, you must proceed with your eyes wide open, especially because of the many questionable men looking for their next piece of ass, rather than love. With online dating comes endless temptation placed enticingly before men—temptation that most find hard to resist. Not only are there way too many players, but my girlfriend and I so often got the same men writing us, literally cutting/pasting the exact same pathetic copy in the hope of seducing us, all the while boastfully claiming to be "different than the rest!" Never have I met so many cowards, as I have online. In addition to the senseless BS that is spewed, they stalk you like prey. Some even steal other men's photos! *Is there no shame?* Obviously not. But, it was the following man that was most frightening: He wrote with seemingly sincere interest. We spoke several times. We planned to meet. But something just—didn't—seem—right. That little voice screamed STOP!! This time, I listened. When I told him I wasn't comfortable, and hence, changed my mind, he went OFF! He then sent me the most vile email, telling me what an "old, ugly, used-up bitch I was, and how women are so fucking gullible, as he, like most other men, were workin' 30 pieces of ass at once!" He went on to give me graphic details, as to where his face would be buried later that night. This man's rage was absolutely terrifying! Even more unnerving, he called back, acted as if nothing happened, and <u>insisted</u> we meet. *Now I knew he was definitely crazy!* Nevertheless, if you want to see if your online love interest is at all sincere in his affections for you—and to help see what he's really made of—you must do a little protective/creative marketing. First, <u>never</u> give out your real name, town that you live in, or other personal business. Next, set up 2 profiles on the same site, using different images and stats. Then sit back and watch who takes the bait. It's sad to see just how many men will attempt to play you! Also, graciously postpone a date. See how the man reacts. Telling a man you're going out alone, with the girls, or even with another man, is also a great character test. If you're not yet serious with him, he should be understanding. But, for those like the man/men above, these precautions may save you grief, if not your very life.

▶ Ladies, do a background check on any man you plan to share your bed with, more so your heart. You need to make sure you know who you're *really* being seduced by. First and foremost, *listen to your inner voice.* If something doesn't feel right, trust me, it <u>isn't</u>! Dare to ask questions. Lots of them. Listen carefully. Take mental notes. Write down his license plate number. File it. You can find out just about all you need with that. Ask for his business card. Verify that info. Discreetly check his glove box for the car registration, as it should confirm his home address. Take notes. File it. In case his car is registered to someone else, you'll need to look at his driver's license. Be sneaky or come right out and ask. Either way, there shouldn't be a problem if the man has nothing to hide. If he refuses, there's your first red flag. Same goes for getting his cell, work, and home number. You've got to be willing to ask for them and see how he responds. Again, if he refuses to give you any of them, especially his home number, WARNING!

That's a huge red flag! If he never answers his cell, but always calls you back, another red flag. Next, get online and type in his name. You'll be surprised what can come up. If you get nothing, there are hundreds of companies who specialize in tracking personal documentation. Now you can, of course, hold off and simply sit tight and see where this relationship takes you, or you can pay a small fee to have them run a search based on the data you've been able to gather. Bottom line, ladies: Do not, *and I repeat,* do NOT take any man on his word alone. Above all, follow your instincts! If your potential love interest is sincere and found to be truthful in all that he claims, great! No problem. But if he's <u>not</u>, this effort, this little bit of research, will save you a lot of heartache, emotional distress, and any potential financial risks. (This mental/emotional health tip was sadly inspired by certain men who have shamelessly played me over the years. Although I consider myself street-smart and sceptical of most men, there are those few who are *sooo smooth and sooo damn charming*, that even I have fallen prey to their tender, but obviously fallacious affections. So, please, ladies, do <u>whatever</u> it takes to protect your heart, your emotions, and your physical well-being!)

▶ As a single woman of 46, and one who is incredibly particular about the men with whom I share my time, it's rare that I even date. But, when I do, I try never to judge a man by the color of his skin, age, physical appearance, or bank account. I've dated men who are much older and those ooooh so much younger, from Caucasian, Black, Italian, and Spanish, from construction worker to CEO, celebrity to starving entrepreneur, etc. While I certainly don't feel I've missed out on dating a variety of men, I must admit I've never done well with long-term relationships. It seems most men fall in "lust" with me, only to then be threatened later by the exact same traits to which they were first attracted. The fact is, I'm a very independent, free-spirited, modestly confident female. One who is equally compassionate, sensitive, and honorable. I'm also keenly aware of my own shortcomings. Regardless, I refuse to hang around for insecure, dominating, manipulative men to abuse me verbally, emotionally, or physically. I also don't do well with men who are never satisfied with one woman's affections, or those less than honest. Look, I don't seek perfection, but there are only so many times I'm willing to forgive—boyfriend or otherwise. And, though, I, like most women, would like to find an extraordinary man to fall profoundly in love with, I've <u>never</u> felt incomplete without a man, nor should any woman. I have, instead, happily and confidently chosen to remain single, rather than ever stay with a man who would treat me less than. My life, and yours, is far too precious to waste on one who does not truly respect, adore, and appreciate all that we are. Therefore, ladies, refuse to settle for less than what you desire—and deserve. And if you're currently in a relationship that leaves you empty and longing for more, or worse yet, if you're in an abusive relationship, please reach within and find the strength, the courage to leave! It could mean life or death. *You are stronger than you'll ever believe!*

▶ To end on a much more positive and empowering thought: "We make a living by what we get, but we make a life by what we give." —Sir Winston Churchill

PART IV

CLOSING

Dear Reader:

Thank you, not only for purchasing my book,
but, more importantly, for having taken the time to read it
from cover to cover. I sincerely hope it helps you on your
journey toward living a much longer, happier, and healthier life,
and achieving those many amazing possibilities without
dieting, depression, ADD, type 2 diabetes, high blood pressure,
cancer, or heart disease—moreover, <u>without</u> having
to risk your life with pharmaceutical drugs!

If you'd like to share how this book has, in any way,
changed your life, I'd love to hear from you.

Wishing you the greatest of health of body, mind, and spirit!

Phoenix Gilman, Founder/CEO
Exacting Nutrition, Inc.
34145 Pacific Coast Hwy #167
Dana Point, CA 92629-2808
USA

To order more copies so as to share the
gift of health with those you love,
please go to
dietfailurethenakedtruth.com
or call
1-877-TRUTHEXPOSED
(1-877-878-8439)

RESEARCH/REFERENCES/RECOMMENDATIONS

Being self-taught, with an insatiable thirst for knowledge, researching has therefore been crucial in my various professional endeavors. Below are a just few of the numerous books, clinical studies, health/wellness subscriptions, and Web sites that have helped me along this extraordinary journey. I encourage you to explore any one of them to even further educate yourself.

Books/Health References:
5-HTP, The Natural Way to Overcome Depression, Obesity, and Insomnia, Michael T. Murray, ND

The Schwarzbein Principle, Diana Schwarzbein, MD, and Nancy Deville

The Cholesterol Myths, Uffe Ravnskov, MD, PhD

Calculated Risks: How to Know When Numbers Deceive You, Gerd Gigerenzer

The Food Revolution: How Your Diet Can Help Save Your Life and Our World, John Robbins

Natural Cures "They" Don't Want You to Know About, Kevin Trudeau

The Shooting Drugs; Prozac and It's Generation Exposed, Donna Smart

Solving the Depression Puzzle, Rita Elkins, MH

The Glucose Revolution, Jennie Miller, PhD; Thomas Wolever, MD, PhD; Stephen Colagiuri, MD; Kaye Powell, M. Nutr., Dietician

Prescription for Nutritional Healing, Phyllis Balch, CNC; James Balch, MD

Natural Hormone Balance for Women, Uzzi Reiss, MD, OB/GYN

Never an Outbreak, William Fharel

Research/Clinical Support:
Wurtman and Wurtman, "Brain serotonin carbohydrate cravings, obesity, and depression." *Advances in Experimental Medicine and Biology* 398 (1996)

J.E. Blundel and M.B. Leshem, "The effect of 5-HTP on food intake and on the anorexic action of amphetamine and fenfluramine," *Journal of Pharmacy and Pharmacology* 27 (1975) 31-37

F. Ceci, "The effects of oral 5-HTP administration on feeding behavior in obese adult female patients." *Journal of Neural Transmission* 76 (1989) 109-17

Wurtman and Wurtman, *The Serotonin Solution*, and *Nutrition and the Brain*

J.J. Alino, J.L. Gutierrez, and M. Iglesias, "5-HTP and an MAOI in the treatment of depression. A double-blind study," *International Pharmacopsychiatry* 11 (1976) 8-15

Benket, "Effect of parachlorophenylalnine and 5-HTP on human sexual behavior." *Monographs in Neural Sciences* 3 (1976) 88-93

R.J. Wyatt, "Effects of 5-HTP on the sleep of normal human subjects." *Electroencephalography and Clinical Neurophysiology* 30 (1971) 505-10

Research in Depression, Advances in Biochemical Psychopharmacology, Vol. 39, pg. 301-313

Gastpar and Wakelin (1988), Selective 5-HTP Reuptake Inhibitors: *Novel or Commonplace Agents?*

Advances in Biological Psychiatry Vol. 19 pg. 18-30 and 52-57

Schwarcz, Young, and Brown (1989), Kynurenine and Seretonin Pathways Progress in Trytophan research Advances in Experimental Medicine and Biology, Vol. 29

Mechanism of Action of Vinpocetine, Acta Pharm Hung, (1996)

Szakall S, et al. Cerebral effects of a single dose of intravenous vinpocetine in chronic stroke patients: a PET study. J Neuroimaging 1998 Oct; 8(4): 197-204

Feigin VL. et al. Vinpocetine treatment in acute ischaemic stroke. a pilot single-blind randomized clinical trial. Eur J Neurol. (2001)

Web Sites:
PETA: peta.com
Viva! USA: vivausa.org
Vegan Outreach: veganoutreach.org
Meet Your Meat: meetyourmeat.com
Centers for Disease Control and Prevention: cdc.gov
National Institutes of Health: nih.gov
nutritiondata.com/index.html
mercola.com/article/statins.htm
thenutritionreporter.com/fructose_dangers.html
usatoday.com/news/health/2004-03-25-hfcs-usat_x.htm
forum.lowcarber.org/showthread.php?p=2297322#post2297322
cspinet.org/sodapop/liquid_candy.htm
upliftprogram.com/depression_stats.html
niddk.nih.gov/health/nutrit/pubs/unders.htm
medical-library.net/sites/framer.html?/sites/_adult_onset_diabetes
4.dr-rath-foundation.org/PHARMACEUTICAL_BUSINESS/laws_of_the_pharmaceutical_industry.htm

Health & Wellness Monthly Subscriptions:
Life Extensions Magazine
1100 West Commercial Blvd.
Ft. Lauderdale, FL 33309
(800) 678-8989

Kevin Trudeau's Natural Cures Newsletter
P.O. Box 342
Elk Grove Village, IL 60009
(847) 777-7131

Alternatives, David G. Williams, MD
P.O. Box 61010
Rockville, MD 20859
(800) 527-3044

Cable TV Show & Documentaries:
HBO's "Real Time with Bill Maher"
"Prescription for Disaster" by Gary Null
"SUPER SIZE ME" by filmmaker Morgan Spurlock

Spiritual/Emotional/Mental Resources:
The following are a few of the many books in which I've found solace in. They are thought-provoking and spiritually inspirational:
The Wisdom of Florence Scovel Shinn, by same
Living the Science of Mind, Ernest Holmes
The Power of Your Subconscious Mind, Dr. Joseph Murphy
The Power of Kabbalah, Yehuda Berg
As a Man Thinketh, James Allen
The Seven Spiritual Laws of Success, Deepak Chopra
Your Erroneous Zones, You'll See It When You Believe It, Real Magic, Dr. Wayne Dyer
The Celestine Prophecy, James Redfield
The Power of Positive Thinking, Norman Vincent Peale
The Power is Within You, Louise L. Hay
Excuse Me, Your Life is Waiting, Lynn Grabhorn
The Other Side and Back, Sylvia Browne
Charlotte's Web, E.B. White

Endocrinology & Metabolism:
Endocrinology Institute
Diana Schwarzbein, MD
5901 Encina Road, Suite A
Goleta, CA 93117
(805) 681-0003

Natural Bioidentical Hormone Replacement Therapy:
Endocrinology Institute
Diana Schwarzbein, MD
5901 Encina Road, Suite A
Goleta, CA 93117
(805) 681-0003

Uzzi Reiss, MD, OB/GYN (Specializes in Natural Bioidentical Hormones & Anti-Aging Therapy)
414 N. Camden Drive, Suite 750
Beverly Hills, CA 90210
(310) 247-1300

Stephanie McClellan, MD, OB/GYN (Plus, Natural Bioidentical Hormone Replacement Therapy)
1601 Avocado Avenue, Suite 100
Newport Beach, CA 92660
(949) 719-3600

California Pharmacy & Compounding Center
Steven Feldman, Pharmacist/Owner
307 Placentia Avenue
Newport Beach, CA 92663
(949) 642-8057

Fitness/Sports Clubs/Spas/Personal Training:
The Sports Club/LA (A Collection of Luxury Sports & Fitness Complexes)
Rex A. Licklider, Vice Chairman/CEO
(Go to thesportsclubla.com to find the club nearest you)

Equinox (World-Class in Both Design & Club Offerings)
Harvey Spevak, CEO/President
(Go to equinox.com to find the club nearest you)

Xclusiv (Excellent Private Training Gym)
Priscilla & Gabe Tuft, Proprietors
(Please go to xclusivfitness.com for location)

Dermatologist:
Stephen Scheinberg, PhD, MD
1441 Avocado Avenue, Suite 806
Newport Beach, CA 92660
(949) 718-1222

Dentists:
William Brownson, DDS
3553 Camino Mira Costa, Suite B
San Clemente, CA 92672
(949) 493-2391

Paul M. Johnson, DDS (Specializing in Cosmetic & Reconstructive Dentistry)
360 San Miguel Drive, Suite 602
Newport Beach, CA 92660
(949) 640-0300

Mentoring:
If you would like to help a child in need by simply giving of yourself, please contact:
Serenity Village
17880 Skypark Circle, Suite 200
Irvine, CA 92614
(949) 643-9942

Dog Adoption:
If you have a sincere/gentle fondness for Rottweilers, please visit Rottweiler Rescue of Los Angeles at rottrescuela.org. Or call Beverly at (818) 765-5997. (And, yes, I adopted my newest baby girl, Ella, from here.) I encourage you, no matter the breed you adore, to please help save lives by adopting!

Custom Couture for Your Pooch
Exceptional Pooch Designs
Designer: Janene Bogardus
Contact: nightbird333b@verizon.net (Web site; exceptionalpoochdesigns.com coming soon!)

Therapy Dogs International, Inc.
88 Bartley Road
Flanders, NJ 07836
(973) 252-9800
tdi-dog.org

EXACTING NUTRITION, INC.
Company profile

Exacting Nutrition's foundation is proudly laid upon solid, scientific, and ethical grounds. As Founder/ CEO, Phoenix spent years pouring through countless medical journals, research abstracts, health books, etc., to discover why 98% of all diets fail—and why depression, type 2 diabetes, ADD, and heart disease are so prevalent. It is this extraordinary research on which her book is based. It is this extraordinary research from which her company's products are developed. Her intentions—through her book, consultations, etc.—are to help others live a much longer, happier, and healthier life.

CONSULTATIONS/WEBINARS/MOTIVATIONAL SPEAKING

Whether as a personal trainer, nutritionist, motivational speaker, or consumer activist, Phoenix's expertise is in high demand. From corporate America, school systems, bariatric centers, to talk radio, educational seminars/webinars, private groups or individuals, her knowledge—along with her relentless devotion to making a difference—can help change and improve lives everywhere. For those interested in securing Phoenix's expertise, please email her at phoenix@dietfailurethenakedtruth.com to confirm availability and fees.

THE PHOENIX WELLNESS & ANTI-AGING CENTER

To further expand her business platform—and passionate reach into the community—Phoenix plans to open The Phoenix Wellness & Anti-Aging Center. The Center's mission would be to teach others how to live longer, look younger, and be healthy for life. (Losing excess weight would be just the beginning!) The Center would cater to those seeking a leaner, younger, more importantly *healthier* body, mind, and spirit. The menu of services would include a unique combination of Phoenix's expertise in nutrition and fitness, as well as anti-aging. She will bring aboard other Wellness experts, from naturopathic and anti-aging doctors, cosmetic dermatologists, to personal trainers, physical and massage therapists, chiropractor, and Science of Mind practitioner. (With regard to cosmetic procedures, no Botox or lipo will be offered/ encouraged. Only non-invasive, non-surgical anti-aging procedures would be performed.) Should you be interested in more information, either as a client, joining her team of experts, or as a potential investor, please email her at phoenix@dietfailurethenakedtruth.com.

THE PHOENIX WELLNESS RETREAT
for body, mind & spirit

Because of her genuine desire to help others, particularly those less fortunate, Phoenix has a vision of one day building a Wellness Retreat in either Southern California or Baja California, Mexico, on the Sea of Cortez. It would be a place where pre-teens and above could go to learn firsthand how to lose the excess weight for good, alleviate depression, anxiety, ADD, reduce their risk for type 2 diabetes and heart disease—and remarkably improve their self-confidence. They would learn, in essence, how to live a healthier lifestyle based on the various teachings found in this book. Phoenix's primary focus would be to give inner city kids and/or those simply in need, a place where they could come to nourish their bodies, minds, and spirits. It would be an environment that would hopefully inspire—and empower them for life.

259

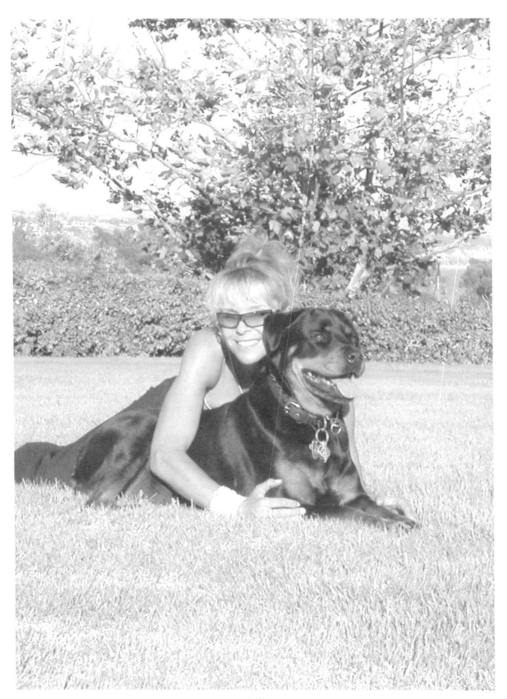

AUTHOR...

Journey of Discovery

Phoenix *(born Phyllis)* Marie Gilman, born May 7, 1959, youngest daughter of Frank and Barbara Gilman, was one of four children. Due to her mother's mental illness and institutionalization, her father took his young children and moved in with his mother. He hired a nanny to help his mother care for the girls, while her baby brother went to live temporarily with her aunt and uncle. Two years later, her dad remarried. Just shy of four, Phoenix was suddenly the sixth of seven kids—and with a stepmother.

Fiercely independent and a tomboy at heart, she grew up in the quaint lakeside community of Gull Lake, Michigan. A natural athlete like her father, Phoenix found tremendous pride in her athletic abilities. But, she was also very much a rebel. It wasn't long before she got bored with high school and the far too controlling, hypocritical surroundings. All the while, her home life was, to say the very least, terribly unsettling. After running away at 16 (her close friend Vicki Gesmundo, and her family, were gracious enough to take her in), Phoenix realized her only way out was to finish school and do it quickly. So, she moved back home, went to summer school, graduated five months early with honors, even earning a State of Michigan Scholarship for her academic achievements. Nevertheless, rather than seek a traditional education—and being a free-spirit who always went against the grain—she chose instead to move to California at barely 18 (but with fake I.D. in hand) to pursue new challenges and adventures. That adventurous spirit had her moving to Florida less than a year later.

However, her adventures were not always positive ones. She endured many personal traumas. Each one, though, only made her stronger, and more determined. And so, with a humble and sincere desire to hopefully inspire other women, be it young girls or adults, Phoenix felt it was important to share a glimpse into her very private world. Her intentions in sharing such personal stories are <u>not</u> for sympathy, but rather to let other females know that they are stronger than they'll ever believe!

Losing her mother was her first tragedy. Being pulled away from her grandmother was equally as traumatic, followed by a stepmother who despised her. This volatile relationship led to years of anguish. From age 12 to 13, she was repeatedly molested (in broad daylight) by two neighborhood men. Deathly afraid of being blamed, she said nothing. Finally, she pulled a butcher knife on one of them. He, backed off. At 17, she was busted for weed at the Canadian/US border. Although it was only a few joints, she was threatened with jail time. Living in Miami, age 24, after several homicidal beatings by her then boyfriend, but with no money to move—and rather than further risk her life at his hands—she chose to live in her car with only a dime in her pocket and her dog at her side. Age 25, living in Palm Beach, she was stalked by an ex-boyfriend for over a year. His reign of terror included various forms of physical/mental assaults, i.e., relentless verbal abuse, choking her until unconscious, stealing/vandalizing her car, breaking into her home, stealing her dog, holding a knife at her throat for hours, and cold sober death threats. She reported this man's violent behavior to the police a dozen times, but it was, appallingly, long before domestic abuse was taken seriously. Ironically, they wouldn't arrest him, but they arrested her for driving under the influence literally days after she *begged them* to protect her.

Personally motivated...

Phoenix not only survived far too many abusive boyfriends—be it viciously cruel verbal bashings or brutal physical beatings—she also *never* backed down. She never allowed anyone to treat her with such low regard, not as a child, a teen, and most assuredly not as a grown woman. And, she did whatever she had to do to survive, no matter how humbling. A few of her proudest personal achievements, though, are the following. She hopes they will inspire women—and make them realize how one person can truly make a difference.

Living in Florida at 19 years of age, Phoenix was pulled over late one night by a policeman who taunted her, threatening to arrest her. Considering she had had a couple of drinks, she felt exceptionally vulnerable. The officer made her drive her car down a darkened alley. He then used his patrol car to block her in. While he continued to taunt her with the idea of taking her to jail, he proceeded to cleverly indulge in his sick, twisted sexual fetish. Upon his departure, he warned her not to say anything because, as far as he was concerned, "They had *never* seen each other!" His mistake, besides having threatened and assaulted her, was that he had called in to run her tags and license. Their encounter was clearly on record. Refusing to *ever* accept such abuse by a man, moreover by the legal system specifically designed to protect her from precisely this type of assault, Phoenix reported the officer to Internal Affairs. She endured the humiliating line of questioning, picked the officer's photo out of dozens of others, and passed a grueling lie detector test. The officer, of course, denied all such claims. When he failed two separate lie detector tests, he was fired.

1988, age 26, and living in West Palm Beach, Kashif, her first beloved Rottweiler, was hit by a UPS truck. The driver knowingly left her on the side of the road to die. Thankfully, a woman witnessed the accident and rushed her to the emergency clinic. The next day Phoenix called UPS's Safety Department to inform them of this tragic incident, moreover the callousness shown by their driver. The Safety Supervisor was extremely apologetic, even offered to pay for Kashif's surgery. Phoenix was moved by his empathy and offer. But, when she called the next day to follow-up, he was no where to be found. He had, in fact, been moved to another department. The company then denied any and all responsibility. Ah, the games were on! But that was only the beginning.

While at the vet's office a few weeks later, a man, along with his hysterical young son in tow, rushed in with his cocker spaniel in his arms. He said their dog had just been hit by a UPS truck in front of their house. Shockingly, the receptionist added that a UPS truck had hit and killed her cat in her driveway a year prior. Later that evening, Phoenix's sister in Michigan told her that her neighbor's dog had been run over in their driveway by a UPS truck a few months earlier. Sadly, the dog was old, and due to her extensive injuries, she had to be put down. *These senseless tragedies were terribly alarming!* Phoenix knew she had to do something, as she believed, without a doubt, the carelessness shown by these drivers was a serious concern *throughout* their national fleet.

Once Kashif was well enough to walk, Phoenix picketed the main UPS branch in West Palm. With her dog faithfully beside her and the rain pouring down, she walked for hours, carrying a sign that read, "Unnecessary Pet Sacrifices!" Within hours, three TV crews and two radio stations arrived, eager to take her story. Her story was, yes, one of desperation for the many animals that had been injured and/or killed by UPS trucks, but it was also about bringing awareness to the frightening reality that if these drivers weren't able to slow down for a dog in residential areas (especially driveways), they sure as hell would never be able to avoid hitting a child chasing a ball. Her goal: Get UPS to change their rushed, unrealistic drop-off policy so their drivers would have ample time to *safely* do their job, encourage safer driving, and all to ultimately help stop the senseless suffering!

Unfortunately, though the news stories aired with great passion, UPS still chose to ignore her. So, Phoenix produced her own video, telling her story in her own way, editing in the various news pieces. She titled the video: *"Today a Dog, Tomorrow a Child. Speaking Out For Those Who Can't."* She mailed copies to 60 Minutes and Dan Rather, along with a copy and letter of intent to UPS's corporate office in Greenwich, Connecticut. Within 24 very short hours, a UPS senior executive called. He apologized profusely, guaranteed an immediate reimbursement of her vet bills, more importantly, he promised he would personally look into the incidents—and the many serious concerns she spoke of. (Phoenix has long regretted that she never got anything in writing that would, in fact, substantiate this VP had indeed made the much-needed policy changes.)

August 1995, age 36, Phoenix was again living in California: A CHP officer requested to come to her home under the ruse of needing to discuss the five-car pileup she had been in earlier that day. She highly questioned his intentions, because he had arrogantly asked her out at the scene of the accident, as she cried over her injuries and smoldering car. But considering he was a "man of the law"—and claiming he needed to discuss the accident—she unwillingly obliged. When she realized it was definitely not an official call, but rather a personal one, she asked him to leave. He refused. He then made several vulgar sexual suggestions. She again asked him to leave. He ignored her. When she refused the officer's continued and aggressive sexual advances, he physically assaulted her. With all that Phoenix had been through in her life, this was the first time she ever truly feared for her life, at the very least, being brutally raped. Staying calm, she eventually convinced him to leave.

Once again, the mistake this man made was to assault her, but to further seal his fate, he called the next day and imprudently left her a message on her answering machine "apologizing for his aggressive, animal-like behavior." He went on to say that she "owed it to him to let him make it up to her." All the while, his police radio could be heard in the background. Phoenix took the priceless recording to Internal Affairs. But, just as before, the officer who took the initial report treated her, as if she was lying, trying to unfairly accuse one of their own. Only when she told them that she had this officer on tape, apologizing for his assault, did they treat her with any consideration or respect. Nevertheless, she endured the same line of humiliating questioning, and even testified twice in court on behalf of the State. The officer was held liable for his actions—at the very minimum, losing his job. Phoenix's intentions in reporting both these assaults was to make sure these men, *men who were horrifically using their badges to assault women,* would NEVER be able to do so again, particularly not while hiding behind a police uniform! With regard to the latter incident, Phoenix received a letter of appreciation from California Attorney General Daniel Lungren.

December 1995, when a man she was dating attempted to con her out of thousands of dollars, she took the assorted documents she had acquired and personally delivered them to the FBI in Los Angeles, only to discover he was a fugitive from Colorado for 7 long years. He had been convicted of defrauding dozens of investors out of several million dollars. Even more frightening, he had also been convicted of kidnapping and rape! Nevertheless, Phoenix demanded her money back. And though this man refused and repeatedly threatened her life, she did not back down. (Her two Rotties, Greta and Gunther, played a huge role in protecting her.) The man finally, yet reluctantly, agreed to give back her money. But that wasn't nearly enough. Phoenix went on to help the FBI and the local police in their investigation. New charges were eventually brought forth. He was indicted and convicted of an investment fraud scheme, resulting in losses to investors exceeding $1,000,000. He was sentenced to 26 months' incarceration, followed by 3 years of supervised release, and was ordered to pay full restitution to the victims of his crime. Phoenix received a letter of sincere gratitude from the FBI. (Phoenix is forever grateful to Linda English, the FBI agent who so vigorously prosecuted this case.)

In 2001, at age 42, a prominent Newport Beach CEO seduced Phoenix into a relationship, a relationship that was based precisely on this man's many wonderfully kind, generous, and what she thought to be *genuine* proposals to win her attention—and ultimately her affections. But, unfortunately, she soon found out that this man (like so many others she had encountered prior) was notorious for playing this game with literally dozens of women. He promised them the world, only to use them, take what he wanted, then kick them to the curb. Be not mistaken. Phoenix was by *no means* naive—but she most definitely wasn't going to let this man exploit her. Whether a written or a verbal contract, this man entered into a mutually binding agreement, an agreement that was based on very defined terms, terms that "he" had proposed, terms that she had lived up to, but terms he felt he could simply default on. Sorry. Wrong lady. She would have loved nothing better than to publicly expose this man to help other unsuspecting women avoid his seductive trappings. And maybe, just maybe, by holding him accountable, he and other men like him, who brazenly use women for their own selfish pleasures, would think twice before they did so again. Though this was nothing compared to prior situations, she had no desire to waste any more time on this man. She chose instead, to have her lawyer quietly negotiate a resolution with his lawyer, which caused this man aggravation, lawyer fees, and a lump sum to cover promised expenses. And hopefully, *imbarazzo!*

Phoenix has certainly been faced with many personal struggles, but her sole purpose in sharing these stories is to hopefully *encourage* other women to rise above such obstacles. To inspire women never to give up on themselves, no matter how tough things may get. To empower women so they are never afraid to stand up for what is right. To make a difference. To not sit in silence, for their sake—and for the other many women who will follow. Dare to hold people accountable for their actions, be it lovers, doctors, lawyers, priests, corporate America, parents, or policemen. If, instead, you choose to simply ignore it, turn your head, and pray it goes away, well, maybe it will. For you. But the next innocent and unsuspecting woman may not be so fortunate. So, please, Phoenix pleads with women everywhere to <u>never</u> accept such abuse—emotional, mental, or physical—and no matter the abuser! You will be far stronger and wiser because of it—in all aspects of your life!

Professionally determined...

As with most entrepreneurial spirits, Phoenix has done various things in her professional life, anxious to find her way. Her struggles are as diverse as her talents: Head cook at 14, personal trainer at 18, Playboy Bunny, gym manager, professional photographer, back to training, to owning and operating her own video production company. All the while supplementing her income with odd jobs as a wait-ress, bartender, pre-school teacher, and veterinarian technician. When she moved back to Southern California at 36, alone, with no friends, no money, no job, but an adorable beach cottage she had to quickly figure out how to pay for, she went down to "Camp OJ" to network with the hundreds of crews. Within weeks, she was freelancing audio/camera for CNN to help cover the murder trial. And, though, Phoenix has done many jobs to stay afloat and widen her experiences, through it all, she has never strayed far from her original passion: helping others stay physically fit.

It's been 28 years since Phoenix first started in the field of Health and Wellness, but the last six years she has come full circle, deciding to devote all of her time, energy, and professional attributes to truly perfecting health—combining all aspects of physical fitness, nutrition, and mental well-being. After all, this is what has always given her the most personal satisfaction. But when it came to the weight loss industry, she refused to settle for the ordinary or accept what this industry was disgracefully market-ing then, and now. She was fed up with the endless deceit—she also wanted to make a difference. It was this, along with her clients' inability to adhere to any diet, i.e., the cravings/emotional eating that were always their downfall, that prompted years of extensive research. And having always questioned authority, this was a very natural progression for her. Hence, Phoenix formed her own corporation and began this amazing journey—researching the science pertaining strictly to brain chemistry, and how it affects eating behaviors, and beyond. It was based on this research that she subsequently developed her body-enhancing supplements.

After nearly four years in R&D, and with her two products showing phenomenal results in the testing stage, Phoenix was eager to launch her national advertising campaign. But how was she possibly going to pay for a million-dollar ad campaign without any investors? To secure investors, angel or venture cap, she didn't even have the required business or marketing plan to secure that kind of funding. Truth be told, considering she had financed this venture on her own—many times not having enough money to pay rent or buy groceries—how was she *ever* going to be able to pay for advertis-ing? Her bigger concern, however, was the opinion most consumers had of the weight-loss industry. She knew most weight-loss consultants and product manufacturers were seen as barely more than snake oil salesmen due to the fact the market was saturated with over-hyped, useless diet products. And with integrity being everything to Phoenix, she wasn't about to risk her reputation, or that of her product. She knew she had to somehow break away from the typical diet arena. More importantly, she realized her product was merely a "bonus" to the extraordinary research, research that could be further complemented by her many years of experience.

Mentally exhausted, financially desperate, she was feeling helpless and terribly frustrated. There had been so many potentially incredible opportunities throughout this journey, but, sadly, most of them either asked her to set aside her integrity and self-respect, or insulted her intelligence as a business-woman. The only thing she knew to do was pray for guidance.

Then, one November day in 2003, while sitting quietly in her home office, it suddenly came to her with such absolute clarity. There was no other way. No other option. With nothing more than a profound inspiration from the Infinite Intelligence, she opted to make her product—a product that took her years to develop, a product that had enhanced so many of her clients' lives—take a back seat and instead focus entirely on writing her book, a book she felt was desperately needed far more than any product, a book she passionately believed could change millions of lives. And thus, the journey continued.

Her private world...

Phoenix has always been an intensely private and independent soul. While she unquestionably enjoys her time alone, she equally cherishes the friendships she's made over her lifetime. She finds tremendous happiness in the rare bond of those extraordinary few.

As a single woman or otherwise, Phoenix never felt motherhood was her role in life. Although she's befriended many neighborhood children, she teasingly admits her "clock" has never ticked. Instead, she's happily fulfilled her maternal instincts through her undying love and devotion to animals. She's done her best to save lives by adopting numerous dogs and cats from homeless shelters' death row. She's also provided a safe haven for snakes, an iguana, even caring for an abandoned horse.

Throughout her adult life, Phoenix has experienced one of the purest forms of friendships with those much older, be it neighbors in need or those she met while visiting local nursing and retirement homes. Those friendships have proven to be some of the most rewarding moments in her life. But, after four of her close friends passed on, she felt the need to give more and decided to seek a slightly different path. She joined an organization called Serenity Village in 2003. Their role is to provide mentors to children who are not as fortunate as most. For the next year and a half she mentored two adorable children—a beautiful 10-year-old girl named Elyse (AKA Cookie), and a handsome yet oh, so wild six-year-old boy named Devonne (AKA Bam Bam).

Late 2004, Phoenix devoted most of her free time to spoiling and training her newest adopted companion: Ella (shown on page 260), a stunning, very lovable three-year-old Rottweiler. Her goal? Getting Ella prepared for becoming a Therapy Dog via TDI (Therapy Dogs International) so she can give the gift of comfort and unconditional love to sick children and seniors at retirement/nursing homes.

Update: November 2005, Phoenix is immensely proud to say that Ella passed the above test with flying colors! Though the TDI evaluators were rather nervous just by the simple fact Ella is a "Rottweiler," Phoenix knew she had trained her well enough to pass their extensive test—and win them over. They indeed gave Ella great praise! And, as such, she is now officially a Therapy Dog! She also earned an AKC Canine Good Citizen certificate. And while Phoenix's desire is for Ella to give love to those in need, as her guardian/handler, she also wants to help change the misconception of Rotties. After all, this is merely another form of prejudice, a prejudice that is perpetuated unfairly by the news media.

Phoenix resides peacefully in a charming, little oceanside town in Southern California, with Ella, her protective canine, Willow, a beautiful, shy feline who was also rescued, and Lily, the iguana, who was adopted years ago from an ex-boyfriend who no longer wanted her.

PERSONAL GOALS

In Loving Memory of
Kashif, Greta, Gunther & Tav

In closing my book, a book that is dedicated to helping others live a longer, happier, and healthier life, I felt it was important to devote this final page to my beloved animals. As much as my soul thrived by loving them, they selflessly gave me more love than mere words can ever express. Although Kashif passed on 11 years ago, I still miss her. Greta, Gunther, and Tav were by my side throughout this journey and many years before. However, it was while writing this book that, sadly, all three got cancer, and all three died within 18 months! While I am *forever grateful* I was able to love them as long as I did, it is *never* a good time to say goodbye to one we love, especially considering I had to put all three down in such a short time! And, while the cycle of life is most certainly not easy to accept, all I know is that I must give back. And so, I reach out, adopting yet another soul in need.

Knowing how much each of these sweet souls gave to me, knowing how each one of them helped me live a more peaceful and meaningful, happier and subsequently *healthier* life, it is, therefore, my sincerest wish that if you have yet to discover this rare and precious bond, please consider adopting an orphan from your local shelter. You will save a life, and they, in turn, will give your life new meaning!